2021

ADVANCES IN PSYCHIATRY AND BEHAVIORAL HEALTH

EDITOR-IN-CHIEF
Deepak Prabhakar

SECTION EDITORS
Jennifer M. Boggs
Aryandokht Fotros
Lauren M. Osborne
Claudia L. Reardon
Eric A. Storch

ELSEVIER

Publishing Director, Medical Reference: Dolores Meloni
Editor: Lauren Boyle
Developmental Editor: Hannah Almira Lopez

Editorial Office:
Elsevier, Inc.
1600 John F. Kennedy Blvd,
Suite 1800
Philadelphia, PA 19103-2899

International Standard Serial Number: 2667-3835
International Standard Book Number: 13: 978-0-323-92013-1

ADVANCES IN PSYCHIATRY AND BEHAVIORAL HEALTH

[illegible]

[illegible], MD, MPH
– Education and Miscellaneous Topics
Chief of Medical Staff
Sheppard Pratt
Associate Professor (Adjunct)
Department of Psychiatry
University of Maryland School of Medicine
Baltimore, MD, USA

SECTION EDITORS

[illegible], MD, [illegible]
[illegible]
Kaiser Permanente Colorado
Institute for Health Research
Aurora, CO, USA

[illegible], MD, MSc
– [illegible]
Assistant Professor of Psychiatry
Department of Psychiatry and Human Behavior
Warren Alpert Medical School of Brown University
Brown University
Providence, RI, USA

LAUREN M. OSBORNE, MD – Women's Mental Health
Associate Professor of Psychiatry & Behavioral Sciences and of Gynecology & Obstetrics
Associate Director, Women's Mood Disorders Center
Fellowship Director, Advanced Research Training Program in Reproductive Psychiatry
The Johns Hopkins University School of Medicine
Baltimore, MD, USA

[illegible], MD, MS – [illegible]
Associate Professor, [illegible] Services
University of Wisconsin School of Medicine and Public Health Department of Psychiatry
Madison, WI, USA

[illegible], PhD – [illegible]
[illegible] Endowed Chair in [illegible]
Vice Chair & Head of Psychology
Department of Psychiatry and Behavioral Sciences
Baylor College of Medicine
Houston, TX, USA

CONTRIBUTORS

BRIAN K. AHMEDANI, PhD, LCSW
Henry Ford Health System, Center for Health Policy & Health Services Research, Detroit, Michigan, USA

ATHANASIOS S. ALEXANDRIS, MBChB
Department of Pathology (Neuropathology), Johns Hopkins University School of Medicine

ANDREA ALTSCHULER, PhD
Division of Research, Kaiser Permanente Northern California, Oakland, California, USA

MOHAMED ABO AOUN, BSc
St. Boniface Hospital Albrechtsen Research Centre, Winnipeg, Manitoba, Canada

BRENDA E. BAILEY, PhD
Rogers Behavioral Health System, Oconomowoc, Wisconsin, USA

LESLIE BARNARD, MPH
Department of Emergency Medicine, University of Colorado School of Medicine, Department of Epidemiology, University of Colorado School of Public Health, Aurora, Colorado, USA

ARNE BECK, PhD
Kaiser Permanente Colorado Institute for Health Research, Aurora, Colorado, USA

ENA BEGOVIC, PhD
Postdoctoral Psychology Resident, Michael E. DeBakey VA Medical Center

MARIAN E. BETZ, MD, MPH
Department of Emergency Medicine, University of Colorado School of Medicine, VA Eastern Colorado Geriatric Research Education and Clinical Center, Aurora, Colorado, USA

JORDAN M. BRACISZEWSKI, PhD
Center for Health Policy & Health Services Research, Henry Ford Health System, Detroit, Michigan, USA

CAMBRIA BRUSCHKE, MSW
Kaiser Permanente Care Management Institute, Oakland, California, USA

KAREN J. COLEMAN, PhD
Department of Research and Evaluation, Kaiser Permanente Southern California, Pasadena, California, USA

NORA COULTIS, MS
Psychology Intern, Behavioral Health, Henry Ford Health System, Detroit, Michigan, USA

ALAN CURRIE, MD
Consultant Psychiatrist, Regional Affective Disorders Service, Cumbria, Northumberland Tyne and Wear NHS Foundation Trust, Wolfson Research Centre, Campus for Ageing and Vitality, Newcastle, United Kingdom

SARAH J. DAVID, PhD
Rogers Behavioral Health System, Oconomowoc, Wisconsin, USA

NICHOLAS R. FARRELL, PhD
Rogers Behavioral Health System, Oconomowoc, Wisconsin, USA

JEAN P. FLORES, DrPH
Kaiser Permanente Care Management Institute, Oakland, California, USA

MOEIN FOROUGHI, MD
Department of Psychiatry and Behavioral Sciences, SUNY Downstate Health Sciences University, Brooklyn, New York, USA

ARYANDOKHT FOTROS, MD
Department of Psychiatry and Human Behavior, Brown University, Providence, Rhode Island, USA

AMVRINE GANGULY, MD
Department of Psychiatry and Behavioral Sciences, SUNY Downstate Health Sciences University, Brooklyn, New York, USA

PAUL GORCZYNSKI, PhD
Senior Lecturer, School of Sport, Health and Exercise Science, University of Portsmouth, Portsmouth, Hampshire, United Kingdom

WILLIAM GRUNEWALD, MA
Miami University, Oxford, Ohio, USA

RISHAB GUPTA, MD
Department of Psychiatry, Brigham and Women's Hospital, Harvard Medical School, Boston, Massachusetts, USA

ANDREW G. GUZICK, PhD
Postdoctoral Fellow, Department of Psychiatry and Behavioral Sciences, Baylor College of Medicine, Houston, Texas, USA

BRITTANY A. HAAGE, MS
Psychology Intern, Behavioral Health, Henry Ford Health System, Detroit, Michigan, USA

BRIAN HAINLINE, MD
Chief Medical Officer, National Collegiate Athletic Association, Indianapolis, Indiana, USA

LIISA HANTSOO, PhD
Assistant Professor, Department of Psychiatry and Behavioral Sciences, Johns Hopkins School of Medicine, Baltimore, Maryland, USA

KRISTINA HARPER, PsyD
Postdoctoral Psychology Resident, Michael E. DeBakey VA Medical Center

ALISON D. HERMANN, MD
Assistant Professor of Clinical Psychiatry, Department of Psychiatry, Weill Cornell Medicine, New York, New York, USA

BRADLEY HILLIER, BM BCh, MA, MFFLM, FRCPsych
Forensic Psychiatrist, West London NHS Trust, Southall, United Kingdom

MARY HITCHCOCK, MA, MS
Senior Academic Librarian, University of Wisconsin-Madison, Ebling Library for the Health Sciences, Madison, Wisconsin, USA

R.I. (VANA) HUTTER, PhD
Assistant Professor, Faculty of Behavioural and Movement Sciences, Vrije Universiteit Amsterdam, Amsterdam, the Netherlands

MICHAEL INGRAM, MD
Department of Psychiatry, University of California Riverside

DANIELLE KAMIS, MD
Stanford University, Palo Alto, California, USA

VASSILIS E. KOLIATSOS, MD
Departments of Pathology (Neuropathology), Neurology, and Psychiatry and Behavioral Sciences, Johns Hopkins School of Medicine, Neuropsychiatry Program, Sheppard Pratt Health System

ALISON KRAUSS, MA
Predoctoral Psychology Intern, Michael E. DeBakey VA Medical Center, Southern Methodist University

FRANCES L. LYNCH, PhD, MSPH
Kaiser Permanente Northwest, Center for Health Research, Portland, Oregon, USA

LISA MacLEAN, MD
Chief Clinical Wellness Officer, Henry Ford Health System, Associate Professor, Wayne State University, School of Medicine, Detroit, Michigan, USA

ANISSA J. MAFFETT, MA
Psychology Intern, Behavioral Health, Henry Ford Health System, Detroit, Michigan, USA

GERALD MAGUIRE, MD
Department of Psychiatry, University of California Riverside

KELLIE M. MARTENS, PhD
Senior Staff Psychologist, Behavioral Health and Bariatric Surgery, Henry Ford Health System, Detroit, Michigan, USA

BENJAMIN P. MEEK, BSc, MA
St. Boniface Hospital Albrechtsen Research Centre, Winnipeg, Manitoba, Canada

LISA R. MILLER-MATERO, PhD, ABPP
Senior Staff Psychologist, Behavioral Health and Center for Health Policy & Health Services Research, Henry Ford Health System, Detroit, Michigan, USA

JUNAID MIRZA, MD
Department of Psychiatry and Behavioral Sciences, SUNY Downstate Health Sciences University, Brooklyn, New York, USA

MANDANA MODIRROUSTA, MD, PhD, FRCPC
Rady Faculty of Health Sciences, University of Manitoba, St. Boniface Hospital Albrechtsen Research Centre, Winnipeg, Manitoba, Canada

SAI B. NAROTAM, MS
Psychology Intern, Behavioral Health, Henry Ford Health System, Detroit, Michigan, USA

ASHLI A. OWEN-SMITH, PhD, SM
Georgia State University and Kaiser Permanente Georgia, Atlanta, Georgia, USA

FILIPPO PASSETTI, MD, PhD, MRCPsych
Addictions Psychiatrist and Addictions Lead, Cognacity, Marylebone, London, United Kingdom

DEEPAK PRABHAKAR, MD, MPH
Chief of Medical Staff, Sheppard Pratt, Associate Professor (Adjunct), Department of Psychiatry, University of Maryland School of Medicine, Baltimore, Maryland, USA

ROSEMARY PURCELL, MPsych, PhD
Professor, Elite Sports and Mental Health, Orygen, Parkville, Victoria, Australia; Director, Research and Translation, Orygen, Centre for Youth Mental Health, The University of Melbourne, Parkville, Melbourne, Australia

DIANA RANCOURT, PhD
University of South Florida, Tampa, Florida, USA

VANI RAO, MD
Department of Psychiatry and Behavioral Sciences, Johns Hopkins School of Medicine

CLAUDIA L. REARDON, MD
Associate Professor, Department of Psychiatry, Associate Professor, University of Wisconsin School of Medicine and Public Health, Madison, Wisconsin, USA

SIMON RICE, MPsych, PhD
Associate Professor, Elite Sports and Mental Health, Orygen, Parkville, Victoria, Australia; Principal Research Fellow, Centre for Youth Mental Health, The University of Melbourne, Orygen, Parkville, Melbourne, Australia

JULIE E. RICHARDS, PhD, MPH
Kaiser Permanente Washington, Health Research Institute, Seattle, Washington, USA

JULIA RIDDLE, MD
Postdoctoral Fellow, Department of Psychiatry and Behavioral Sciences, Johns Hopkins School of Medicine, Baltimore, Maryland, USA

BRADLEY C. RIEMANN, PhD
Rogers Behavioral Health System, Oconomowoc, Wisconsin, USA

REBECCA ROSSOM, MD, MS
HealthPartners Institute, Minneapolis, Minnesota, USA

ALI ROWHANI-RAHBAR, MD, MPH, PhD
Department of Epidemiology, University of Washington School of Public Health, Harborview Injury Prevention and Research Center, University of Washington, Seattle, Washington, USA

GREGORY E. SIMON, MD, MPH
Kaiser Permanente Washington, Health Research Institute, Seattle, Washington, USA

APRIL R. SMITH, PhD
Miami University, Oxford, Ohio, USA

ANJU SONI, MB, BS, MRCPsych
Forensic Psychiatrist, Broadmoor Hospital, West London NHS Trust and Imperial College London, Southall, United Kingdom

STEPHEN M. STAHL MD, PhD, DSC (HON)
Department of Psychiatry, University of California Riverside, Department of Psychiatry, University of California San Diego, Department of Psychiatry, University of Cambridge, Neuroscience Education Institute

CODY STAPLES, BS
University of South Florida, Tampa, Florida, USA

STACY STERLING, DrPH, MSW
Division of Research, Kaiser Permanente Northern California, Oakland, California, USA

CHRISTINE C. STEWART, PhD
Kaiser Permanente Washington, Health Research Institute, Seattle, Washington, USA

ERIC A. STORCH, PhD
Professor of Psychiatry, McIngvale Presidential Endowed Chair, Department of Psychiatry and Behavioral Sciences, Baylor College of Medicine, Houston, Texas, USA

LEAH C. SUSSER, MD
Assistant Professor of Clinical Psychiatry, Department of Psychiatry, Weill Cornell Medicine, White Plains, New York, USA

CLARE SWANSON, MD
Psychiatry Resident, Department of Psychiatry, NewYork-Presbyterian Hospital/Weill Cornell, New York, New York, USA

ELLEN J. TENG, PhD
Clinical Research Psychologist, Michael E. DeBakey VA Medical Center, Associate Professor, Menninger Department of Psychiatry and Behavioral Sciences, Baylor College of Medicine

IAN TREASADEN, MB, BS, LRCP, MRCS, FRCPsych, LLM
Forensic Psychiatrist, West London NHS Trust and Bucks New University, Southall, United Kingdom

ERIKA S. TRENT, MA
Doctoral Candidate, Department of Psychology, University of Houston, Houston, Texas, USA

ANDRES G. VIANA, PhD, ABPP
Associate Professor, Department of Psychology, University of Houston, Associate Professor, Texas Institute of Measurement, Evaluation, and Statistics, University of Houston, Houston, Texas, USA

PAMELA WALTERS, MB BCh, MRCPysch
Clinical Director, Substance Misuse and Mental Health Services, The Forward Trust Edinburgh House, London, United Kingdom; NHS Forensic and Addictions Psychiatrist, HMP Wandsworth, Wandsworth, United Kingdom

COURTNEY C. WALTON, MPsych, PhD
Postdoctoral Research Fellow, Elite Sports and Mental Health, Orygen, Parkville, Victoria, Australia; Postdoctoral Research Fellow, Centre for Youth Mental Health, The University of Melbourne, Orygen, Parkville, Melbourne, Australia

CONTENTS

VOLUME 1 • 2021

Advances in Psychiatry and Behavioral Health 1 (2021) xv–xvi

ADVANCES IN PSYCHIATRY AND BEHAVIORAL HEALTH

Preface

Onwards and upwards

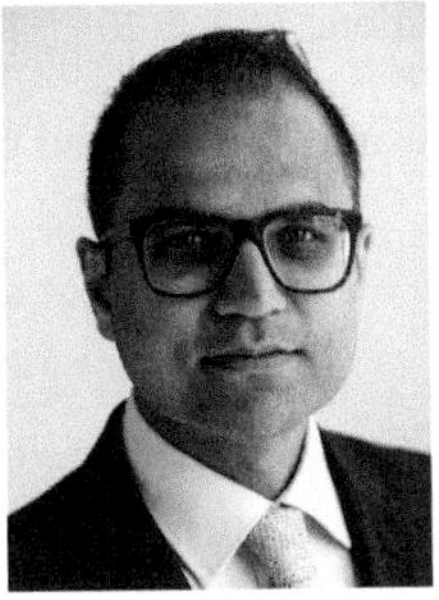

Deepak Prabhakar, MD, MPH
Editor

It's an honor to serve as the first Editor-in-Chief of *Advances in Psychiatry and Behavioral Health*. Work on the inaugural issue of *Advances in Psychiatry and Behavioral Health* started in late 2019; at that time, the phrase "onwards and upwards" had a different meaning to me personally, and perhaps to us collectively. When I started recruiting a distinguished panel of editors for our first issue of *Advances in Psychiatry and Behavioral Health*, we all stepped into this endeavor with a goal to help facilitate dissemination of topics geared toward translational application of scientific advances in our field. Since most of the topics were solicited prior to or during the early phase of the pandemic, barring one article, this issue does not delve into clinical, research, and educational aspects of the pandemic. However, all of us have been impacted by the pandemic, in one way or the other, some more than the others, and perhaps adversely.

Grief and loss during the pandemic has brought a different depth and meaning to our shared humanity and collective empathy. Pandemic has served as a reminder of the natural environment and limited resources we all share. On one hand, this awareness has connected individuals, society, and countries like never before; however, this has also exposed our fault lines, and some have not shied away from creating a "fear of the other" to further their own agenda. Psychiatry stands at this unique moment, in my opinion, best suited to take on and help manage the pandemic and its multiple sequelae, both medical and societal. Let's take this opportunity to address depression, anxiety, substance use, and suicide in our communities. But, let's not stop there, let's also address rising disparities in school outcomes, food insecurity, unemployment, racism, gender-inequity, lack of affordable housing, and clean environment. This is where our collective wisdom, gained after years of learning and applying holistic models, such as bio-psycho-social, wrap-around, and integrated care, can offer practical help, and above all, hope to a postpandemic world. Let's also do this with an eye toward self-care, as one may not be able to or is not needed to take on all that needs fixing.

The first issue of *Advances in Psychiatry and Behavioral Health* is a step toward advancing our field in a way that

https://doi.org/10.1016/j.ypsc.2021.06.003
2667-3827/21/

will bring not only late-breaking research findings but also articles on application of these findings in a real-world setting. Our editors are a diverse group of individuals at different stages of their career. All are experts in their areas and have a unique perspective as well as have their fingers on the pulse of frontline needs. Broadly, the content is divided into six sections: Aryan Fotros has edited the Neurosciences section; Eric Storch has edited the section on advances in Psychotherapy; Jennifer Boggs has edited the section on Suicide; Lauren Osborne has edited the section on Women's Mental Health; Claudia Reardon has edited the section on Sports Psychiatry; and I have edited the section on Education. I can't even begin to thank our editors, contributors, and the Elsevier staff, who have worked diligently through the ever-changing dynamic of the pandemic and have helped deliver this first issue for our readers. Their hard work and perseverance have made this inaugural issue a possibility and truly a step toward a hopeful message of onwards and upwards!

Deepak Prabhakar, MD, MPH
Sheppard Pratt
6501 North Charles Street
Baltimore, MD 21204, USA

E-mail address: dprabhakar@sheppardpratt.org

Psychotherapeuthics

Advances in Psychiatry and Behavioral Health 1 (2021) 1–12

ADVANCES IN PSYCHIATRY AND BEHAVIORAL HEALTH

Advances in Psychotherapy for Posttraumatic Stress Disorder

Alison Krauss, MA[a,b,c], Ena Begovic, PhD[a,b], Kristina Harper, PsyD[a,b], Ellen J. Teng, PhD[a,b,d,*]

[a]Michael E. DeBakey VA Medical Center, 2002 Holcombe Boulevard, Houston, TX 77030, USA; [b]Center for Innovative Treatment of Anxiety and Stress; [c]Southern Methodist University, 6425 Boaz Lane, Dallas, TX 75205, USA; [d]Menninger Department of Psychiatry and Behavioral Sciences at Baylor College of Medicine, 1977 Butler Boulevard, Suite E4.400, Houston, TX 77030, USA

KEYWORDS

- Cognitive behavioral therapy • Cognitive processing • Intensive treatment • Massed treatment
- Prolonged exposure • Technology

KEY POINTS

- A significant body of research supports the efficacy of several trauma-focused psychotherapies in addressing PTSD, including prolonged exposure therapy, cognitive processing therapy, eye movement desensitization and reprocessing, brief eclectic psychotherapy for PTSD, narrative exposure therapy, cognitive behavioral therapy for PTSD, and written exposure therapy.
- Intensive delivery of these treatments, which allows clients to receive TF-EBPs across a short period, appears just as efficacious in reducing PTSD symptoms as standard delivery formats.
- Brief TF-EBPs, such as written exposure therapy, also demonstrate promising results in ameliorating PTSD symptoms, suggesting that significant symptom reduction can be gained in as few as 5 sessions of psychotherapy.
- Technology-facilitated deliveries of PTSD treatments, including video telehealth, represent a promising approach to increase the accessibility of gold-standard treatments for PTSD.

INTRODUCTION

The psychotherapy literature for treating posttraumatic stress disorder (PTSD) has proliferated over the last several years, largely due to advances in neuroscience. Translational research incorporating the roles of neural circuitry, biomarkers, and epigenetics in PTSD has helped elucidate the mechanisms involved in fear conditioning—a key process in developing and maintaining PTSD [1]. These approaches provide a framework for understanding how specific psychotherapy approaches for PTSD work and why they are effective. To date, cognitive-behavioral approaches remain the first-line treatment for people with PTSD [2]. Although unique differences exist in their approach to treatment, these treatments specifically target the reduction of factors that maintain the fear-conditioning process, and they promote memory reconsolidation, both of which are critical to the recovery process.

Despite the effectiveness of these evidence-based treatments, not all individuals respond similarly to these therapies, with some showing little to no symptom improvement [3]. Initiation and engagement in psychotherapy for PTSD is also low, as many are unable to either access these treatments or complete a full course of treatment because of the time commitments required of these treatments [4]. In response to these barriers, researchers have begun to investigate the efficacy of using different approaches to deliver psychotherapy that

*Corresponding author. Michael E. DeBakey VA Medical Center, 116 MHCL, 2002 Holcombe Boulevard, Houston, TX 77030. *E-mail address:* Ellen.Teng@va.gov

https://doi.org/10.1016/j.ypsc.2021.05.005
2667-3827/21/ Published by Elsevier Inc.

reduces the overall amount of time needed to complete treatments. Often referred to as "intensive" or "massed" treatments, individuals can complete a full course of a gold-standard therapy over several weeks [5,6]. To improve access to care for persons living in rural communities, clinicians and researchers have also incorporated the use of clinical video telehealth (CVT) in delivering psychotherapy directly into clients' homes or a nearby clinic [7]. There is also a growing literature base on incorporating other forms of technology such as Internet-based interventions (IBIs) and mobile smartphone applications to increase access and engagement in care [8,9]. Each of these approaches offers advantages and disadvantages, which will be discussed in this article.

This article briefly reviews the current gold-standard behavioral treatments for PTSD, including prolonged exposure (PE), cognitive processing, and eye movement desensitization and reprocessing (EMDR) therapies. This is followed by a brief overview of other specific cognitive behavioral therapies (CBTs) for PTSD with a strong evidence base, including brief eclectic psychotherapy (BEPP), narrative exposure therapy (NET), and written narrative exposure. Next is an overview of intensive and brief treatment approaches, including accelerated resolution therapy (ART), a newly emerging brief treatment. This is followed by a review of the evidence for technology-based interventions, including IBIs, mobile applications, and CVT. The article concludes with practice considerations.

OVERVIEW OF EVIDENCE-BASED TREATMENTS FOR POSTTRAUMATIC STRESS DISORDER

According to clinical practice guidelines from the American Psychological Association [10], the International Society for Traumatic Stress Studies [11], and the Department of Veterans Affairs [2], trauma-focused (TF) therapies are the most effective psychotherapies for PTSD. PE [12], cognitive processing therapy (CPT) [13], and EMDR [14] have demonstrated effectiveness in various populations and are recommended as first-line treatments. Other specific CBTs have also been found to be efficacious and are recommended for the treatment of PTSD (Table 1). TF treatments are generally designed to be time-limited and involve working through thoughts, feelings, and memories associated with traumatic events. Despite common underlying mechanisms, there are substantial differences in how these therapies are delivered and the required engagement of the client.

Prolonged Exposure Therapy

PE is grounded in emotional processing theory (EPT), which suggests that fear is represented in memory as a cognitive structure that includes representations of feared stimuli, fear responses, and associated meanings [15,16]. Normal fear structures represent stimuli that are realistic threats (eg, the combat zone), and when activated, result in an adaptive response (eg, preparing a weapon). However, a pathologic fear structure is one that has become overgeneralized and is activated in response to innocuous stimuli (eg, loud noises), and when triggered, results in maladaptive responses (eg, escape).

According to EPT, natural recovery following a trauma occurs when the fear structure is repeatedly activated in the absence of feared consequences leading to a reduction in negative affect (ie, habituation) [17]. Pathologic fear structures inherent in PTSD occur because of avoidance and the development of cognitive biases [10]. Such fear structures are characterized by (1) representations of trauma reminders erroneously associated with danger, (2) avoidance behaviors or intense physiologic responses, and (3) beliefs that these are dangerous.

PE consists of 8 to 15 individual 90-minute weekly sessions and includes psychoeducation followed by both imaginal and in vivo exposure to activate the fear structure while confronting feared consequences, thereby altering threat meaning and trauma-related cognitions [12,18]. Postexposure processing helps to emphasize changes in trauma-related beliefs and habituation. Clients listen to recordings of the trauma narrative between sessions and complete graduated in vivo exposure to previously avoided situations [19].

Treatment outcomes suggest that PE often results in a clinically meaningful reduction in PTSD symptoms by session 8, and treatment completers show more improvement than 86% of patients in control conditions at posttreatment [20]. Based on intent-to-treat analyses, 41% to 95% of those who initiate PE no longer meet diagnostic criteria for PTSD, with rates averaging 68% among treatment completers [21]. These treatment gains are maintained up to 5 years posttreatment [22–24]. PE effectively reduces comorbid depressive and anxiety symptoms [21,25] and is associated with increased quality of life among those with PTSD [26].

Cognitive Processing Therapy

CPT [13] draws from EPT and social cognitive theory (SCT). SCT indicates that individual behavior and beliefs are influenced by direct experiences, observation

TABLE 1
Summary of Empirically Supported Trauma-Focused Treatments

Treatment	Number/Duration/ Frequency of Sessions	Key Components	Recommendation Status
BEPP	16 weekly sessions, 45–60 min per session	Psychoeducation; imaginal exposure; writings tasks and mementos; meaning-making and integration; farewell ritual	APA: *Conditional for* ISTSS: *Insufficient evidence* VA/DoD: *Strong for*
CBT for PTSD	9–12 weekly sessions, 60–90 min per session	Psychoeducation; cognitive restructuring; exposure; distress management (eg, relaxation exercises)	APA: *Strong for* ISTSS: *Strong recommendation* VA/DoD: *Strong for*
CPT	12 weekly sessions, 50–60 min per session	Psychoeducation; cognitive restructuring; imaginal exposure[a]	APA: *Strong for* ISTSS: *Strong recommendation* VA/DoD: *Strong for*
EMDR	8-phase treatment typically completed over the course of 5–15 weekly sessions, 60–90 min per sessions	Imaginal exposure; horizontal eye movements	APA: *Conditional for*[b] ISTSS: *Strong recommendation* VA/DoD: *Strong for*
NET	4–12 weekly sessions, 90 min per session	Imaginal exposure; meaning-making	APA: *Conditional for*[b] ISTSS: Standard recommendation VA/DoD: *Strong for*
PE	8–15 weekly sessions, 90 min per session	Psychoeducation; breathing retraining; imaginal exposure; in-vivo exposure	APA: *Strong for* ISTSS: *Strong recommendation* VA/DoD: *Strong for*
WET	5 weekly sessions, 60 min for first session and 40 min for subsequent sessions	Psychoeducation; imaginal exposure	APA: n/a ISTSS: *Emerging evidence* VA/DoD: *Strong for*

Abbreviations: APA, American Psychological Association; BEPP, brief eclectic psychotherapy for PTSD; CBT, cognitive behavioral therapy; CPT, cognitive processing therapy; EMDR, eye movement desensitization and reprocessing; ISTSS, International Society for Traumatic Stress Studies; NET, narrative exposure therapy; PE, prolonged exposure; VA/DoD, Veterans Affairs/ Department of Defense; WET, written exposure therapy.

[a] Imaginal exposure is only included in cognitive processing therapy with a written trauma account.

[b] The APA (2017) clinical practice guidelines note that the recommendation statuses for EMDR and NET may be upgraded to "strong" on the basis of an updated search that includes studies published between 2012 and 2016.

of others, and environmental influences [27]. CPT postulates that following a trauma, individuals attempt to make sense of the event, often resulting in distorted beliefs about themselves, the world, and others. Such beliefs arise from 2 primary processes: (1) assimilation, which involves altering new information to confirm prior beliefs, and (2) overaccommodation when existing beliefs are altered such that they become extreme or overgeneralized [28]. CPT dictates that engaging in assimilation and overaccommodation creates maladaptive patterns of thinking (ie, "stuck points") that interfere with natural recovery [29]. Thus, CPT aims to shift beliefs toward accommodation, the process of altering existing beliefs sufficiently to incorporate new learning [28].

CPT is a manualized treatment consisting of 12 weekly individual or group sessions of 60 to 90 minutes each. It includes psychoeducation and the development of an impact statement detailing why the traumatic event occurred and how it affected one's beliefs related to domains of safety, intimacy, trust, power/control, and esteem. Clients work to identify stuck points and learn cognitive techniques to challenge assimilated and overaccommodated thoughts.

A recent meta-analysis of CPT found large effect sizes in the reduction of negative cognitions from pretreatment to posttreatment [30], and evidence supports the maintenance of these cognitive shifts at 5 and 10 years posttreatment [31]. CPT is an effective treatment for PTSD across a broad range of trauma types [32,33], including sexual traumas [28], combat-related trauma among veterans [32], and individuals with comorbid PTSD and TBI [34]. Meta-analyses suggest that CPT results in significant reductions in PTSD symptoms that are sustained up to 10 years posttreatment [35,36], and the rates for participants who no longer meet PTSD diagnostic criteria following CPT treatment range from 30% to 97% [37].

Eye Movement Desensitization and Reprocessing

EMDR was developed as a psychological treatment for PTSD following observations that the intensity of traumatic memories was reduced through eye movements.[38] EMDR is based on adaptive information processing (AIP) [14,39,40], which theorizes that humans have a physiologically based information-processing system that processes new experiences by integrating them with preexisting memory networks. PTSD purportedly develops from incomplete processing of traumatic events that prevents connections to more adaptive information held in other memory networks. Thus, the goal of EMDR is to access the inadequately processed information using bilateral stimulation to integrate the information into the client's larger memory system.

EMDR is completed in an 8-step standardized protocol; sessions last 60 to 90 minutes, and the number of sessions per phase can vary [14,38]. During the course of treatment, the client is instructed to retrieve a distressing memory of the traumatic event and focus on related thoughts and feelings while simultaneously performing bilateral eye movements [41]. Additionally, the client elicits currently held negative beliefs, desired positive beliefs, and physical sensations to activate different aspects of stored memory. Consistent with the AIP model, this recall process is thought to facilitate integration into the client's larger memory system.

Several meta-analyses indicate that EMDR is an effective treatment for PTSD compared with inactive control conditions and produces effects similar to those of other CBTs [36,42,43]. In 1 recent meta-analysis [44] comparing EMDR with other PTSD treatments, the differential effect of EMDR was significant, and this was true in follow-up analyses comparing EMDR with *only* CBT and PE therapies. However, in subgroup analyses that only included studies with lower risk of bias, there were no significant differences between EMDR and other therapies. Following EMDR, 36% to 95% of individuals no longer meet diagnostic criteria for PTSD [45,46], and EMDR may be particularly efficacious for individuals with severe forms of PTSD or who have comorbid severe psychiatric disorders (eg, psychosis) [47,48]. Although there is some controversy as to whether EMDR effects are due to bilateral eye movement or PE [49], some research points to the added utility of this technique [42].

Cognitive Behavioral Therapy

CBT refers to a broad category of treatments that employ psychoeducation, cognitive restructuring, exposure, or stress management in varying degrees [50]. These treatments encompass programs using a specific CBT-based protocol (eg, PE, CPT, EMDR) as well as treatments that apply general CBT techniques to treat PTSD (henceforth referred to as "CBT for PTSD"). Treatments often subsumed under CBT for PTSD include cognitive therapy (CT) [51] and treatments that use cognitive behavioral techniques but "don't quite fit cleanly into one of the other categories." [36](p131) CBT for PTSD is typically delivered in 9 to 12 sessions of 60 to 90 minutes each.

Numerous randomized control trials have investigated the efficacy of CBT-based treatments for PTSD in civilians and US service members/veterans with various trauma types. Meta-analyses of these studies demonstrate that CBT treatments are more efficacious than wait list and many non-TF interventions [24,36,52,53].

Brief Eclectic Psychotherapy for Posttraumatic Stress Disorder

BEPP [54,55] is an individual, manualized TF treatment that draws from a combination of theoretic frameworks, including psychodynamic, cognitive behavioral, and directive. BEPP is delivered in 16 weekly sessions lasting 45 to 60 minutes, and the protocol consists of 5 key components: (1) psychoeducation about PTSD; (2) imaginal exposure; (3) writing tasks and mementos; (4) meaning and integration; and (5) farewell ritual. Imaginal exposures entail orally recounting the traumatic event for 15 to 20 minutes followed by a brief discussion of the exposure. Writing tasks are used outside of sessions to facilitate further emotional expression. Unlike other exposure interventions, the goal of imaginal exposure in BEPP is to promote emotional catharsis rather than habituation. Treatment commences with a "farewell ritual" as a way to symbolically leave the traumatic event in the past.

BEPP was originally developed to treat PTSD in police officers, and a randomized controlled trial with this population demonstrated significant reduction in PTSD symptoms [56]. Subsequent studies conducted with a general population of adults with various traumas have further supported the efficacy of BEPP [46,57]. BEPP significantly reduced PTSD symptoms compared with wait list controls and had similar efficacy to EMDR (although the response rate was more gradual for BEPP). Across these 3 trials, PTSD symptom reduction resulted in small to medium effect sizes [36].

Narrative Exposure Therapy

NET [58] is a manualized, individual TF treatment delivered in 4 to 12 sessions of 90 to 120 minutes each. The treatment was specifically developed for demographically and culturally diverse individuals who have experienced complex trauma. NET uses imaginal exposure via oral narration to organize and coherently integrate traumatic events within one's broader life story. Individuals receive a transcription of their life story at the end of treatment, which can serve as an empowering testimonial.

The efficacy of NET has been examined in multiple randomized control trials with various populations, most commonly refugees and asylum seekers [59]. In a recent review and meta-analysis, Lely and colleagues [60] found a large effect of treatment on the reduction of PTSD symptoms at posttreatment and follow-up (also see Lewis and colleagues [52]). Further, NET was more efficacious than non-TF treatments and wait list conditions but comparable to other TF treatments [60].

INTENSIVE AND BRIEF POSTTRAUMATIC STRESS DISORDER TREATMENT APPROACHES

Intensive Trauma-Focused Treatments

Unlike the standard delivery format of TF-EBPs, which typically consist of 1 to 2 sessions per week over the course of 2 to 4 months in an outpatient setting, intensive TF-EBPs are delivered in the same setting over a significantly shorter period. The frequency and duration of sessions and treatment modalities (ie, individual, group, or combination) can vary considerably among intensive TF-EBPs. Typically, however, individual therapy is delivered daily for 1 to 3 weeks.

Although still in its infancy, research on intensive TF EBPs shows promising results. To date, studies have examined the efficacy of intensive delivery of a single TF-EBP (PE, CPT, CT, or EMDR) [61,62] or a combined treatment consisting of a TF-EBP and an adjunctive intervention [63]. Several uncontrolled studies of intensive TF-EBPs have demonstrated significant decreases in PTSD symptoms at posttreatment and follow-up among US military service members/veterans and civilians with various trauma types [64,65]. Presently, only 2 randomized controlled trials of intensive TF-EBPs have been published (intensive CT [6], intensive PE) [5]. Results from both trials showed that intensively delivered TF-EBP was equally as efficacious as the standard weekly format and more efficacious than a non-TF therapy or control condition [5,6]. A recent systematic review of intensive TF-EBPs [66] reported a large reduction in PTSD symptoms. The pooled dropout rate of participants across studies was 5.51%, whereas the dropout rates seen in standard, weekly TF-EBPs are approximately 3.25 to 7 times higher [66]. In addition to the demonstrated efficacy and lower dropout rate, participants' experiences and overall satisfaction with an intensive TF treatment were overwhelmingly positive [67].

Brief Treatments

Written exposure therapy (WET) [68] is a brief TF treatment recommended by the *VA/DOD Clinical Practice Guideline* for PTSD. WET is an individual, manualized treatment that consists of 5 weekly sessions. Sessions are 40 minutes long except for the first session, which lasts 60 minutes. The protocol consists of 2 main components: (1) psychoeducation about PTSD and (2) imaginal exposure via a written narrative. Clients are initially instructed to write about the traumatic event, including sensory-perceptual details of the event and thoughts and feelings experienced at the time of the event. In the latter stages, individuals shift to writing about the meaning of the trauma event and its impact on their lives. Approximately 30 minutes of each session are spent writing about the traumatic event, followed by processing clients' experiences of the process. Unlike PE and CPT, WET does not include homework assignments. However, individuals are encouraged to experience and not avoid any thoughts and feelings that may emerge between sessions.

The efficacy of WET has been examined in individuals with motor vehicle accident-related PTSD [68] and US military veterans with combat or military sexual trauma-related PTSD [69]. A significant reduction in PTSD symptoms was observed at follow-up, with many participants no longer meeting the full criteria for a PTSD diagnosis. Research also shows that WET is noninferior to standard weekly CPT among veterans and nonveterans with various traumas [70], and treatment effects were maintained 60 weeks posttreatment [71]. In addition to being efficacious, WET showed low dropout rates and high levels of client satisfaction [68–70].

Emerging brief treatments

ART [72,73] is an emerging brief TF treatment derived from EMDR. ART is a manualized, individual TF treatment delivered in 1 to 5 sessions of 60 to 75 minutes each. The 2 key components of the protocol are imaginal exposure and imaginal rescripting of the traumatic event, both of which are coupled with horizontal smooth pursuit eye movements. While ART retains the main elements found in EMDR, there is some variation in the overall protocol (eg, ART places a greater emphasis on bodily sensations, and eye movement sets are more standardized) [74]. Similar to WET, homework assignments are not included in the treatment protocol. In initial evaluations, ART appears to significantly reduce PTSD symptoms [75,76] and address comorbid depressive symptoms [77]. Additional investigations of ART are underway to bolster these promising findings.

TECHNOLOGY-ASSISTED DELIVERY OF POSTTRAUMATIC STRESS DISORDER TREATMENT

Internet-Based Interventions

Over the years, researchers have begun to examine ways for PTSD treatment to be facilitated or delivered via technology. The use of technology in treatment delivery presents a unique opportunity to provide a more convenient and accessible way for clients to engage in psychotherapy. A relatively recent advance in the delivery of PTSD treatments includes IBIs. Such programs are self-managed interventions, allowing clients to access and progress through an intervention with little to no guidance from a clinician. Several such programs exist, including *interapy* [9], *survivor to thriver* (*S to T*) [78], and *iCBT* [8]. The majority of these programs are founded on cognitive-behavioral or expressive writing principles [79].

Overall, these Internet programs appear well accepted by clients, as most studies reported moderate to high acceptability responses from patients [80]. However, the reported use of these programs is low. Several studies report program completion rates of between 35% to 40% [81,82]. Although dropout rates are similar between TF-IBIs and non-TF-IBI control programs, dropout rates from TB-IBIs appear higher compared with control conditions (such as treatment as usual)

Although IBIs are more efficacious in reducing PTSD symptoms than no treatment control conditions [79], Several meta-analytic reviews of IBIs indicate that such programs demonstrate few if any reductions in PTSD symptoms. IBIs appear to be more effective when they include more than 8 sessions and clinician support as needed. Thus, IBIs currently seem limited in their efficacy to reduce PTSD symptoms, although these findings may be due to poor engagement.

Mobile Applications

Similar to IBIs, mobile applications (or apps) have emerged as another promising tool in addressing PTSD symptoms. In fact, VA and DoD have developed several psychotherapy mobile apps in recent years in an attempt to increase the reach and engagement of veterans in mental health services [83]. Such mobile apps generally fall into 2 categories: (1) self-managed apps focused on providing skills for symptom reduction and (2) treatment companion apps focused on aiding the client/clinician during a course of treatment.

To date, almost 70 apps have been developed to target PTSD symptoms, but few have undergone empirical investigation [84]. The most researched app is *PTSD Coach*, a self-managed app aimed at providing psychoeducation and skills to manage symptoms of PTSD. Empirical research supports the acceptability of the app by patients, with most users finding the app helpful in managing symptoms [85,86]. Source code for the *PTSD Coach* app has been openly shared, allowing implementation of this app across several different countries [87].

Similar to IBIs, use of the *PTSD Coach* app appears low [86]. In addition, the app alone seems to have little to no effect on PTSD symptoms compared with control conditions across several evaluations [85–88]. However, *PTSD Coach* has demonstrated improvements in other areas of functioning, including depressive symptoms, psychosocial functioning, and quality of life [87,89]. Taken together, the extent to which these apps aid in managing symptoms or complement existing treatments remains unclear.

Within the realm of treatment companion apps, 2 are commonly used: *PE Coach* and *CPT Coach*. Despite the growing empirical work on *PTSD Coach*, relatively little empirical study has been conducted with *PE Coach*, and no work to date has investigated the effects of *CPT Coach* [90]. *PE Coach* and *CPT Coach* are similar in that they were created specifically to facilitate administration of traditional PE or CPT. Both apps include tools such as symptom assessments, homework tracking, consolidation of treatment materials, and appointment reminders. Within the *PE Coach* app, clients can also can audio record imaginal exposures.

Investigations of *PE Coach* have been limited to case studies and qualitative examinations of the feasibility of using the app [91,92]. Based on these few studies, *PE Coach* appears acceptable to clients, with users reporting high levels of satisfaction when engaging in PE plus use of *PE Coach* compared with PE alone [91]. Providers also report high satisfaction with the app, noting that the app aids in mimicking the structure of the session and increases the perceived credibility of treatment among clients. Clinicians also highlighted the audio recording feature of the app in recording imaginal exposures, noting that the app includes additional privacy measures that other audio recorders may not (eg, the ability for the client's phone to lock and the addition of a PIN to access the *PE Coach* app). The primary disadvantage of the app is a lack of technology literacy among some clients and providers.

Despite the promising work detailing the strengths of the *PE Coach* app, no research has examined the efficacy of using the *PE Coach* app compared with the administration of PE without its companion app. *CPT Coach* also has yet to be empirically evaluated. Thus, the evidence to date suggests that these apps are promising in their potential utility and are well-accepted by clients. Future research is warranted as these apps hold potential for improving treatment engagement, increasing homework compliance, and decreasing the number of missed sessions.

Video Telehealth

A final area of technology-assisted care receiving growing attention includes video telehealth interventions, sometimes referred to as clinical video telehealth. In CVT, a provider and client meet synchronously through a video platform. Mental health professionals have used such technology for many years to better serve communities with limited access to psychotherapy services (eg, rural communities). More recently, home-based CVT has become a necessity for providing continued health care to clients during the COVID-19 pandemic [93].

A recent systematic review suggests that CVT administration of PTSD treatment is well accepted by clients [94]. Studies show that around half of clients report a preference for CVT over in-person care. Persons who received psychotherapy via CVT show comparable rates of improvement in PTSD symptoms as those receiving in-person care, with gains maintained at 3 and 6 months posttreatment [94,95]. In 1 study evaluating CVT and in-person administration of CPT, clients were less likely to decline CVT administration than in-person administration [96]. Treatment dropout was also lower among those assigned to CVT administration compared with in-person administration. Several studies document the efficacy of CVT administration of CPT, suggesting clients experience similar declines in PTSD symptoms compared with in-person administration in posttreatment, 3-month, and 6-month assessments [97].

Similar to CVT-administered CPT, CVT-administered PE is noninferior to in-person administration at posttreatment, 3-month, and 6-month follow-up assessments [98]. However, dropout rates for CVT administration of PE are higher than those for in-person administration [94,98]. This may be attributed to technology difficulties experienced with CVT administration. Another theory posits that the decreased amount of time and effort required to attend CVT sessions compared with in-person sessions may devalue psychotherapy [99]. Despite this, client and provider satisfaction of PE appear similar across administration formats [100,101], and some data suggest clients may prefer CVT administration of PE over in-person PE [94].

PRACTICE CONSIDERATIONS

When considering the gold-standard interventions for PTSD, some factors (eg, unmanaged symptoms of mania or psychosis, imminent suicidality, severe nonsuicidal self-injurious behavior) may preclude clients from experiencing significant symptom reduction. Recommendations for CPT and PE are to delay treatment until these concerns are addressed [12,13]. Evidence indicates that gold-standard treatments for PTSD can be effectively administered in the context of comorbidity, including personality disorders, anger, dissociation, anxiety disorders, and traumatic brain injury.

Many PTSD treatments require homework assignments to be completed outside of sessions. Clients completing CPT and PE can expect to spend 1 to 2 hours daily on therapy-related work, including completing homework forms, listening to session audio recordings, and completing *in vivo* exposures. Although such daily work may appear time-consuming, empirical evidence suggests that homework adherence in both CPT and PE is associated with greater symptom reduction posttreatment [101–103]. Clients unwilling to commit to daily homework assignments are unlikely to derive maximum benefit from these interventions.

In addition to clinical considerations for traditional administration of PTSD treatments, providers should assess a client's access and familiarity with technology before deciding to implement these tools. Clients with limited access or significant discomfort in using technology may experience more benefit from traditional in-person treatment rather than technology-facilitated treatment. Few guidelines are currently available to determine when it may be most appropriate to use IBIs or mobile applications. Current knowledge indicates that IBIs and self-managed mobile applications alone show little improvement in PTSD symptoms. Similarly, there is limited research on the additive effectiveness of treatment companion applications. Thus, these programs should not be used as a first-line treatment for clients but instead at a clinician's discretion in conjunction with gold-standard treatments.

In considering advances in the treatment of PTSD, some novel approaches require additional resources to implement. This is especially true for delivery formats that use technology. These delivery approaches often require that the client or provider has access to appropriate equipment to facilitate treatment. Specifically, when using mobile applications, clients need access to a smartphone and familiarity with the phone's functions (eg, how to download, access, and use the specific mobile application).

When using CVT, the client and provider require devices that allow for a secure video connection; such devices could include a smartphone, tablet, or computer. Some healthcare settings may be able to lend clients devices to facilitate CVT [94]. However, in settings with limited resources, a lack of appropriate equipment may be a barrier to conducting CVT sessions. Another important consideration when using CVT is access to secure and HIPAA-compliant video platforms [94]. Clinicians may require access to more than 1 secure video platform if a client is unable to connect to the primary platform. Additional equipment may also be needed to provide and obtain sensitive clinical materials (eg, homework assignments or consent forms) [94].

Although intensive and massed treatment approaches address many barriers to traditional forms of therapy, the cost-effectiveness of these approaches needs to be examined further, as these treatments may sometimes require additional resources [104]. For example, these treatments may take place outside of normal operation hours, such as in the evenings or weekends. Additional staff may be required when therapeutic services are offered, including administrative staff assisting in contacting and scheduling clients and facility security. Furthermore, some insurance programs may not provide coverage for prolonged services; thus, treatment formats that require such services may place a financial burden on clients.

CLINICS CARE POINTS

- Intensive and brief treatment formats have been developed to address treatment barriers, where individuals complete a full course of treatment in as little as 1 week.
- Preliminary evidence supports the efficacy of intensive and brief treatments for PTSD.
- Technology helps increase the accessibility of PTSD psychotherapies.
- IBIs and mobile applications are also being used to increase treatment engagement and augment standard therapy approaches.
- Although incorporating technology in treatment shows high acceptability ratings from users, more work is needed to evaluate the effectiveness of these approaches in improving PTSD symptoms.
- It is important to ensure that resources to conduct video telehealth are available, including the development of safety protocols.

REFERENCES

[1] Michopoulos V, Norrholm SD, Jovanovic T. Diagnostic biomarkers for posttraumatic stress disorder (PTSD): promising horizons from translational neuroscience research. Biol Psychiatry 2015;78(5):344–53.

[2] VA/DoD Clinical Practice Guideline Working Group. VA/DoD clinical practice guideline for the management of posttraumatic stress disorder and acute stress disorder. Washington, DC: VA Office of Quality and Performance; 2017.

[3] Steenkamp MM, Litz BT, Hoge CW, et al. Psychotherapy for military-related PTSD: a review of randomized clinical trials. JAMA 2015;314(5):489–500.

[4] Stecker T, Shiner B, Watts BV, et al. Treatment-seeking barriers for veterans of the Iraq and Afghanistan conflicts who screen positive for PTSD. Psychiatr Serv 2013;64(3):280–3.

[5] Foa EB, McLean CP, Zang Y, et al. Effect of prolonged exposure therapy delivered over 2 weeks vs 8 weeks vs present-centered therapy on PTSD symptom severity in military personnel: a randomized clinical trial. JAMA 2018;319(4):354–64.

[6] Ehlers A, Hackmann A, Grey N, et al. A randomized controlled trial of 7-day intensive and standard weekly cognitive therapy for PTSD and emotion-focused supportive therapy. Am J Psychiatry 2014;171(3):294–304.

[7] Morland LA, Mackintosh MA, Rosen CS, et al. Telemedicine versus in-person delivery of Cognitive Processing Therapy for women with posttraumatic stress disorder: a randomized noninferiority trial. Depress Anxiety 2015;32(11):811–20.

[8] Spence J, Titov N, Dear BF, et al. Randomized controlled trial of Internet-delivered cognitive behavioral therapy for posttraumatic stress disorder. Depress Anxiety 2011;28(7):541–50.

[9] Lange A, Schricken B, van de Ven J, et al. "Interapy": the effects of a short protocolled treatment of posttraumatic stress and pathological grief through the internet. Behav Cogn Psychother 2000;28(2):175–92.

[10] American Psychological Association. Clinical practice guideline for the treatment of posttraumatic stress disorder (PTSD) in adults 2017 Washington, DC.

[11] Forbes D, Bisson JI, Monson CM, et al. Effective treatments for PTSD: practice guidelines from the International Society for traumatic stress studies. 3rd edition. New York: The Guildford Press; 2020.

[12] Foa E, Hembree E, Rothbaum BO, et al. Prolonged exposure therapy for PTSD: emotional processing of traumatic experiences therapist guide. 2nd edition. New York: Oxford University Press; 2019.

[13] Resick PA, Monson CM, Chard KM. Cognitive processing therapy for PTSD: a comprehensive manual. New York: Oxford University Press; 2017.

[14] Shapiro F. Eye movement desensitization and reprocessing (EMDR) therapy: basic principles, protocols and procedures. 3rd edition. New York: The Guildford Press; 2017.

[15] Foa EB, Kozak MJ. Treatment of anxiety disorders: implications for psychopathology. In: Tuma AH, Maser JD, editors. Anxiety and the anxiety disorders. New Jersey: Lawrence Erlbaum Associates; 1985. p. 421–52.

[16] Foa EB, Kozak MJ. Emotional processing of fear: exposure to corrective information. Psychol Bull 1986; 99(1):20–35.

[17] Foa EB, Cahill SP. Emotional processing in psychological therapies. In: Smelser NJ, Bates PB, editors. International encyclopedia of the social and behavioral sciences. Oxford (United Kingdom): Elsevier; 2001. p. 12363–9.

[18] Foa EB, Huppert JD, Cahill SP. Emotional processing theory: an update. In: Rothbaum BO, editor. Pathological anxiety: emotional processing in etiology and treatment. New York: The Guilford Press; 2006. p. 3–24.

[19] McLean CP, Foa EB. Prolonged exposure therapy for post-traumatic stress disorder: a review of evidence and dissemination. Expert Rev Neurother 2011;11(8): 1151–63.

[20] Clapp JD, Kemp JJ, Cox KS, et al. Patterns of change in response to prolonged exposure: implications for treatment outcome. Depress Anxiety 2016;33(9):807–15.

[21] Foa EB, Hembree EA, Cahill SP, et al. Randomized trial of prolonged exposure for posttraumatic stress disorder with and without cognitive restructuring: outcome at academic and community clinics. J Consult Clin Psychol 2005;73(5):953–64.

[22] Powers MB, Halpern JM, Ferenschak MP, et al. A meta-analytic review of prolonged exposure for posttraumatic stress disorder. Clin Psychol Rev 2010;30(6):635–41.

[23] Resick PA, Williams LF, Suvak MK, et al. Long-term outcomes of cognitive–behavioral treatments for posttraumatic stress disorder among female rape survivors. J Consult Clin Psychol 2012;80(2):201.

[24] Bradley R, Greene J, Russ E, et al. A multidimensional meta-analysis of psychotherapy for PTSD. Am J Psychiatry 2005;162(2):214–27.

[25] Rothbaum BO, Astin MC, Marsteller F. Prolonged exposure versus eye movement desensitization and reprocessing (EMDR) for PTSD rape victims. J Trauma Stress 2005;18(6):607–16.

[26] Schnurr PP, Friedman MJ, Engel CC, et al. Cognitive behavioral therapy for posttraumatic stress disorder in women: a randomized controlled trial. JAMA 2007; 297(8):820–30.

[27] Bandura A. Human agency in social cognitive theory. Am Psychol 1989;44(9):1175–84.

[28] Resick PA, Schnicke MK. Cognitive processing therapy for sexual assault victims. J Consult Clin Psychol 1992;60(5):748–56.

[29] Sobel AA, Resick PA, Rabalais AE. The effect of cognitive processing therapy on cognitions: impact statement coding. J Trauma Stress 2009;22(3):205–11.

[30] Holliday R, Holder N, Surís A. A single-arm meta-analysis of cognitive processing therapy in addressing trauma-related negative cognitions. J Aggress Maltreat Trauma 2018;27(10):1145–53.

[31] Iverson KM, King MW, Cunningham KC, et al. Rape survivors' trauma-related beliefs before and after cognitive processing therapy: associations with PTSD and depression symptoms. Behav Res Ther 2015;66:49–55.

[32] Chard KM, Ricksecker EG, Healy ET, et al. Dissemination and experience with cognitive processing therapy. J Rehabil Res Dev 2012;49:667–78.

[33] Chard KM, Schumm JA, Owens GP, et al. A comparison of OEF and OIF veterans and Vietnam veterans receiving cognitive processing therapy. J Trauma Stress 2010;23(1):25–32.

[34] Chard KM, Schumm JA, McIlvain SM, et al. Exploring the efficacy of a residential treatment program incorporating cognitive processing therapy-cognitive for veterans with PTSD and traumatic brain injury. J Trauma Stress 2011;24(3):347–51.

[35] Asmundson GJG, Thorisdottir AS, Roden-Foreman JW, et al. A meta-analytic review of cognitive processing therapy for adults with posttraumatic stress disorder. Cogn Behav Ther 2019;48(1):1–14.

[36] Cusack K, Jonas DE, Forneris CA, et al. Psychological treatments for adults with posttraumatic stress disorder:

a systematic review and meta-analysis. Clin Psychol Rev 2016;43:128–41.
[37] Jonas DE, Cusack K, Forneris CA, et al. Psychological and pharmacological treatments for adults with post-traumatic stress disorder (PTSD). Maryland: Agency for Healthcare Research and Quality; Comparative effectiveness review No. 92 2013.
[38] Shapiro F. Efficacy of the eye movement desensitization procedure in the treatment of traumatic memories. J Trauma Stress 1989;2:199–223.
[39] Shapiro F, Forrest MS. EMDR: eye movement desensitization and reprocessing. New York: Guilford; 2001.
[40] Shapiro F. New notes on adaptive information processing. Hamden (CT): EMDR Humanitarian Assistance Programs; 2006.
[41] Shapiro F, Maxfield L. Eye movement desensitization and reprocessing (EMDR): information processing in the treatment of trauma. J Clin Psychol 2002;58(8):933–46.
[42] Lee CW, Cuijpers P. A meta-analysis of the contribution of eye movements in processing emotional memories. J Behav Ther Exp Psychiatry 2013;44(2):231–9.
[43] Chen L, Zhang G, Hu M, et al. Eye movement desensitization and reprocessing versus cognitive-behavioral therapy for adult posttraumatic stress disorder: systematic review and meta-analysis. J Nerv Ment Dis 2015; 203(6):443–51.
[44] Cuijpers P, van Veen SC, Sijbrandij M, et al. Eye movement desensitization and reprocessing for mental health problems: a systematic review and meta-analysis. Cogn Behav Ther 2020;49(3):165–80.
[45] Capezzani L, Ostacoli L, Cavallo M, et al. EMDR and CBT for cancer patients: comparative study of effects on PTSD, anxiety, and depression. J EMDR Pract Res 2013;7(3):134–43.
[46] Nijdam MJ, Gersons BPR, Reitsma JB, et al. Brief eclectic psychotherapy v. eye movement desensitisation and reprocessing therapy for post-traumatic stress disorder: randomised controlled trial. Br J Psychiatry 2012; 200(3):224–31.
[47] van den Berg DPG, de Bont PAJM, van der Vleugel BM, et al. Prolonged exposure vs eye movement desensitization and reprocessing vs waiting list for posttraumatic stress disorder in patients with a psychotic disorder: a randomized clinical trial. JAMA Psychiatry 2015; 72(3):259–67.
[48] van den Berg D, de Bont PAJM, van der Vleugel BM, et al. Long-term outcomes of trauma-focused treatment in psychosis. Br J Psychiatry 2018;212(3):180–2.
[49] McNally RJ. The evolving conceptualization and treatment of PTSD: a very brief history. Trauma Psychology Newsletter 2013;7–11.
[50] Harvey AG, Bryant RA, Tarrier N. Cognitive behaviour therapy for posttraumatic stress disorder. Clin Psychol Rev 2003;23(3):501–22.
[51] Ehlers A, Clark DM. A cognitive model of posttraumatic stress disorder. Behav Res Ther 2000;38(4): 319–45.
[52] Lewis C, Roberts NP, Andrew M, et al. Psychological therapies for post-traumatic stress disorder in adults: systematic review and meta-analysis. Eur J Psychotraumatol 2020;11(1):1729633.
[53] Kline AC, Cooper AA, Rytwinksi NK, et al. Long-term efficacy of psychotherapy for posttraumatic stress disorder: a meta-analysis of randomized controlled trials. Clin Psychol Rev 2018;59:30–40.
[54] Gersons BPR, Carlier IVE, Olff M. Protocol brief eclectic psychotherapy for posttraumatic stress disorder. Amsterdam: Academic Medical Center, University of Amsterdam; 2004.
[55] Gersons BPR, Meewisse ML, Nijdam MJ, et al. Protocol: brief eclectic psychotherapy for posttraumatic stress disorder (BEPP). 3rd edition. Amsterdam: Academic Medical Centre, University of Amsterdam; 2011 Maul-Phillips J, trans.
[56] Gersons BP, Carlier IV, Lamberts RD, et al. Randomized clinical trial of brief eclectic psychotherapy for police officers with posttraumatic stress disorder. J Trauma Stress 2000;13(2):333–47.
[57] Lindauer RJ, Gersons BP, van Meijel EP, et al. Effects of brief eclectic psychotherapy in patients with posttraumatic stress disorder: randomized clinical trial. J Trauma Stress 2005;18(3):205–12.
[58] Schauer M, Neuner F, Elbert T. Narrative exposure therapy: a short-term treatment for traumatic stress disorders. 2nd edition. Cambridge (MA): Hogrefe Publishing; 2011.
[59] Neuner F, Elbert T, Schauer M. Narrative Exposure Therapy (NET) as a treatment for traumatized refugees and post-conflict populations. In: Morina N, Nickerson A, editors. Mental health of refugee and conflict-affected populations: theory, research and clinical practice. Cham (Switzerland): Spring Nature; 2018. p. 183–99.
[60] Lely JC, Smid GE, Jongedijk RA, et al. The effectiveness of narrative exposure therapy: a review, meta-analysis and meta-regression analysis. Eur J Psychotraumatol 2019;10(1):1550344.
[61] Ehlers A, Clark DM, Hackmann A, et al. Intensive cognitive therapy for PTSD: a feasibility study. Behav Cogn Psychother 2010;38(4):383–98.
[62] Hendriks L, Kleine RA, Broekman TG, et al. Intensive prolonged exposure therapy for chronic PTSD patients following multiple trauma and multiple treatment attempts. Eur J Psychotraumatol 2018;9(1):1425574.
[63] Harvey MM, Petersen TJ, Sager JC, et al. An intensive outpatient program for veterans with posttraumatic stress disorder and traumatic brain injury. Cogn Behav Pract 2019;26(2):323–34.
[64] Zalta AK, Held P, Smith DL, et al. Evaluating patterns and predictors of symptom change during a three-week intensive outpatient treatment for veterans with PTSD. BMC Psychiatry 2018;18(1):242.
[65] Van Woudenberg C, Voorendonk EM, Bongaerts EM, et al. Effectiveness of an intensive treatment programme

combining prolonged exposure and eye movement desensitixation and reprocessing for severe post-traumatic stress disorder. Eur J Psychotraumatol 2018;9(1): 1467225.
[66] Sciarrino NA, Warnecke AJ, Teng EJ. A systematic review of intensive empirically supported treatments for post-traumatic stress disorder. J Trauma Stress 2020;33(4): 443–54.
[67] Sherrill AM, Maples-Keller JL, Yasinski CW, et al. Perceived benefits and drawbacks of massed prolonged exposure: a qualitative thematic analysis of reactions from treatment completers. Psychol Trauma 2020. https://doi.org/10.1037/tra0000548.
[68] Sloan DM, Marx BP, Bovin MJ, et al. Written exposure as an intervention for PTSD: a randomized clinical trial with motor vehicle accident survivors. Behav Res Ther 2012;50(10):627–35.
[69] Sloan DM, Lee DJ, Litwack SD, et al. Written exposure therapy for veterans diagnosed with PTSD: a pilot study. J Trauma Stress 2013;26(6):776–9.
[70] Sloan DM, Marx BP, Lee DJ, et al. A brief exposure-based treatment vs cognitive processing therapy for posttraumatic stress disorder: a randomized noninferiority clinical trial. JAMA Psychiatry 2018;75(3):233–9.
[71] Thompson-Hollands J, Marx BP, Lee DJ, et al. Long-term treatment gains of a brief exposure-based treatment for PTSD. Depress Anxiety 2018;35(10):985–91.
[72] Kip KE, Elk CA, Sullivan KL, et al. Brief treatment of symptoms of post-traumatic stress disorder (PTSD) by use of accelerated resolution therapy (ART®). Behav Sci (Basel) 2012;2(2):115–34.
[73] Kip KE, Rosenzweig L, Hernandez DF, et al. Randomized controlled trial of accelerated resolution therapy (ART) for symptoms of combat-related post-traumatic stress disorder (PTSD). Mil Med 2013;178(12): 1298–309.
[74] Kip KE, Diamond DM. Clinical, empirical, and theoretical rationale for selection of accelerated resolution therapy for treatment of post-traumatic stress disorder in VA and DoD facilities. Mil Med 2018;183(9–10): e314–21.
[75] Kip KE, D'Aoust RF, Hernandez DF, et al. Evaluation of brief treatment of symptoms of psychological trauma among veterans residing in a homeless shelter by use of Accelerated Resolution Therapy. Nurs Outlook 2016;64(5):411–23.
[76] Rossiter AG, D'Aoust RF, Shafer MR, et al. Accelerated resolution therapy for women veterans experiencing military sexual trauma related to posttraumatic stress disorder. Ann Psychiatry Ment Health 2017;5(4):1–6.
[77] Kip K, Sullivan KL, Lengacher CA, et al. Brief treatment of co-occurring post-traumatic stress and depressive symptoms by use of accelerated resolution therapy®. Front Psychiatry 2013;4:11.
[78] Littleton H, Buck K, Rosman L, et al. From survivor to thriver: a pilot study of an online program for rape victims. Cogn Behav Pract 2012;19(2):315–27.
[79] Kuester A, Niemeyer H, Knaevelsrud C. Internet-based interventions for posttraumatic stress: a meta-analysis of randomized controlled trials. Clin Psychol Rev 2016;43:1–16.
[80] Simon N, McGillivray L, Roberts NO, et al. Acceptability of internet-based cognitive behavioural therapy (i-CBT) for post-traumatic stress disorder (PTSD): a systematic review. Eur J Psychotraumatol 2019;10(1): 164092.
[81] Ivarsson D, Blom M, Hesser H, et al. Guided internet-delivered cognitive behavior therapy for post-traumatic stress disorder: a randomized controlled trial. Internet Interv 2014;1(1):33–40.
[82] Lewis CE, Farewell D, Groves V, et al. Internet-based guided self-help for posttraumatic stress disorder (PTSD): randomized controlled trial. Depress Anxiety 2017;34(6):555–65.
[83] Gould CE, Kok BC, Ma VK, et al. Veterans affairs and the department of defense mental health apps: a systematic literature review. Psychol Serv 2018;16(2): 196–208.
[84] Sander LB, Schorndanner J, Terhorst Y, et al. 'Help for trauma from the app stores?' A systematic review and standardized rating of apps for Post-Traumatic Stress Disorder (PTSD). Eur J Psychotraumatol 2020;11: 1701788.
[85] Miner A, Kuhn E, Hoffman JE, et al. Feasibility, acceptability, and potential efficacy of the PTSD Coach App: a randomized controlled trial with community trauma survivors. Psychol Trauma 2016;8(3):384–92.
[86] Pacella-Labarbara ML, Suffoletto BP, Kuhn E, et al. A pilot randomized controlled trial of the PTSD Coach app following motor vehicle crash-related injury. J Acad Emerg Med 2020. https://doi.org/10.1111/acem.14000.
[87] Kuhn E, Kanuri N, Hoffman JE, et al. A randomized controlled trial of a smartphone app for posttraumatic stress disorder symptoms. J Consult Clin Psychol 2017;85(3):267–73.
[88] Possemato K, Kuhn E, Johnson E, et al. Using PTSD Coach in primary care with and without clinician support: a pilot randomized controlled trail. Gen Hosp Psychiatry 2016;38:94–8.
[89] Tiet QQ, Duong H, Davis L, et al. PTSD Coach mobile application with brief telephone support: a pilot study. Psychol Serv 2019;16(2):227–32.
[90] Rodriguez-Paras C, Tippey K, Brown E, et al. Posttraumatic stress disorder and mobile health: app investigation and scoping literature review. JMIR Mhealth Uhealth 2017;5(10):e156.
[91] Reger GM, Skoop NA, Edwards-Stewart W, et al. Comparison of Prolonged Exposure (PE) Coach to treatment as usual: a case series with two active duty soldiers. Mil Psychol 2015;27(50):287–96.
[92] Reger GM, Browne KC, Campellone TR, et al. Barriers and facilitators to mobile application use during PTSD treatment: clinician adoption of PE Coach. Prof Psychol Res Pr 2017;48(6):510–7.

[93] Hagerty SL, Wielgosz J, Kraemer J, et al. Best practices for approaching cognitive processing therapy and prolonged exposure during the COVID-19 pandemic. J Trauma Stress 2020;33:623–33.

[94] Morland LA, Wells SY, Glassman LH, et al. Advances in PTSD treatment delivery: review of findings and clinical considerations for the use of telehealth interventions for PTSD. Curr Treat Options Psychiatry 2020;7: 221–41.

[95] Olthuis JV, Wozney L, Asmundson GJG, et al. Distance-delivered interventions for PTSD: a systematic review and meta-analysis. J Anxiety Disord 2016;44:9–26.

[96] Peterson AL, Mintz J, Moring JC, et al. In-office, in-home, and telebehavioral health cognitive processing therapy for combat-related PTSD: Preliminary results of a randomized clinical trial. Paper presented at the San Antonio Combat PTSD Conference, San Antonio, TX; 2019.

[97] Moring JC, Dondanville KA, Rina BA, et al. Cognitive processing therapy for posttraumatic stress disorder via telehealth: practical considerations during the COVID-19 pandemic. J Trauma Stress 2020;33:371–9.

[98] Gros DF, Allan NP, Lancaster CL, et al. Predictors of treatment discontinuation during prolonged exposure for PTSD. Behav Cogn Psychother 2018;46:35–49.

[99] Clark P, Kimberly C. Impact of fees among low-income clients in a training clinic. Contemp Fam Ther 2014;36: 363–8.

[100] Gros DF, Lancaster CL, López CM, et al. Treatment satisfaction of home-based telehealth versus in-person delivery of prolonged exposure for combat-related PTSD in veterans. J Telemed Telecare 2018;24(1):51–5.

[101] Hernandez-Tejada MA, Zoller JS, Ruggiero KJ, et al. Early treatment withdrawal from evidence-based psychotherapy for PTSD: telemedicine and in-person parameters. Int J Psychiatry Med 2014;48(1):33–55.

[102] Cooper AA, Kline AC, Graham B, et al. Homework "dose," type, and helpfulness as predictors of clinical outcomes in prolonged exposure for PTSD. Behav Ther 2017;48(2):182–94.

[103] Wiltsey Stirman S, Gutner CA, Suvak MK, et al. Homework completion, patient characteristics, and symptom change in cognitive processing therapy for PTSD. Behav Ther 2018;49(5):741–55.

[104] Deacon B, Abramowitz J. A pilot study of two-day cognitive0behavioral therapy for panic disorder. Behav Res Ther 2006;44(6):807–17.

Advances in Psychiatry and Behavioral Health 1 (2021) 13–23
ADVANCES IN PSYCHIATRY AND BEHAVIORAL HEALTH

Advances in Psychotherapy for Eating Disorders

Cody Staples, BS[a], William Grunewald, MA[b], April R. Smith, PhD[b], Diana Rancourt, PhD[a,*]
[a]University of South Florida, 4202 East Fowler Avenue, Tampa, FL 33620, USA; [b]Miami University, 90 North Patterson Avenue, Oxford, OH 45056, USA

KEYWORDS
• Feeding and eating disorders • Humans • Male • Minority groups • Psychotherapy • Treatment outcome

KEY POINTS

- Cognitive behavior therapy-enhanced remains the primary psychotherapy for all eating disorders, though third-wave approaches may be useful adjuncts.
- A unified protocol for eating disorders, cue exposure and response prevention, appetite awareness training, and biofeedback-focused approaches shows promise.
- Limited research examines the efficacy of eating disorder psychotherapy for men, members of sexual minority groups, members of racial/ethnic minority groups, and individuals with excess weight who present with restriction/compensatory behaviors.

BACKGROUND

Eating disorders (EDs) are serious mental illnesses associated with increased morbidity and mortality. For instance, anorexia nervosa (AN) has the highest mortality rate of any psychiatric illness, with suicide as the second-leading cause of death [1]. Without treatment, EDs tend to have a chronic course and exact significant mental and physical tolls. Unfortunately, despite decades of research, the effectiveness of ED treatment remains limited for many individuals, particularly adults with AN. Further, ED treatments have been vastly understudied in a variety of populations, including men, racial/ethnic minorities, individuals with excess weight, and LGBTQ+ populations. This review summarizes the past 5 years of ED psychotherapy treatment research across ED diagnoses and concludes with avenues for future research. Understanding which treatments work and for whom can allow for more personalized treatment selection and improve outcomes for individuals with EDs.

CURRENT EVIDENCE

Cognitive behavior therapy—enhanced (CBT-E) is a transdiagnostic treatment for eating disorders. CBT-E has the strongest empirical support of any psychotherapy for EDs and is more effective than third-wave therapies, including acceptance and commitment therapy (ACT), dialectical behavioral therapy (DBT), mindfulness-based interventions (MBIs), and compassion-focused therapy (CFT) [2]. Because of the efficacy of CBT-E, research has shifted to investigate the mechanisms underlying the success of this treatment approach and its utility for treating understudied/severe forms of eating psychology.

The authors have nothing to disclose.

*Corresponding author, *E-mail address:* drancourt@usf.edu

https://doi.org/10.1016/j.ypsc.2021.05.007
2667-3827/21/

None of the third-wave behavior therapies (ACT, DBT, MBIs, and CFT) were superior to CBT-E in randomized controlled trials. Furthermore, none met the criteria for an empirically supported treatment (ie, outperforming an alternate evidence-based treatment in multiple randomized controlled trials conducted by different groups of researchers) [2], though they are more efficacious than wait-list controls [3]. Among third-wave interventions, DBT-based interventions showed the largest effects on pre–post treatment improvements in disordered eating and body image [3]. The Stanford model of DBT, which posits that binge eating and purging occur as a means to regulate negative affect, is currently the most common form of DBT used to treat bulimia nervosa (BN) and binge eating disorder (BED) [4]. It is important to note that many studies examining the utility of DBT for eating disorders employ DBT skills along with another treatment modality, such as family-based treatment (FBT).

Interpersonal therapy (IPT) and ACT may be useful as adjuncts to CBT-E. IPT is often used with individuals who do not show significant improvements with CBT-E [2]. Preliminary research supports ACT as a supplemental treatment modality to CBT-E or another third-wave approach [3]. Additional research on the sequential application of treatment modalities is needed. See Table 1 for the empirically supported treatment status of psychotherapies for EDs.

Psychotherapy for Anorexia Nervosa

CBT-E is a well-documented treatment for AN among adults; however, recent data suggest similar outcomes for the Maudsley model (ie, family-based treatment), specialist supportive clinical management (ie, management of AN symptoms with supportive psychotherapy), and CBT-E, suggesting the need for further comparison studies [5]. IPT was less effective than either CBT-E or specialist supportive clinical management [6], suggesting that IPT may not be an effective treatment choice for AN. Mechanisms of CBT-E include reducing starvation symptoms and decreasing body image concern and body checking behaviors [7–9].

Among adolescents, FBT is the most well-established and supported treatment for AN [10]. FBT shows comparable outcomes in single- and multi-family settings [11] and is associated with fewer hospitalizations than other parent-focused interventions [12,13]. Efforts to enhance outcomes include integrating aspects of CBT-E and skills from DBT [14] and testing the utility of sequential treatment with CBT-E and FBT [15]. Notably, these enhancement efforts seem to primarily impact weight gain and not disordered eating behaviors. For example, FBT combined with DBT improves weight but does not decrease disordered eating behaviors [16], and both direct and indirect parental prompts are associated with weight gain but not changes in eating pathology [17]. Consistent with these findings, integrations of FBT and DBT show small to medium effect sizes for decreased binge eating and small effect sizes for decreased restriction and depressive symptoms [18]. The sequential use of CBT-E followed by FBT shows promise and is associated with increased weight and decreased ED symptoms among adolescents [15]. Interestingly, acceptance-based separated family treatment (ie, the therapist meets with the adolescent and parents separately) yielded significant changes in disordered eating symptoms and weight gain from baseline to completion of treatment [19], suggesting the utility of providing both family and individual treatment modalities to adolescents with AN.

Third-wave treatments (eg, ACT and DBT) have little data to support their effectiveness for decreasing disordered eating behaviors in individuals with AN, primarily due to a lack of randomized controlled trials. Applications of DBT to treat AN have specifically targeted emotion regulation and overcontrol and demonstrate increases in body mass index (BMI) and decreases in broad ED symptoms [20,21]. Radically open DBT (RO-DBT) is a novel adaptation of DBT for AN that focuses on social skills and connectedness [22], but RO-DBT is in the early phases of testing, precluding definitive conclusions about its effectiveness [4]. Few studies have tested the utility of ACT, with generally nonsignificant findings. In an inpatient setting, ACT showed slightly better treatment outcomes than treatment as usual, but these group differences were not statistically significant [23]. Similarly, a comparison of acceptance/mindfulness strategies, cognitive restructuring, and distraction tasks to address body image concerns among individuals with AN or Body Dysmorphic Disorder suggested that cognitive restructuring was the most effective [23], lending additional support for the use of CBT-E with individuals with AN.

Psychotherapy for Bulimia Nervosa

Interventions incorporating CBT-E demonstrate the highest remission rates for BN among adults [24], and CBT-E routinely outperforms integrative cognitive-affective therapy for BN in reducing bulimic symptomology [25,26]. Notably, while FBT is associated with higher binge eating and purging abstinence rates than CBT-E at 6 months, these differences do not persist at 12 months posttreatment [27]. While not specifically targeted as part of CBT-E, improvements in emotion

TABLE 1
Status of Most Common Treatment Modalities

Treatment	Empirically Supported Treatment?	Evidence Regarding Effectiveness
Cognitive behavior therapy — enhanced (CBT-E)	Yes	• The gold-standard of psychotherapy for all eating disorders
Interpersonal therapy (IPT)	Yes (for BN and BED)	• Efficacious treatment alternative to CBT-E • Less evidence supports effectiveness for individuals with AN
Family-based treatment	Yes (for AN and BN)	• Most well-supported treatment for adolescents with AN, BN, and ARFID • Often coupled with CBT-E for adolescents
Dialectical behavior therapy (DBT)	No	• Early evidence suggests DBT may be the most effective third-wave treatment approaches
Acceptance and commitment therapy (ACT)	No	• May be most effective as an adjunct to CBT-E
Cue Exposure and Response Prevention (CERP)	No	• Preliminary evidence suggests ED-specific CERP may be effective in increasing caloric intake (AN) and decreasing binge eating and purging (BN)
Mindfulness-Based Interventions (MBIs)	No	• Often utilized in the treatment of individuals with binge eating • Frequently paired with other therapies

Abbreviations: AN, anorexia nervosa; ARFID, avoidance/restrictive food intake disorder; BED, binge eating disorder; BN, bulimia nervosa; OSFED, other specified feeding or eating disorder.

regulation may be a salient mechanism for CBT-E for BN [28,29].

DBT for BN places emphasis on emotion regulation, as changes in emotion regulation are related to changes in disordered eating symptomology over time [20]. DBT integrated into FBT yielded decreased overall eating pathology, objective binge episodes, and self-induced vomiting [30]. Despite emotion regulation being the theorized mechanism, the integration of DBT and FBT did not result in statistically significant improvements in self-reported emotion regulation [30]. It may be that while emotion regulation remains unchanged, individuals are using more adaptive and non-BN behaviors to regulate their emotional distress.

Interventions that address interpersonal processes show promise for treating BN. Client-centered group therapy with a focus on interpersonal problems decreased global eating pathology [31]. Although short-term effects may be less robust, IPT demonstrates comparable long-term effects to CBT-E [32]. In a treatment study involving women with BN and comorbid depressive symptoms, IPT-BN improved both disordered eating and depressive symptoms [33]. Notably, individuals who display a more domineering interpersonal style may do better with IPT than CBT-E [34].

Though little recent work has focused on the utility of ACT for BN, a randomized pilot study of 140 women with a diagnosis of AN, BN, and other specified feeding or eating disorder (OSFED) suggested that ACT may be associated with larger decreases in eating pathology, as well as fewer rehospitalizations 6-month posttreatment compared with treatment as usual [35].

Psychotherapy for Binge Eating Disorder

In general, IPT performs comparably to CBT-E for BED [32]. One study reported that CBT-E produced better treatment outcomes than IPT; however, the sample included individuals with a range of eating disorder diagnoses (ie, BN, BED, OSFED) [36]. Notably, rapid responders to CBT guided self-help (GSH) showed greater remission rates than individuals who received IPT, and it is suggested that IPT be used as a second treatment option for non–rapid responders to CBT GSH [37]. No recent work has tested the utility of FBT for BED; however, emotion-focused family therapy may be a future direction for the application of FBT to binge eating [38].

The Stanford model of DBT, which largely focuses on emotion regulation, is efficacious for BED and is recommended for individuals who do not respond to CBT-E [4]. Group DBT is associated with decreased binge eating but does not contribute to improved mood [39]. Currently, efforts are being made to extend the availability of DBT for BED through GSH, with positive early evidence [40]. Of note, 1 study suggested comparable decreases in eating pathology across a DBT-based intervention and a weight management treatment [41], underscoring the importance of comparative BED treatment studies and investigating mechanisms of treatment-related change.

ACT yielded decreases in global eating pathology, frequency of binge eating, and depression, as well as improved quality of life among individuals with excess weight and binge eating [42]. A brief acceptance-based intervention focused on compassion also yielded reductions in eating pathology, binge eating, and self-criticism [43]. Incorporating elements of self-compassion into ACT could enhance treatment outcomes for individuals with BED.

Psychotherapy for Avoidant/Restrictive Food Intake Disorder

FBT is the primary treatment modality for children and adolescents with avoidant restrictive food intake disorder (ARFID) and is associated with weight gain and decreased clinical severity compared to usual care [44]. CBT-E has been identified as an efficacious treatment for ARFID that reduces key symptoms in pre-post designs and is associated with significant increases in BMI over the course of treatment [45–47]. Additionally, preliminary data suggest CBT-E may be utilized in conjunction with family therapy to treat ARFID in adolescents [48]. However, additional long-term outcome research and controlled trials are needed to compare the effects of family-based and cognitive-based treatment approaches targeting ARFID.

Factors Predicting Treatment Outcomes

Varied factors (eg, client motivation, symptom severity) influence the success of psychotherapy, and these factors may impact individuals differently based on their ED diagnosis. See Table 2 for information regarding specific factors that predict ED treatment outcomes.

Telehealth, Online Interventions, and Just-in-Time-Adaptive Interventions

While few online adaptations for AN treatment/prevention have been tested, the shift to telehealth due to the COVID-19 pandemic has led to an interest in testing FBT via telepsychology [49]. Online FBT with GSH elements was associated with increases in BMI and decreases in ED symptoms posttreatment in multiple samples of adolescents [50,51]. Results for these studies are promising, but limited research prevents definitive claims about the efficacy of online AN treatment.

Treatments incorporating virtual reality (VR) to generate immersive artificial experiences (eg, a restaurant setting) show promise for treating BN and BED. VR-enhanced cognitive behavioral therapy (VR-CBT) was comparable to standard CBT-E and multimodal treatment, but only VR-CBT also promoted weight

TABLE 2
Factors Predicting Treatment Outcomes by Eating Disorder

Eating Disorder	Factors Related to Positive Outcomes	Factors Related to Negative Outcomes
Anorexia Nervosa	• Higher motivation for recovery at baseline [91] • For adolescents, better functioning in family relationships [92]	• More severe eating pathology • Lower motivation • Lower BMI and having binge-purge subtype predict treatment dropout [91]
Bulimia Nervosa	• CBT-E for those with low baseline self-esteem [93] • Better emotion regulation [20]	• Worse global functioning • Higher age at treatment • Higher drive for thinness [94]
Binge Eating Disorder	• Higher pretreatment relative functioning [95] • Higher adaptive defense mechanisms (eg, humor, affiliation, self-assertion) [96]	• Higher negative urgency [97] • Increased rumination [98]

Abbreviations: BMI, body mass index; CBT-E, cognitive behavior therapy-enhanced.

loss over the course of treatment for BED [52]. Similarly, VR applied specifically as part of cue-exposure therapy (VR-CET; eg, exposing the individual to a feared or strongly craved food) demonstrated superior outcomes compared with standard CBT-E in reducing binge/purge episodes, behavioral/attitudinal features of BED/BN, and food cravings [53–55]. VR demonstrates promising results for the treatment of BN and BED and in weight reduction.

Just-in-time-adaptive-interventions (JITAIs) show theoretic promise in preventing 'relapses' of disordered eating behaviors, but empirically, these programs need refinement, as they show only moderate levels of sensitivity/specificity, with inflated negative predictive values [56].

OTHER PROMISING APPROACHES

Cue exposure and response prevention

Cue exposure and response prevention (CERP) has been adapted for relevance to eating disorders. For ED treatment, food and weight gain are conceptualized as the feared stimuli, and changes in weight and shape, loss of control, and various negative emotions (eg, embarrassment, rejection, abandonment, appearing/feeling disgusting) are the feared outcomes [57]. Among individuals with AN, a small randomized controlled pilot study demonstrated increased caloric intake and decreased eating-related anxiety [58]. In addition, CERP specific to either purging or binge eating was more successful at promoting long-term abstinence among individuals with BN compared with relaxation training [59], and CERP may decrease the frequency of binge eating [60]. While ED-specific CERP shows promise, additional research with larger samples, rigorous methodology, and long-term follow-up is needed.

Appetite awareness training

Limited literature supports appetite awareness training to prevent [61] and treat binge eating and BED [62,63]. There is evidence for its application as a childhood obesity intervention [64–66], but its utility has yet to be tested across other eating disorder presentations (eg, AN, BN, OSFED, ARFID). Of note, appetite awareness training conceptually overlaps with intuitive eating (rejecting diet mentality, accepting all foods, using hunger and satiety cues to guide eating behaviors) and mindful eating approaches (paying full attention to eating experience without judgment). Preliminary evidence suggests an intuitive eating approach associated with improvements in disordered eating attitudes and behaviors, body image, and quality of life among residential patients across all eating disorder diagnoses [67]. An uncontrolled pilot feasibility trial showed that an intuitive eating intervention yielded reductions in disordered eating behavior when delivered both in a group setting and via GSH [68]. Mindfulness-based approaches have primarily been tested with individuals with excess weight and binge eating and show promise for decreasing binge eating disorder symptoms [69].

Biofeedback-focused approaches

Recent efforts have focused on whether physiologic changes, such as heart rate, could be used to predict disordered eating behaviors. This work is nascent but shows promise that heart rate variability may indicate emotion regulation and binge eating severity [70]. Further, heart rate variability may demonstrate acceptable sensitivity and specificity for predicting emotional eating episodes [71]. This work is limited, however, by its use of small samples of adults with excess weight and overeating behaviors (eg, emotional eating, loss of control eating, binge eating) and its exclusive focus on heart rate variability. Blood glucose monitoring also demonstrates the potential for use as a physiologic indicator of hunger that may be useful for hunger and satiety training [72,73]; however, this work has only been conducted with adults with excess weight. Nonetheless, biologically based indicators show promise, especially given the feasibly of collecting these types of data with increasingly ubiquitous wrist-worn sensors (eg, Fitbit, Apple Watch, Garmin) [74].

Unified protocol

A unified protocol (UP) for ED treatment that integrates treatment strategies from various modalities has been proposed for treating severe/comorbid ED cases [75]. Preliminary data from an uncontrolled pre–post study suggest the UP for ED was effective in reducing ED symptomology and various indicators of general psychopathology in complex/severe ED cases [76]. Additional treatment outcome data are needed to understand the promise of UP for ED as being efficacious for the treatment of severe/comorbid EDs.

UNDERSTUDIED POPULATIONS

Studies on ED treatment outcomes almost exclusively include samples of heterosexual White women. Although research suggests that men represent up to a third of ED cases [77], only 2 studies on ED treatments in men currently exist [78,79]. It is possible that findings of ED treatment studies using samples of women might not generalize to men experiencing disordered eating, as males often exhibit different symptom presentations than females (eg, muscularity-oriented disordered eating, compulsive exercise as a primary compensatory behavior, binge eating episodes in the form of "cheat meals," etc) [77]. Additionally, despite overwhelming evidence that sexual minority populations are at disproportionate risk of developing EDs [80–82], research on ED treatment outcomes in this vulnerable population was nonexistent until very recently. Ethnic/racial minority individuals have also been overwhelmingly neglected in ED treatment research [83]. Lastly, individuals with excess weight who present with restrictive eating and compensatory behaviors are underassessed and underidentified in ED treatment studies despite shared risk factors, including dieting behaviors, overvaluation of weight and shape/body dissatisfaction, and low self-esteem [84–86]. Specific findings concerning the limited ED treatment research among these populations are presented in Table 3. It is imperative that future research incorporates these groups into rigorous ED treatment research to understand if existing treatments are appropriate for use with these vulnerable populations.

DISCUSSION

This review highlights that ED treatments for certain populations are more established and effective than for others. Overall, CBT-E is the primary treatment for AN, CBT-E and IPT are promising choices for BN and BED, FBT is effective for treating adolescent AN, and CBT-E and FBT appear to work well for ARFID. However, there are still sizable numbers of individuals for whom many treatments are not effective (eg, adults with chronic AN) or current treatment protocols may not be relevant/appropriate (ie, men). Future research must test interventions within these groups as well as with other neglected populations (eg, LGBTQ+, racial/ethnic minorities). An additional difficulty the field must contend with is that only 1 in 4 individuals with an ED is estimated to seek treatment [87,88]. Thus, work aimed at minimizing treatment barriers (eg, access, expertise, affordability) is also imperative [87].

This review also highlighted several promising new therapies. Online GSH interventions seem promising, and scholars have argued for the economic utility that these programs could provide [89]. Due to their infancy, further replication/validation is required. Similarly, JITAIs show promise in reducing binge/purge behaviors, but additional refinement is necessary to reduce the negative predictive values these programs produce. Concerns regarding JITAI may be assuaged upon results of current pre-registered projects [90]. The delivery of ED treatments online/virtually, especially those incorporating cue exposure, has made

TABLE 3
Understudied Populations in Eating Disorder Treatment Research

Understudied Population	Finding(s)
Men	• Elevated crude and standardized mortality rates [78] • Higher remission rates from other specified feeding or eating disorders (OSFED) • Lower scores on Eating Disorder Inventory subscales, obsessive-compulsive symptoms, and depressive symptoms [79]
Sexual Minorities	• Greater levels of eating disorder/general psychopathology [82] • Early evidence suggests treatment outcomes do not differ [81]
Racial/Ethnic Minorities	• Evidence suggests differences in body esteem and appearance comparison between ethnic groups [99] • There are currently *no data* available on treatment outcomes
Individuals with Excess Weight	• Little research examining restrictive or compensatory eating pathology • *H*ealthy *AP*proach to we*I*ght management and *F*ood in *E*ating *D*isorders (HAPIFED) shows promising results in addressing eating disorder symptoms and weight loss [100,101]

Abbreviation: OSFED, other specified feeding or eating disorder.

progress in the past 5 years, which hopefully will continue to expand treatment access as well as contribute to improved treatment outcomes.

SUMMARY

CBT-E is the leading psychotherapy modality for eating disorders, with IPT, ACT, and DBT serving as potential treatment adjuncts. Promising treatment approaches include the UP for eating disorders, appetite awareness, cue-exposure, and biofeedback-focused approaches. Novel treatment approaches with preliminary evidence include virtual reality interventions. Additional research is needed regarding psychotherapy for eating disorders in men, members of sexual, racial, and ethnic minority groups, and individuals with excess weight suffering from restrictive or compensatory eating pathology.

CLINICS CARE POINTS

- The effectiveness of CBT-E may be enhanced when combined with other treatment approaches (eg, DBT skills, IPT, ACT, and CERP).
- Adolescents may benefit from combined individual and family-based interventions.
- Early evidence suggests that online guided self-help approaches may be useful for individuals who are unable to attend in-person treatment.
- Existing treatments are understudied in their effectiveness for males, racial/ethnic minorities, and intersectional populations and may require adaptations.

REFERENCES

[1] Arcelus J, Mitchell AJ, Wales J, et al. Mortality rates in patients with anorexia nervosa and other eating disorders: a meta-analysis of 36 studies. Arch Gen Psychiatry 2011;68(7):724–31.
[2] Linardon J, Fairburn CG, Fitzsimmons-Craft EE, et al. The empirical status of the third-wave behaviour therapies for the treatment of eating disorders: a systematic review. Clin Psychol Rev 2017;58:125–40.
[3] Linardon J, Gleeson J, Yap K, et al. Meta-analysis of the effects of third-wave behavioural interventions on disordered eating and body image concerns: Implications for eating disorder prevention. Cogn Behav Ther 2019;48(1):15–38.
[4] Ben-Porath D, Duthu F, Luo T, et al. Dialectical behavioral therapy: an update and review of the existing treatment models adapted for adults with eating disorders. Eat Disord 2020;28(2):101–21.
[5] Byrne S, Wade T, Hay P, et al. A randomised controlled trial of three psychological treatments for anorexia nervosa. Psychol Med 2017;47(16):2823–33.
[6] McIntosh VV, Jordan J, Carter JD, et al. Assessing the distinctiveness of psychotherapies and examining change over treatment for anorexia nervosa with cognitive-behavior therapy, interpersonal psychotherapy, and specialist supportive clinical management. Int J Eat Disord 2016;49(10):958–62.
[7] Calugi S, Chignola E, El Ghoch M, et al. Starvation symptoms in patients with anorexia nervosa: a longitudinal study. Eat Disord 2018;26(6):523–37.
[8] Calugi S, El Ghoch M, Conti M, et al. Preoccupation with shape or weight, fear of weight gain, feeling fat and treatment outcomes in patients with anorexia nervosa: a longitudinal study. Behav Res Ther 2018;105: 63–8.
[9] Calugi S, El Ghoch M, Dalle Grave R. Body checking behaviors in anorexia nervosa. Int J Eat Disord 2017; 50(4):437–41.
[10] Lock J. An update on evidence-based psychosocial treatments for eating disorders in children and adolescents. J Clin Child Adolesc Psychol 2015;44(5):707–21.
[11] Marzola E, Knatz S, Murray SB, et al. Short-term intensive family therapy for adolescent eating disorders: 30-month outcome. Eur Eat Disord Rev 2015;23(3): 210–8.
[12] Lock J, Agras WS, Bryson S, et al. Does family-based treatment reduce the need for hospitalization in adolescent anorexia nervosa? Int J Eat Disord 2016;49(9): 891–4.
[13] Lock J, Le Grange D, Agras WS, et al. Can adaptive treatment improve outcomes in family-based therapy for adolescents with anorexia nervosa? Feasibility and treatment effects of a multi-site treatment study. Behav Res Ther 2015;73:90–5.
[14] Johnston JA, O'Gara JS, Koman SL, et al. A pilot study of Maudsley family therapy with group dialectical behavior therapy skills training in an intensive outpatient program for adolescent eating disorders. J Clin Psychol 2015;71(6):527–43.
[15] Hurst K, Zimmer-Gembeck M. Family-based treatment with cognitive behavioural therapy for anorexia. Clin Psychol 2019;23(1):61–70.
[16] Accurso EC, Astrachan-Fletcher E, O'Brien S, et al. Adaptation and implementation of family-based treatment enhanced with dialectical behavior therapy skills for anorexia nervosa in community-based specialist clinics. Eat Disord 2018;26(2):149–63.
[17] White HJ, Haycraft E, Madden S, et al. Parental strategies used in the family meal session of family-based treatment for adolescent anorexia nervosa: links with

treatment outcomes. Int J Eat Disord 2017;50(4): 433–6.
[18] Peterson CM, Van Diest AMK, Mara CA, et al. Dialectical behavioral therapy skills group as an adjunct to family-based therapy in adolescents with restrictive eating disorders. Eat Disord 2020;28(1):67–79.
[19] Timko CA, Zucker NL, Herbert JD, et al. An open trial of Acceptance-based Separated Family Treatment (ASFT) for adolescents with anorexia nervosa. Behav Res Ther 2015;69:63–74.
[20] Brown TA, Cusack A, Berner LA, et al. Emotion regulation difficulties during and after partial hospitalization treatment across eating disorders. Behav Ther 2020; 51(3):401–12.
[21] Chen EY, Segal K, Weissman J, et al. Adapting dialectical behavior therapy for outpatient adult anorexia nervosa—A pilot study. Int J Eat Disord 2015;48(1): 123–32.
[22] Hempel R, Vanderbleek E, Lynch TR. Radically open DBT: targeting emotional loneliness in anorexia nervosa. Eat Disord 2018;26(1):92–104.
[23] Hartmann AS, Thomas JJ, Greenberg JL, et al. Accept, distract, or reframe? An exploratory experimental comparison of strategies for coping with intrusive body image thoughts in anorexia nervosa and body dysmorphic disorder. Psychiatry Res 2015;225(3):643–50.
[24] Linardon J, Wade TD. How many individuals achieve symptom abstinence following psychological treatments for bulimia nervosa? A meta-analytic review. Int J Eat Disord 2018;51(4):287–94.
[25] Accurso EC, Fitzsimmons-Craft EE, Ciao A, et al. Therapeutic alliance in a randomized clinical trial for bulimia nervosa. J Consult Clin Psychol 2015;83(3):637.
[26] Haynos AF, Pearson CM, Utzinger LM, et al. Empirically derived personality subtyping for predicting clinical symptoms and treatment response in bulimia nervosa. Int J Eat Disord 2017;50(5):506–14.
[27] Le Grange D, Lock J, Agras WS, et al. Randomized clinical trial of family-based treatment and cognitive-behavioral therapy for adolescent bulimia nervosa. J Am Acad Child Adolesc Psychiatry 2015;54(11): 886–94, e882.
[28] MacDonald DE, Trottier K, Olmsted MP. Rapid improvements in emotion regulation predict intensive treatment outcome for patients with bulimia nervosa and purging disorder. Int J Eat Disord 2017;50(10): 1152–61.
[29] Peterson CB, Berg KC, Crosby RD, et al. The effects of psychotherapy treatment on outcome in bulimia nervosa: examining indirect effects through emotion regulation, self-directed behavior, and self-discrepancy within the mediation model. Int J Eat Disord 2017;50(6): 636–47.
[30] Murray SB, Anderson LK, Cusack A, et al. Integrating family-based treatment and dialectical behavior therapy for adolescent bulimia nervosa: preliminary outcomes of an open pilot trial. Eat Disord 2015;23(4):336–44.
[31] Ung EM, Erichsen CB, Poulsen S, et al. The association between interpersonal problems and treatment outcome in patients with eating disorders. J Eat Disord 2017;5(1):1–9.
[32] Miniati M, Callari A, Maglio A, et al. Interpersonal psychotherapy for eating disorders: current perspectives. Psychol Res Behav Manag 2018;11:353–69.
[33] Bäck M, Falkenström F, Gustafsson SA, et al. Reduction in depressive symptoms predicts improvement in eating disorder symptoms in interpersonal psychotherapy: results from a naturalistic study. J Eat Disord 2020;8(1): 1–10.
[34] Gomez Penedo JM, Constantino MJ, Coyne AE, et al. Patient baseline interpersonal problems as moderators of outcome in two psychotherapies for bulimia nervosa. Psychother Res 2019;29(6):799–811.
[35] Juarascio A, Shaw J, Forman E, et al. Acceptance and commitment therapy as a novel treatment for eating disorders: an initial test of efficacy and mediation. Behav Modif 2013;37(4):459–89.
[36] Fairburn CG, Bailey-Straebler S, Basden S, et al. A transdiagnostic comparison of enhanced cognitive behaviour therapy (CBT-E) and interpersonal psychotherapy in the treatment of eating disorders. Behav Res Ther 2015;70:64–71.
[37] Hilbert A, Hildebrandt T, Agras WS, et al. Rapid response in psychological treatments for binge eating disorder. J Consult Clin Psychol 2015;83(3):649.
[38] Robinson AL, Dolhanty J, Greenberg L. Emotion-focused family therapy for eating disorders in children and adolescents. Clin Psychol Psychother 2015;22(1): 75–82.
[39] Blood L, Adams G, Turner H, et al. Group dialectical behavioral therapy for binge-eating disorder: outcomes from a community case series. Int J Eat Disord 2020; 53(11):1863–7.
[40] Kenny TE, Carter JC, Safer DL. Dialectical behavior therapy guided self-help for binge-eating disorder. Eat Disord 2020;28(2):202–11.
[41] Mazzeo SE, Lydecker J, Harney M, et al. Development and preliminary effectiveness of an innovative treatment for binge eating in racially diverse adolescent girls. Eat Behav 2016;22:199–205.
[42] Juarascio AS, Manasse SM, Schumacher L, et al. Developing an acceptance-based behavioral treatment for binge eating disorder: rationale and challenges. Cogn Behav Pract 2017;24(1):1–13.
[43] Duarte C, Pinto-Gouveia J, Stubbs RJ. Compassionate attention and regulation of eating behaviour: a pilot study of a brief low-intensity intervention for binge eating. Clin Psychol Psychother 2017;24(6):O1437–47.
[44] Lock J, Sadeh-Sharvit S, L'Insalata A. Feasibility of conducting a randomized clinical trial using family-based treatment for avoidant/restrictive food intake disorder. Int J Eat Disord 2019;52(6):746–51.
[45] Dumont E, Jansen A, Kroes D, et al. A new cognitive behavior therapy for adolescents with avoidant/

restrictive food intake disorder in a day treatment setting: a clinical case series. Int J Eat Disord 2019; 52(4):447–58.

[46] Lane-Loney SE, Zickgraf HF, Ornstein RM, et al. A cognitive-behavioral family-based protocol for the primary presentations of Avoidant/Restrictive Food Intake Disorder (ARFID): case examples and clinical research findings. Cogn Behav Pract 2020.

[47] Thomas JJ, Becker KR, Kuhnle MC, et al. Cognitive-behavioral therapy for avoidant/restrictive food intake disorder: feasibility, acceptability, and proof-of-concept for children and adolescents. Int J Eat Disord 2020; 53(10):1636–46.

[48] Spettigue W, Norris ML, Santos A, et al. Treatment of children and adolescents with avoidant/restrictive food intake disorder: a case series examining the feasibility of family therapy and adjunctive treatments. J Eat Disord 2018;6(1):20.

[49] Matheson BE, Bohon C, Lock J. Family-based treatment via videoconference: clinical recommendations for treatment providers during COVID-19 and beyond. Int J Eat Disord 2020;53(7):1142–54.

[50] Anderson KE, Byrne CE, Crosby RD, et al. Utilizing telehealth to deliver family-based treatment for adolescent anorexia nervosa. Int J Eat Disord 2017;50(10):1235–8.

[51] Lock J, Darcy A, Fitzpatrick KK, et al. Parental guided self-help family based treatment for adolescents with anorexia nervosa: a feasibility study. Int J Eat Disord 2017;50(9):1104–8.

[52] Cesa GL, Manzoni GM, Bacchetta M, et al. Virtual reality for enhancing the cognitive behavioral treatment of obesity with binge eating disorder: randomized controlled study with one-year follow-up. J Med Internet Res 2013;15(6):e113.

[53] Ferrer-García M, Gutiérrez-Maldonado J, Pla-Sanjuanelo J, et al. A randomised controlled comparison of second-level treatment approaches for treatment-resistant adults with bulimia nervosa and binge eating disorder: assessing the benefits of virtual reality cue exposure therapy. Eur Eat Disord Rev 2017;25(6):479–90.

[54] Ferrer-Garcia M, Pla-Sanjuanelo J, Dakanalis A, et al. A randomized trial of virtual reality-based cue exposure second-level therapy and cognitive behavior second-level therapy for bulimia nervosa and binge-eating disorder: outcome at six-month followup. Cyberpsychol Behav Soc Netw 2019;22(1):60–8.

[55] Pla-Sanjuanelo J, Ferrer-Garcia M, Vilalta-Abella F, et al. VR-based cue-exposure therapy (VR-CET) versus VR-CET plus pharmacotherapy in the treatment of bulimic-type eating disorders. Annual Review of CyberTherapy and Telemedicine 2017;15:116–22.

[56] Forman EM, Goldstein SP, Zhang F, et al. OnTrack: development and feasibility of a smartphone app designed to predict and prevent dietary lapses. Transl Behav Med 2019;9(2):236–45.

[57] Butler RM, Heimberg RG. Exposure therapy for eating disorders: a systematic review. Clin Psychol Rev 2020; 78:101851.

[58] Steinglass JE, Albano AM, Simpson HB, et al. Confronting fear using exposure and response prevention for anorexia nervosa: a randomized controlled pilot study. Int J Eat Disord 2014;47(2):174–80.

[59] McIntosh V, Carter F, Bulik C, et al. Five-year outcome of cognitive behavioral therapy and exposure with response prevention for bulimia nervosa. Psychol Med 2011;41(5):1061.

[60] Magson NR, Handford CM, Norberg MM. The empirical status of cue exposure and response prevention treatment for binge eating: a systematic review. Behav Ther 2020;52(2):442–54.

[61] Brown AJ, Smith LT, Craighead LW. Appetite awareness as a mediator in an eating disorders prevention program. Eat Disord 2010;18(4):286–301.

[62] Allen HN, Craighead LW. Appetite monitoring in the treatment of binge eating disorder. Behav Ther 1999; 30(2):253–72.

[63] Craighead LW, Allen HN. Appetite awareness training: a cognitive behavioral intervention for binge eating. Cogn Behav Pract 1995;2(2):249–70.

[64] Bloom T, Sharpe L, Mullan B, et al. A pilot evaluation of appetite-awareness training in the treatment of childhood overweight and obesity: a preliminary investigation. Int J Eat Disord 2013;46(1):47–51.

[65] Boutelle KN, Zucker NL, Peterson CB, et al. Two novel treatments to reduce overeating in overweight children: a randomized controlled trial. J Consult Clin Psychol 2011;79(6):759.

[66] Marx LS, Reddy SD, Welsh JA, et al. Pilot study of appetite monitoring at a family-based camp for obese youth. Clin Pract Pediatr Psychol 2015;3(1):59.

[67] Richards PS, Crowton S, Berrett ME, et al. Can patients with eating disorders learn to eat intuitively? A 2-year pilot study. Eat Disord 2017;25(2):99–113.

[68] Burnette CB, Mazzeo SE. An uncontrolled pilot feasibility trial of an intuitive eating intervention for college women with disordered eating delivered through group and guided self-help modalities. Int J Eat Disord 2020; 53(9):1405–17.

[69] Kristeller J, Wolever RQ, Sheets V. Mindfulness-based eating awareness training (MB-EAT) for binge eating: a randomized clinical trial. Mindfulness 2014;5(3): 282–97.

[70] Godfrey KM, Juarascio A, Manasse S, et al. Heart rate variability and emotion regulation among individuals with obesity and loss of control eating. Physiol Behav 2019;199:73–8.

[71] Juarascio AS, Crochiere RJ, Tapera TM, et al. Momentary changes in heart rate variability can detect risk for emotional eating episodes. Appetite 2020;152:104698.

[72] Jospe MR, de Bruin WE, Haszard JJ, et al. Teaching people to eat according to appetite–Does the method of glucose measurement matter? Appetite 2020;151:104691.
[73] Jospe MR, Taylor RW, Athens J, et al. Adherence to hunger training over 6 months and the effect on weight and eating behaviour: Secondary analysis of a randomised controlled trial. Nutrients 2017;9(11):1260.
[74] Smith KE, Mason TB, Juarascio A, et al. Moving beyond self-report data collection in the natural environment: a review of the past and future directions for ambulatory assessment in eating disorders. Int J Eat Disord 2019;52(10):1157–75.
[75] Thompson-Brenner H, Brooks GE, Boswell JF, et al. Evidence-based implementation practices applied to the intensive treatment of eating disorders: Summary of research and illustration of principles using a case example. Clin Psychol 2018;25(1):e12221.
[76] Thompson-Brenner H, Boswell JF, Espel-Huynh H, et al. Implementation of transdiagnostic treatment for emotional disorders in residential eating disorder programs: a preliminary pre-post evaluation. Psychother Res 2019;29(8):1045–61.
[77] Murray SB, Nagata JM, Griffiths S, et al. The enigma of male eating disorders: a critical review and synthesis. Clin Psychol Rev 2017;57:1–11.
[78] Quadflieg N, Strobel C, Naab S, et al. Mortality in males treated for an eating disorder—A large prospective study. Int J Eat Disord 2019;52(12):1365–9.
[79] Strobel C, Quadflieg N, Naab S, et al. Long-term outcomes in treated males with anorexia nervosa and bulimia nervosa—A prospective, gender-matched study. Int J Eat Disord 2019;52(12):1353–64.
[80] Calzo JP, Blashill AJ, Brown TA, et al. Eating disorders and disordered weight and shape control behaviors in sexual minority populations. Curr Psychiatry Rep 2017;19(8):49.
[81] Donahue JM, DeBenedetto AM, Wierenga CE, et al. Examining day hospital treatment outcomes for sexual minority patients with eating disorders. Int J Eat Disord 2020;53(10):1657–66.
[82] Mensinger JL, Granche JL, Cox SA, et al. Sexual and gender minority individuals report higher rates of abuse and more severe eating disorder symptoms than cisgender heterosexual individuals at admission to eating disorder treatment. Int J Eat Disord 2020;53(4):541–54.
[83] Reyes-Rodríguez ML, Bulik CM. Hacia una adaptación cultural del tratamiento de trastornos alimentarios para Latinos residentes en Estados Unidos. Rev Mex Trastor Aliment 2010;1(1):27–35.
[84] Goldschmidt AB, Wall MM, Zhang J, et al. Overeating and binge eating in emerging adulthood: 10-year stability and risk factors. Dev Psychol 2016;52(3):475.
[85] Haines J, Kleinman KP, Rifas-Shiman SL, et al. Examination of shared risk and protective factors for overweight and disordered eating among adolescents. Arch Pediatr Adolesc Med 2010;164(4):336–43.
[86] Neumark-Sztainer D. Higher weight status and restrictive eating disorders: an overlooked concern. J Adolesc Health 2015;56(1):1–2.
[87] Forrest LN, Smith AR, Swanson SA. Characteristics of seeking treatment among US adolescents with eating disorders. Int J Eat Disord 2017;50(7):826–33.
[88] Merikangas KR, Avenevoli S, Costello EJ, et al. National comorbidity survey replication adolescent supplement (NCS-A): I. Background and measures. J Am Acad Child Adolesc Psychiatry 2009;48(4):367–79.
[89] Kass AE, Balantekin KN, Fitzsimmons-Craft EE, et al. The economic case for digital interventions for eating disorders among United States college students. Int J Eat Disord 2017;50(3):250–8.
[90] van den Berg E, Melisse B, Koenders J, et al. Online cognitive behavioral therapy enhanced for binge eating disorder: study protocol for a randomized controlled trial. BMC Psychiatry 2020;20:1–11.
[91] Gregertsen EC, Mandy W, Kanakam N, et al. Pre-treatment patient characteristics as predictors of drop-out and treatment outcome in individual and family therapy for adolescents and adults with anorexia nervosa: a systematic review and meta-analysis. Psychiatry Res 2019;271:484–501.
[92] Balottin L, Mannarini S, Mensi MM, et al. Are family relations connected to the quality of the outcome in adolescent anorexia nervosa? An observational study with the Lausanne Trilogue Play. Clin Psychol Psychother 2018;25(6):785–96.
[93] Cooper Z, Allen E, Bailey-Straebler S, et al. Predictors and moderators of response to enhanced cognitive behaviour therapy and interpersonal psychotherapy for the treatment of eating disorders. Behav Res Ther 2016;84:9–13.
[94] Quadflieg N, Fichter MM. Long-term outcome of inpatients with bulimia nervosa—Results from the Christina Barz Study. Int J Eat Disord 2019;52(7):834–45.
[95] Maxwell H, Tasca GA, Grenon R, et al. Change in attachment dimensions in women with binge-eating disorder following group psychodynamic interpersonal psychotherapy. Psychother Res 2018;28(6):887–901.
[96] Hill R, Tasca GA, Presniak M, et al. Changes in defense mechanism functioning during group therapy for binge-eating disorder. Psychiatry 2015;78(1):75–88.
[97] Manasse SM, Espel HM, Schumacher LM, et al. Does impulsivity predict outcome in treatment for binge eating disorder? A multimodal investigation. Appetite 2016;105:172–9.

[98] Smith KE, Mason TB, Lavender JM. Rumination and eating disorder psychopathology: a meta-analysis. Clin Psychol Rev 2018;61:9–23.

[99] Rodgers RF, Donovan E, Cousineau TM, et al. Ethnic and racial diversity in eating disorder prevention trials. Eat Disord 2019;27(2):168–82.

[100] da Luz FQ, Swinbourne J, Sainsbury A, et al. Hapifed: a healthy approach to weight management and food in eating disorders: a case series and manual development. J Eat Disord 2017;5(1):29.

[101] Sainsbury-Salis A. The don't go hungry diet. Random House Australia; 2011.

Advances in Psychiatry and Behavioral Health 1 (2021) 25–35

ADVANCES IN PSYCHIATRY AND BEHAVIORAL HEALTH

Is Less Really More? Analysis of Brief, Intensive Treatments for Obsessive-Compulsive Disorder

Bradley C. Riemann, PhD*, Sarah J. David, PhD, Nicholas R. Farrell, PhD, Brenda E. Bailey, PhD

Rogers Behavioral Health System, Oconomowoc, WI, USA

KEYWORDS

- Anxiety disorders • Brief intensive treatments • Cognitive behavioral therapy
- Exposure and response prevention • Inhibitory learning • Obsessive-compulsive disorder

KEY POINTS

- Traditional intensive treatment (IT) models of exposure and response prevention (ERP) (with daily sessions over 3 weeks) and traditional outpatient spaced-treatment (ST) models of ERP (with twice-weekly sessions over 8 weeks or weekly sessions spaced out over a longer period) are highly effective in treating obsessive-compulsive disorder (OCD).
- Open trials of brief intensive treatment (BIT) models (with daily sessions over a few days or 1 week) have produced impressive results; however, concerns related to the strength of data and lack of theoretic support (eg, from an inhibitory learning model) exist.
- Additional research is needed to directly compare BIT approaches with IT and ST models and determine the ideal candidates for this type of intervention.

OCD is a common and debilitating psychiatric disorder characterized by recurrent obsessions or compulsions that interfere substantially with functioning in a variety of life domains (eg, occupational, social, recreational; DSM-5, [1]). OCD has also been found to lead to a significant decrease in the quality of life in adult (eg, [2]) and pediatric samples (eg, [3]). Additionally, one-third of a clinical sample of individuals with OCD reported an inability to work due to the disorder [4], and OCD has also been associated with increases in the use of health-care services [5].

Fortunately, effective treatment in the form of ERP is available. ERP for OCD involves systematic, repeated, and prolonged exposure to situations that provoke obsessional fear while refraining from performing compulsive behaviors (that is, response prevention; for example, [6]). ERP has been found to be effective in ameliorating OCD symptoms in outpatients [7,8] and residential samples [9,10]. It also produces durable gains following treatment completion [8,11–13]. In addition, ERP leads to significant improvement in functional impairment and quality of life for those diagnosed with OCD [14–16].

Depending on a variety of factors, including symptom severity and patient preference, ERP can be effectively delivered in a variety of formats with a varying number of sessions (ie, doses), session durations, and session frequencies (ie, intensities; [8,17,18]). The most studied intensive form of ERP treatment for OCD includes fifteen 2-hour sessions administered daily over 3 weeks (30 total hours of ERP; [7,19]). This model of IT has been considered the "gold standard" for OCD. In a double-blind,

*Corresponding author. Rogers Behavioral Health System, 34700 Valley Road, Oconomowoc, WI 53066. *E-mail address:* bradley.riemann@rogersbh.org

https://doi.org/10.1016/j.ypsc.2021.05.006

randomized, placebo-controlled trial comparing ERP with clomipramine and their combination, Foa and colleagues [20] found that IT was not only effective in reducing OCD symptoms (pretreatment Yale-Brown Obsessive Compulsive Scale [Y-BOCS; [21]] $M = 24.6$; posttreatment $M = 11.0$), but also superior to clomipramine on all measures. The combination of IT and clomipramine was also superior to clomipramine alone, and IT performance did not differ significantly from that of IT and clomipramine combined. In addition to several randomized controlled trials (RCTs) establishing the efficacy of IT for OCD (eg, [22]), the effectiveness of this regimen has been found to significantly reduce OCD symptoms—effect size (ES) = 3.26—in clinical populations without stringent inclusion or exclusion criteria [23]. In pediatric patients who were partial or nonresponders to previous trials of pharmacotherapy [24], IT led to a 54% reduction in OCD symptom severity, which was maintained at a 3-month follow-up. Collectively, there is strong empirical support for IT delivered daily for 3 weeks in adult and pediatric populations [20,22,24].

Unfortunately, the IT model may not be feasible or accessible for many with OCD. The quick symptom reduction experienced over a relatively short period may be offset by the inability to devote the concentrated time necessary to participate in treatment. Some may not be able to rearrange work or school schedules to accommodate this type of treatment format. In addition to the logistics of seeking this type of care, the financial cost of missing work or the academic "cost" of missing school may be prohibitive. The lack of programs and trained clinicians offering this service also produces issues related to access. As a result, patients and families may also incur costs associated with travel (eg, lodging), and the limited number of programs available can mean substantial wait times before one can begin this type of treatment. Therefore, despite being very effective, the 3-week IT format may not be accessible or feasible for all.

As a result, researchers have investigated different versions of this model. Some have kept the dose constant but spaced the treatment out over time (ST; for example, [17]), whereas others have created BIT models (for example, [25]), in both cases in an attempt to address the gaps associated with access and feasibility. In BIT models, essential components of ERP are "compressed" into a truncated schedule. Patients receive less dose of ERP but in a more intensive manner, completing treatment in a matter of days or within a week. The purpose of this article is to review the literature exploring the use of BIT models of ERP for OCD. To better understand these models and their generalizability, we will first briefly review relevant studies investigating the use of traditional, massed IT versus ST models of ERP.

EXPOSURE-BASED TREATMENT FOR OBSESSIVE-COMPULSIVE DISORDER: MASSED VERSUS SPACED MODELS

As discussed above, the 3-week IT model of ERP for OCD is highly effective (eg, [7]). However, due to the logistical challenges, investigators have explored the effects of similar doses of ERP (ie, 30 hours) but spread out over longer periods (ie, reducing the intensity of sessions). These studies explored the notions of "massed" versus "spaced" learning as applied to OCD treatment response. Massed practice maximizes immediate performance at the expense of deteriorating performance when conditions are removed, whereas spaced learning may delay learning during acquisition but enhance long-term retention [26]. Schmidt and Bjork found that while comparing random versus blocked schedules of practice in verbal and motor domains, random conditions were less effective during the acquisition phase but ultimately led to better outcomes than the blocked conditions on a random retention test (ie, the difference between studying for an exam over time vs "cramming" the night before). So what impact, if any, would spacing out the delivery intervals of the same or similar doses of ERP have on OCD outcomes?

Abramowitz and colleagues [17] investigated using an IT versus ST model consisting of 15 twice-weekly sessions over 8 weeks in adults with OCD. They found clinically significant improvement on the Y-BOCS in both conditions at posttreatment (IT ES = 2.70; ST ES = 1.80) and at 3-month follow-up (IT ES = 2.55; ST ES = 2.12). Although a trend at posttreatment was observed in Y-BOCS change, no significant differences between groups at posttreatment or follow-up were found. However, using the Jacobsen and Truax [27] methodology to determine clinically significant change, more patients in the IT condition were found to be recovered than those in the ST condition at posttreatment, but no significant difference was found at a 3-month follow-up. Notably, the lack of between-group differences at 3-month follow-up was seemingly due to the deterioration of treatment gains under the IT condition as well as continued improvement in the ST group. The authors noted that this could have been due to massed versus spaced learning differences [17].

In a nonrandomized comparison, Storch and colleagues [28] examined massed versus spaced delivery of intensive treatment of ERP in adults using fourteen 75-minute to 90-minute sessions delivered daily for

3 weeks (IT) versus once per week (ST), thus spacing the treatment out even further than Abramowitz and colleagues had [17]. Investigators found that both conditions were associated with large ESs based on Y-BOCS at the end of treatment (IT ES = 2.94, ST ES = 2.04) and at a 3-month follow-up (IT ES = 2.41, ST ES = 2.23). There was no main effect for treatment condition (ie, IT vs ST), suggesting that both forms of treatment were equally efficacious. There was also no significant difference between IT or ST in remission status at posttreatment or follow-up, thus supporting the use of either massed or spaced models of ERP. Although nonsignificant, the trends of degradation in IT gains and continued improvement in ST at 3-month follow-up were similar to those found by Abramowitz and colleagues [17].

In a pediatric population, Storch and colleagues [18] conducted an RCT comparing an intensive ERP treatment of fourteen 90-minute daily sessions (IT) with fourteen 90-minute sessions delivered weekly (ST). At least 1 parent attended each session. Both IT (ES = 2.62) and ST (ES = 1.73) produced significant reductions in OCD symptoms at posttreatment based on the Childhood Yale-Brown Obsessive Compulsive Scale (CY-BOCS [29]), but no between-group differences were found at posttreatment nor at 3-month follow-up (IT ES = 2.20; ST ES = 2.33). However, on the Clinical Global Impressions-Severity Scale (CGI-S; [30]), IT was found to have an immediate advantage (mean change 2.8 vs 1.6) over ST. This advantage was lost at follow-up, with no significant group × time interaction on CGI-S. Interestingly, the identical pattern of nonsignificant Y-BOCS/CY-BOCS trends continued with IT losing gains at follow-up and ST showing improvement.

These studies, taken collectively, support the use of IT or ST in the treatment of OCD. Perhaps indicating that dose (ie, number of ERP sessions) is more important than intensity (ie, frequency of ERP sessions). However, there were also indications that IT produced posttreatment results superior to those of ST (eg, clinically significant change; CGI-S) that were lost at 3-month follow-up. In addition, a consistent, nonsignificant trend of IT producing superior Y-BOCS/CY-BOCS reductions at posttreatment and subsequent regression at follow-up and ST producing inferior results posttreatment but continued gains at follow-up was exhibited in all 3 studies. Although nonsignificant trends, one wonders what the effects of larger sample sizes or longer follow-up periods (eg, 6 or 12 months) would have had on the results. Is it possible that ST would have outperformed IT in the long run, consistent with Schmidt and Bjork's [26] massed versus spaced learning theory? Clearly, this is an area for further research. In any event, at a minimum, it appears that those with OCD have a choice between engaging in IT or ST and the logistical pros and cons of each and can expect roughly equivalent results in short-term follow-up.

But what would the result be if, rather than spacing out the ERP sessions, one were to reduce the dose (ie, number of hours of ERP) and deliver ERP hours in a compressed, "super" massed version for a week or less (ie, increasing session intensity)? Would this result in lower, the same, or higher posttreatment gains? At follow-up, would we see the familiar pattern of advantage lost, or possibly even exaggerated losses as Schmidt and Bjork [26] might suggest? Or could super-massed treatment somehow override this phenomenon? Clearly, if ERP could be effectively delivered in a 1-week package, patients would be provided with not only a third viable option but also one they might find preferable to IT or ST. The genesis of brief intensive models was the pioneering single-session, exposure-based interventions by Öst and colleagues for specific phobias (for example, [31]). This concept has also been successfully applied to panic disorder using a 2-day intensive treatment model [32,33]. We will now turn our attention to BIT models of ERP for OCD.

BRIEF INTENSIVE TREATMENTS FOR PEDIATRIC OBSESSIVE-COMPULSIVE DISORDER

Whiteside and colleagues were the first to explore BIT models of ERP for OCD [25]. In an initial case series study, 3 adolescents and their parents received an intensive 5-day ERP treatment for OCD. Emphasis was not only on in-session ERP but also on educating parents to continue to conduct exposures with their children following treatment. This treatment comprised ten 50–75-minute sessions (a total of 8 to 10 hours of ERP) over 5 days. For 2 of the 3 patients, substantial improvement (ie, 40% reduction in symptoms on CY-BOCS) had occurred by posttreatment. For the other, a reduction in OCD symptoms did not occur until after the patient returned home and applied the skills learned during the 5-day treatment [25].

Whiteside and Jacobsen [34] delivered their BIT model to 16 children and adolescents (included in the sample were the 3 from the original case series study) ages 10 to 18 with severe OCD (pretreatment CY-BOCS M = 28.4). Results showed this brief treatment significantly decreased OCD symptoms at posttreatment (ES = 2.07) and 5-month follow-up (ES = 2.77). The mean total posttreatment CY-BOCS was significantly different from the pretreatment mean score and follow-up total mean score, indicating that participants continued to improve after treatment.

In a sample of 22 children and adolescents ages 7 to 18 with severe OCD (pretreatment CY-BOCS *M* = 25.0), Whiteside and colleagues [35] delivered their BIT model using multiple therapists across 2 sites. They also provided key data related to participant "selection." Eighty-five families had received information on the study. Thirty-five (41%) declined to participate for a variety of reasons, 23 (27%) failed the phone screen related to inclusion/exclusion study criteria, and 5 (5.8%) failed the baseline assessment. After these exclusions, only 22 of the original 85 (26%) participants were still enrolled in the study, and 2 more dropped out when they declined to participate in the follow-up assessment. Nevertheless, the authors found additional support for their 5-day BIT model at posttreatment (ES = 1.37) and 3-month follow-up (ES = 1.98). The difference between posttreatment and follow-up was significant, once again showing that patients continued to improve during the follow-up period. Moreover, parental accommodation of OCD decreased significantly at posttreatment (ES = 1.04) and at follow-up (ES = 1.27).

Riise and colleagues [36] administered a 4-day BIT version of blended individual and group ERP (ie, referred to as the Bergen 4-day treatment or B4DT) to children and adolescents (ages 11–17) with severe OCD (pretreatment CY-BOCS *M* = 28.0). Sixty-five individuals were "referred" for treatment, with only 22 being "offered" it for a variety of reasons (eg, did not have OCD, outside of age range). Only 7 (10.8%) individuals eligible chose not to participate (2 did not want group treatment, 4 declined, and 1 asked to postpone treatment). However, it is not clear how many may have "self-selected" out before the referral stage (ie, refused a referral for this type of treatment). Treatment was delivered to 2 to 4 participants and their parents at a time with patient-therapist ratios of 1:1. Two patients discontinued treatment. One experienced motivational issues (the individual's data remained in the intent-to-treat data set), and the other experienced psychotic symptoms, ultimately resulting in 21 participants being analyzed.

Following 1 to 3 assessment sessions, day 1 of treatment consisted of a 3-hour session of psychoeducation, with the first hour combining parents and patients. Parents then met in an individual session with a therapist, focusing on externalizing OCD and providing encouragement to stop all forms of family accommodation, while the adolescent had a concurrent small-group session and began the formulation of a treatment plan. The treatment plan was then completed in a family session, and at the end of the first day, the group met again for a summary. The patients presented their treatment plans to other patients in their groups. On day 2, patients and parents met in a group for a brief repetition of psychoeducation, followed by 5 hours of ERP. In the last 30 minutes of the day, patients and parents met in a group to summarize. Self-administered ERP tasks continued in the evening with a detailed plan for these tasks that covered every hour. On day 3, patients and parents met for a group to summarize homework, followed by a short repetition of psychoeducation on ERP and then 5 hours of ERP (total of 10 hours of in-session ERP). At the end of the day, patients again met in a group to summarize, followed by self-administered ERP tasks in the evening. On day 4, the patients met for 3 hours in a group, summarized their self-administered ERP, received psychoeducation focused on relapse prevention, followed by planning for daily self-administered ERP tasks for the next 3 weeks. Results from this study found that in those that participated, OCD symptoms were substantially reduced after 4 days (ES = 4.67), and their improvements were maintained at both 3-month (ES = 4.98) and 6-month follow-up (ES = 5.20; *n* = 19).

A replication study was conducted by Riise and colleagues [37]. They received 116 patient referrals that ultimately resulted in a sample of 41 adolescents (35.3% of those referred) with severe OCD (pretreatment CY-BOCS *M* = 25.7). Fifty-five patients were excluded for reasons similar to those documented by Risse and colleagues [36] (eg, did not have OCD, outside of age range). Twenty (17.2%) eligible individuals chose not to participate (13 declined any treatment, 6 did not want group treatment, one asked to postpone treatment). Following 3 assessment sessions, Riise and colleagues found that the B4DT model resulted in a significant reduction in OCD symptoms at posttreatment (ES = 4.15) and maintenance of gains at 3-month (ES = 3.24) and 6-month follow-ups (ES = 3.95). The authors noted that "no patients declined due to the concentration of sessions." However, it is not clear how many may have "self-selected" out of this type of treatment to begin with, perhaps related to the intensity of the treatment or the belief that 4 days of treatment would not be beneficial for them.

BRIEF INTENSIVE TREATMENT FOR ADULT OBSESSIVE-COMPULSIVE DISORDER

The initial pilot study [38] of what would become the B4DT model was conducted with 6 adults and involved

2 preliminary sessions for assessment and treatment information gathering, followed by the delivery of the concentrated group treatment over 4 consecutive days. Participants completed a 4-hour psychoeducation session on day 1, a 10-hour ERP session on day 2, an 8-hour ERP session on day 3 (18 hours total of ERP), and a 5-hour relapse prevention and exposure planning session on day 4, followed by a 2-hour booster session 3 months later. Results indicated the mean score on the clinician-rated Y-BOCS decreased from 23.5 points pretreatment to 5.7 at 1-week following posttreatment. The mean Y-BOCS score was 6.5 at 1-month follow-up, 5.8 at 3-month follow-up, and 6.3 at 6-month follow-up, thus illustrating maintenance of gains.

In a larger sample of 37 adults (2 declined to participate) receiving the B4DT [39], results showed a significant decrease in Y-BOCS from pretreatment ($M = 26.14$) to posttreatment ($M = 9.00$; ES = 2.60), with no significant changes in scores from posttreatment to 3-month ($M = 10.63$; ES = 2.20) or 6-month follow-up ($M = 10.26$; $n = 30$; ES = 2.37). The recovery rate (ie, defined as a pretreatment to posttreatment or follow-up reduction in Y-BOCS of 10 points or more and a Y-BOCS score of 14 points or below at posttreatment or follow-up) following treatment was high, with 77% classified as recovered at posttreatment and 74% recovered at follow-up. No additional information was provided regarding referrals to the treatment center other than participants were "consecutively referred to the OCD outpatient clinic."

Havnen and colleagues [40] conducted a replication study with another 42 adults to determine whether the effects from Havnen [39] were repeatable with a different set of therapists. No information was provided about how these 42 participants presented to the treatment center or how this resulted in the final sample. Results indicated a significant decrease from pretreatment ($M = 25.71$) to posttreatment ($M = 10.79$) on Y-BOCS with no significant changes found from posttreatment to 6-month follow-up ($M = 12.21$). The recovery rate following treatment was high, with 74% recovered at posttreatment and 60% recovered at 6-month follow-up.

Kvale and colleagues [41] enrolled 97 adult OCD patients waiting for access to treatment at another Norwegian site to receive the B4DT model. Seven were "removed" from the study for various reasons leaving a final sample of 90 participants. Pretreatment OCD was severe based on Y-BOCS ($M = 26.12$). A large ES on OCD symptoms (ES = 4.63; $n = 86$) was found at posttreatment and 3-month follow-up (ES = 4.59; $n = 78$). At posttreatment, 91% of patients had responded (ie, defined as ≥35% Y-BOCS improvement), and 72.2% were in remission (≥35% reduction and Y-BOCS score ≤12). At 3-month follow-up, 84.4% had responded, and 67.8% were in remission.

Hansen and colleagues [42] examined follow-up results of the B4DT model at 12 months posttreatment. They offered treatment to 69 of 95 patients referred for treatment, of which 65 (68.4% of referred) started the program. They reported an ES of 3.31 ($n = 63$) at 3-month follow-up and an ES of 3.27 ($n = 59$) at 12-month follow-up. Hansen and colleagues [43] explored the benefits of the B4DT model at 3-month, 6-month, and on-average 4-year follow-up (34–60 months). Their sample was the 77 combined participants of Havnen and colleagues [39] and Havnen and colleagues [40]. Remarkably, 76/77 (98.7%) patients provided follow-up data at 3 months, 60/77 (77.9%) at 6 months, and 58/77 (75.3%) at on-average 4 years posttreatment. Participant symptoms at baseline on the Y-BOCS were severe ($M = 25.9$). Significant reductions were found at posttreatment ($M = 10.0$; ES = 3.65), 3-month follow-up ($M = 10.7$; ES = 2.73), 6-month follow-up ($M = 10.3$; ES = 2.69), and 4-year follow-up ($M = 9.9$; ES = not provided), with no differences found between follow-up conditions.

Finally, in an RCT with adults, Launes and colleagues [44] compared B4DT ($n = 16$) with a 3-month self-help (SH; $n = 16$) or 3-month wait list (WL; $n = 16$) condition. Forty-eight of 66 individuals considered for the study actually participated. Fourteen were excluded for not fulfilling inclusion criteria or for fulfilling exclusion criteria. Study participants had severe OCD based on pretreatment Y-BOCS scores ($M = 27.17$). Launes and colleagues found that those receiving B4DT experienced significant decreases in OCD symptoms pretreatment to posttreatment (ES = 3.75), at 3-month follow-up (ES = 4.30), and at 6-month follow-up (ES = 4.16) compared with those in the control conditions.

In summary, BIT models for pediatric and adult OCD proved highly effective in a series of open trials conducted by the creators of each of the specific treatment protocols. In a series of pediatric studies, Whiteside and colleagues provided 8 to 10 hours of ERP over 5 days and found ESs at posttreatment and short-term follow-up (ie, 3 to 5 months) slightly lower but roughly equivalent to what has been found with IT and ST models (30 hours of ERP). In a different series of pediatric studies, the B4DT model (10–18 hours of ERP over 4 days) has produced extremely large treatment effects at posttreatment and in short-term follow-up (ie, 3 to 6 months). In fact, ESs reported are considerably larger than what has typically been reported for IT or ST studies, as well as those found by Whiteside and colleagues. The B4DT model has also been found to be very effective in adult populations, producing ESs far exceeding those typically found with traditional IT and ST models. These improvements have also been robust, with maintenance of gains exhibited at 4-year follow-up.

So what are we to conclude regarding BIT, supermassed ERP models for OCD? Data strongly support their use as a third treatment option for individuals with OCD, and one that some might prefer. However, it behooves us to evaluate these findings related to the strength of the data obtained and what theoretic basis we may or may not have to support their effectiveness, and in the case of the B4DT model, its apparent superiority over IT and ST models.

STRENGTH OF DATA

All but 1 of the studies described above in support of BIT ERP interventions for OCD were open trials. Although useful, open trials have significant weaknesses [45]. Both the participants and the investigators know the experimental treatment, and this can lead to biases for both groups. Participants may be desperate for relief and be overly optimistic about the treatment's effect. Researchers may be biased in their ratings of participants' progress.

In addition, the open trial studies above did not include a comparison group. It is difficult to draw conclusions about the effectiveness of an intervention when we have nothing to compare [45]. The purpose of a comparison or control group is to allow researchers the ability to conclude that any effects observed in the treatment group are due solely to that treatment and no other factors (eg, time spent with a clinician). A by-product of having no comparison groups is having no randomization. Randomization is another key to eliminating selection bias and other potential unknown, confounding study variables [45]. The single RCT conducted for B4DT [44] addressed these issues but only compared their intervention with a self-help group or a wait list control, both of which are considered generally weak comparisons. A control condition with matched therapist interaction, or an active treatment condition that receives the same treatment time as those who receive BIT, would provide stronger conclusions regarding the treatment. Additionally, a series of blinded studies that involve those with no affiliation with the researchers who created the BIT intervention used may reduce the potential of bias and strengthen possible conclusions.

In light of the limitations described above, another important issue is the generalizability of these findings. Some information was provided about how participants were referred or recruited but not enough to gain a full understanding of who they were, and perhaps more importantly, who they were not. Particularly important is potential "self-selection" bias. Knowing the intervention parameters (eg, 4 or 5 days of intensive treatment) may cause some to "opt out" of even attempting this form of treatment. Such voluntary exclusions may be motivated by participant concerns about the prospect of facing their top OCD fears in a matter of days or a "face validity" issue of not believing they would benefit from such an abbreviated treatment. The latter could be related to the level of impairment they experience and a "too good to be true" mentality. Who chooses BITs and who does not, and who is deemed appropriate or not, are very important issues related to the overall impact and generalizability of these models. In future studies, more information is needed on methods related to referrals made to these research or clinical centers as well as how participants are selected. These issues would not be as problematic if the conclusions drawn recognized these potential limitations (eg, "this model worked for these types of individuals with OCD"). But it is much more relevant when this point seems to be diminished or even ignored, and a "one size fits all" treatment stance is taken. This issue seems to be of particular relevance for the B4DT model. Indeed, Hansen and colleagues [42] concluded, "Since the 4-day approach is developed within an ordinary outpatient clinic, the relevance of the approach is undisputable" (p. 8) implying that all patients presenting to an outpatient clinic with OCD would respond to this treatment model.

Those who were "referred" to the clinics used in the B4DT studies but not enrolled in their studies were described as not being appropriate for any model of ERP (eg, did not have OCD) rather than not for B4DT. However, OCD patients are unique in many ways, including the severity and complexity of OCD, possible comorbidity, motivation, insight, personality factors, how much support one needs to engage in ERP, and how long support will be needed. It is likely that anyone who has treated OCD has had cases that were unwilling or unable to comply with exposure assignments or ritual prevention expectations despite having significant, life-interfering symptoms. It is common to find patients who are noncompliant with homework assignments or parents who will not limit accommodations. Yet the B4DT models seem impervious to these realities. Clearly, these models work for those who engage in these programs, but it is critically important to know the moderators of that benefit.

In addition to the strength-of-data concerns discussed, we also need to understand how BIT models' findings are or are not supported by massed versus spaced learning theory and more recent inhibitory learning models of OCD treatment [46,47]. These models must also be tested in populations that are diverse, from various geographic regions, and in different cultures with nontreatment developers in order to examine the generalizability of these interventions and determine who may be candidates for BIT models.

THEORETIC BASIS FOR FINDINGS OF BRIEF EXPOSURE AND RESPONSE PREVENTION MODELS

Schmidt and Bjork [26] suggest that massed learning allows for greater gains in the short run, but spaced learning produces more lasting benefit. As reviewed above, some indicators that IT produced posttreatment results superior to those of ST were lost at short-term follow-up. In addition, some trends indicated that ST continued to improve at follow-up. A series of pediatric studies by Whiteside and colleagues produced different results. They found that massed treatment provided over 5 days produced strong posttreatment results, but unlike the case with IT, their patients continued to improve in follow-up (ie, after 3 to 5 months). It is unclear why less treatment provided in less time would nullify the losses typically seen in massed treatment and produce continued improvement in follow-up. Whiteside's model emphasized continuing posttreatment exposure and thus may have mimicked "spaced" models more than one would think, which could explain the continued improvement seen in follow-up.

The B4DT model has also produced very strong posttreatment results that are maintained in short-term and long-term follow-up. How does compressing ERP to fewer sessions and delivering less overall ERP produce seemingly the "perfect" treatment environment? That perfect environment results in extremely high initial symptom reduction exceeding that of IT models and the Whiteside model but somehow also overrides the tendency of the return of fear associated with typical massed models at follow-up.

Using Schmidt and Bjork's [26] views on massed learning, we could possibly make a case for the B4DT model to produce superior immediate results due to its great massed intensity. But we would also expect those benefits to be short-lived and regress in follow-up, perhaps even more severely than in IT models. By that, we mean we would expect that the B4DT's greatest strength, its super-massed format, would also be its greatest weakness and result in a lack of maintenance of gains. However, this is not what has been found. The B4DT model also emphasizes homework during and after the 4-day treatment period. Is this emphasis alone responsible for the maintenance of observed gains? Unfortunately, the answer is unclear and is therefore an important area for future investigation and may require much more stringent research models than have been used to date.

More recently, inhibitory learning principles have been examined to enhance the results of exposure-based treatments [46], including those for OCD [48]. Is it possible that BITs have maximized the use of these principles to achieve the unexpected long-term success of these massed treatment models? In the inhibitory learning model, fear acquisition, or learned fear, is based on the association between a conditioned stimulus (CS) and an unconditioned stimulus (US). Fear extinction is the basis for exposure therapy; over the course of exposure therapy, the CS is presented without the US, and the fear is extinguished. An inhibitory learning model of extinction posits that the original CS–US association learned during fear acquisition is not "erased" during the process of extinction, but is left intact as a new, secondary inhibitory learning about the CS–US develops; the CS no longer predicts the US [49,50].

According to Abramowitz and colleagues [48], the 2 most critical treatment goals of an inhibitory learning approach for OCD are (1) violation of negative expectations and (2) generalization of inhibitory associations across multiple contexts. Several clinical strategies for optimizing inhibitory learning to maximize ERP outcomes for OCD have been proposed (see [47,51–53]). How might these principles be utilized and affect results found with BIT models of ERP?

Expectancy violation is a core strategy of inhibitory learning. It involves designing exposures that maximally violate expectancies regarding feared outcomes. The primary purpose of violating expectancies is to increase the element of "surprise" during extinction, or the degree of mismatch between a patient's expectation regarding a feared outcome and what actually occurs during an exposure [54]. The greater the degree of surprise, the greater the hypothesized inhibitory learning. Compressing ERP allows for violating expectancies, but it seems that the more repetition one would get with expectancy violation, the stronger the inhibitory learning would be, not the opposite. In addition, BITs would not be able to violate any expected results that would exceed the treatment time frame of 4 or 5 days (eg, *"What if I get sick next week because I touched that door handle?"*).

Conducting exposures in multiple contexts is also a key to inhibitory learning. From an inhibitory learning model, original fear associations are not erased during extinction (ie, during exposure practice); thus, reencounters with the CS (eg, obsessional thoughts and cues) in a context different from the extinction context can lead to a reinstatement of fear [55,56]. Context renewal effects are believed to account for a sizable portion of lapses following exposure treatment; offsetting these effects can enhance long-term exposure outcomes [54]. Conducting exposures in multiple contexts has been shown to offset context renewal [57]. In the treatment of OCD, ERP needs to be conducted in as many different contexts and situations as possible to enhance the accessibility and retrieval of newly learned nonthreat associations and to reduce relapse. As such, exposure-based treatments emphasize the need to practice exposure outside the therapy session to improve the generalization of exposure-based learning to address the immense gap between treatment context and living context [58,59]. Providing treatment over a 4-day or 5-day period greatly reduces the opportunity to conduct exposures in more than 1 context, thus proving to be a hindrance and not an asset. Completing out-of-session exposures (ie, homework) is an important component of any ERP model and helps strengthen and generalize learning across contexts. Nightly homework is assigned during BITs, but due to the shortened time frame, it does not seem to explain the superiority of the B4DT model at posttreatment nor its ability to avoid relapse. Continuing ERP posttreatment is emphasized in both Whiteside's model and B4DT but not to a greater degree than in the IT or ST approaches, and therefore, it seems unlikely that it can explain the maintenance of gains seen in BIT models.

In addition to concerns related to expectancy violation and conducting exposures in multiple contexts, BIT models also appear to have potential difficulties with other inhibitory learning principles. Because safety signals or safety behaviors can interfere with inhibitory learning, ERP models aim is to eliminate safety signals, safety behaviors, and accommodation [52]. This inhibitory learning strategy may be implemented into BIT models, although adequately assessing and eliminating all safety signals, safety behaviors, and accommodation in such a short time span would prove to be very challenging. As many ERP clinicians are aware, even the most highly motivated patients may struggle to completely discontinue their safety behaviors and other avoidance strategies, especially early in treatment.

Expanding spaced sessions (expanding the intersession interval) may be ideal when patients demonstrate that they are capable of refraining or substantially reducing rituals between sessions. Bjork and Bjork's "A New Theory of Disuse" [60,61] states that progressively increasing the amount of time between learning sessions creates the most durable long-term learning. For inhibitory learning to be maximized, initial sessions may be close together (as in the case of BITs), and then intersession intervals are suggested to be gradually expanded (eg, 2x weekly sessions, 1x weekly sessions, 2x monthly sessions, 1x monthly sessions) with booster sessions at increasing intervals to help further consolidate what the patient has learned. Evidence suggests that gradually expanding the interval between therapist-guided exposure sessions so that exposures can be conducted when retrieval is difficult but still possible leads to enhanced long-term learning [62,63]. Integration of this type of expansion of the intersession interval in BITs is not possible and thus points to another limitation of these models. Other inhibitory learning principles made more difficult in BIT models include deepened extinction [64], variability in exposures, intermittent reinforcement of extinction [52,65], and mental reinstatement of what is learned during exposures.

In short, the enhanced, immediate posttreatment findings of the B4DT model, continued improvement in the follow-up of Whiteside's model, and long-term maintenance of gains found for the B4DT model do not appear to be supported by Schmidt and Bjork's [26] massed versus spaced learning theory nor by inhibitory learning principles of exposure therapy [46]. Regarding the latter, the very nature of BITs makes many of the inhibitory learning principles difficult if not impossible to apply. Thus, based on these learning models, we would expect BITs to be outperformed by IT and ST models rather than vice versa. As a result, we are left with a limited understanding of the theoretic basis underlying the data produced by BITs.

SUMMARY AND FUTURE DIRECTIONS IN BRIEF, INTENSIVE TREATMENTS FOR OBSESSIVE-COMPULSIVE DISORDER

The optimal dose and intensity of ERP sessions have yet to be established and represent an important area in need of further research. IT and ST models of ERP have been widely and routinely supported (eg, [7,17]) and appear to be equally effective in the long run, thus providing patients with treatment options. The effects of both models appear rooted in Schmidt and Bjork's massed versus spaced model of learning (1992). Outcomes of both models also seem to be enhanced when inhibitory learning principles are applied, especially expectancy violation and conducting exposures in multiple contexts. The principles of inhibitory learning seem to require time, however—time to have expectancies violated and to conduct exposures in as many contexts as possible, and time to eliminate all safety signals, behaviors, and family accommodation as well as spacing out the sessions. All these principles are difficult to impossible to implement with BIT models of ERP. If following inhibitory learning principles enhances treatment outcomes, and if the very nature of BITs does not allow for these principles to be somewhat or fully applied, what then explains the treatment enhancements found using these brief models?

One explanation could be self-selection bias in who does and does not participate in BIT open trials and what effects this bias may have on the resulting outcomes. If true, this bias would also have a tremendous impact on the generalizability of these results. The B4DT model has produced extremely large ESs with few to no participants declining or dropping out of treatment. In addition, the effects it produces are maintained over long periods with very high participation rates in follow-up data collection. It appears that the B4DT model provides the optimal treatment environment. The model seems to treat those with severe OCD and comorbidity, yet something seems to be missing from the samples. Gone are the patients who routinely refuse or drop out of ERP or are noncompliant with exposures or response-prevention expectations. Gone are the parents who refuse to reduce accommodation or make excuses for their child's noncompliance with homework assignments. It seems that the B4DT model either has found a special way to overcome these common obstacles or has not been treating these patients.

Assuming the latter does not take away from the fact that the B4DT model produces extremely strong outcomes and has helped hundreds of individuals with OCD. A hurdle B4DT must overcome before becoming a third viable treatment option and perhaps even a preferred one for some, is more rigorous investigation. Research into the effectiveness of B4DT to date has included mostly open trials with 1 RCT. There is a great need to directly compare BIT approaches with IT and ST models. Additionally, studies geared toward identifying moderators related to BIT ERP models are critical to combat the "one size fits all" mentality that appears to be contrary to the overall push for individualized medicine. Finally, future research is needed to explore the effects of combining the best elements of IT, ST, and BIT models to maximize patient outcomes and provide more treatment options, and therefore, more access to effective care.

DISCLOSURE

The authors declare that they have no conflict of interest to disclose. No funding or other support was received for this review.

REFERENCES

[1] American Psychiatric Association. Diagnostic and statistical manual of mental disorders, 5th edition: DSM-5. 5th edition. American Psychiatric Publishing; 2013.
[2] Jacoby RJ, Leonard RC, Riemann BC, et al. Predictors of quality of life and functional impairment in obsessive–compulsive disorder. Compr Psychiatry 2014;55(5):1195–202.
[3] Molinari AD, Andrews JL, Zaboski BA, et al. Quality of life and anxiety in children and adolescents in residential treatment facilities. Residential Treat Child Youth 2019;36(3):220–34.
[4] Eisen JL, Mancebo MA, Pinto A, et al. Impact of obsessive-compulsive disorder on quality of life. Comprehensive Psychiatry 2006;47(4):270–5.
[5] Bobes J, González MP, Bascarán MT, et al. Quality of life and disability in patients with obsessive-compulsive disorder. Eur Psychiatry 2001;16(4):239–45.
[6] Foa EB, Steketee G, Grayson JB, et al. Deliberate exposure and blocking of obsessive-compulsive rituals: Immediate and long-term effects. Behav Ther 1984;15(5):450–72.
[7] Foa EB, Kozak MJ, Steketee GS, et al. Treatment of depressive and obsessive-compulsive symptoms in OCD by imipramine and behaviour therapy. Br J Clin Psychol 1992;31(3):279–92.
[8] Olatunji BO, Davis ML, Powers MB, et al. Cognitive-behavioral therapy for obsessive-compulsive disorder: A meta-analysis of treatment outcome and moderators. J Psychiatr Res 2013;47(1):33–41.
[9] Kay B, Eken S, Jacobi D, et al. Outcome of multidisciplinary, CBT-focused treatment for pediatric OCD. Gen Hosp Psychiatry 2016;42:7–8.
[10] Leonard RC, Franklin ME, Wetterneck CT, et al. Residential treatment outcomes for adolescents with obsessive-compulsive disorder. Psychotherapy Res 2015;26(6):727–36.
[11] DiMauro J, Domingues J, Fernandez G, et al. Long-term effectiveness of CBT for anxiety disorders in an adult outpatient clinic sample: A follow-up study. Behav Res Ther 2013;51(2):82–6.
[12] Eisen JL, Sibrava NJ, Boisseau CL, et al. Five-year course of obsessive-compulsive disorder. J Clin Psychiatry 2013;74(03):233–9.

[13] Rosa-Alcázar AI, Sánchez-Meca J, Gómez-Conesa A, et al. Psychological treatment of obsessive–compulsive disorder: A meta-analysis. Clin Psychol Rev 2008;28(8): 1310–25.

[14] Macy AS, Theo JN, Kaufmann SCV, et al. Quality of life in obsessive compulsive disorder. CNS Spectrums 2013; 18(1):21–33.

[15] Moritz S, Rufer M, Fricke S, et al. Quality of life in obsessive-compulsive disorder before and after treatment. Compr Psychiatry 2005;46(6):453–9.

[16] Subramaniam M, Soh P, Vaingankar JA, et al. Quality of life in obsessive-compulsive disorder: Impact of the disorder and of treatment. CNS Drugs 2013;27(5):367–83.

[17] Abramowitz JS, Foa EB, Franklin ME. Exposure and ritual prevention for obsessive-compulsive disorder: Effects of intensive versus twice-weekly sessions. J Consulting Clin Psychol 2003;71(2):394–8.

[18] Storch EA, Geffken GR, Merlo LJ, et al. Family-based cognitive-behavioral therapy for pediatric obsessive-compulsive disorder: Comparison of intensive and weekly approaches. J Am Acad Child Adolesc Psychiatry 2007;46(4):469–78.

[19] Kozak MJ, Foa EB. Mastery of obsessive– compulsive disorder: a cognitive– behavioral approach. San Antonio, TX: The Psychological Corporation; 1997.

[20] Foa EB, Liebowitz MR, Kozak MJ, et al. Randomized, placebo-controlled trial of exposure and ritual prevention, clomipramine, and their combination in the treatment of obsessive-compulsive disorder. Am J Psychiatry 2005;162(1):151–61.

[21] Goodman WK, Price LH, Rasmussen SA, et al. The Yale-Brown obsessive compulsive scale. I. Development, use, and reliability. Arch Gen Psychiatry 1989;46(11): 1006–11.

[22] Lindsay M, Crino R, Andrews G. Controlled trial of exposure and response prevention in obsessive–compulsive disorder. Br J Psychiatry 1997;171(2):135–9.

[23] Franklin ME, Abramowitz JS, Kozak MJ, et al. Effectiveness of exposure and ritual prevention for obsessive-compulsive disorder: Randomized compared with nonrandomized samples. J Consult Clin Psychol 2000; 68(4):594–602.

[24] Storch EA, Lehmkuhl HD, Ricketts E, et al. An open trial of intensive family based cognitive-behavioral therapy in youth with obsessive-compulsive disorder who are medication partial responders or nonresponders. J Clin Child Adolesc Psychol 2010;39(2):260–8.

[25] Whiteside SP, Brown AM, Abramowitz JS. Five-day intensive treatment for adolescent OCD: A case series. J Anxiety Disord 2008;22(3):495–504.

[26] Schmidt RA, Bjork RA. New conceptualizations of practice: Common principles in three paradigms suggest new concepts for training. Psychol Sci 1992;3(4): 207–18.

[27] Jacobson NS, Truax P. Clinical significance: A statistical approach to defining meaningful change in psychotherapy research. J Consult Clin Psychol 1991;59(1):12–9.

[28] Storch EA, Merlo LJ, Lehmkuhl H, et al. Cognitive-behavioral therapy for obsessive–compulsive disorder: A non-randomized comparison of intensive and weekly approaches. J Anxiety Disord 2008;22(7): 1146–58.

[29] Scahill L, Riddle MA, McSwiggin-Hardin M, et al. Children's Yale-Brown Obsessive Compulsive Scale: Reliability and validity. J Am Child Adolesc Psychiatry 1997;36:844–52.

[30] National Institute of Mental Health. Rating scales and assessment instruments for use in pediatric psychopharmacology research. Psychopharmacol Bull 1985;21: 839–43.

[31] Öst L-G. One-session treatment for specific phobias. Behav Res Ther 1989;27(1):1–7.

[32] Deacon B. Two-day, intensive cognitive-behavioral therapy for panic disorder. Behav Modif 2007;31(5): 595–615.

[33] Deacon B, Abramowitz J. A pilot study of two-day cognitive-behavioral therapy for panic disorder. Behav Res Ther 2006;44(6):807–17.

[34] Whiteside SP, Jacobsen AB. An uncontrolled examination of a 5-day intensive treatment for pediatric OCD. Behav Ther 2010;41(3):414–22.

[35] Whiteside SP, McKay D, De Nadai AS, et al. A baseline controlled examination of a 5-day intensive treatment for pediatric obsessive-compulsive disorder. Psychiatry Res 2014;220(1–2):441–6.

[36] Riise EN, Kvale G, Öst L-G, et al. Concentrated exposure and response prevention for adolescents with obsessive-compulsive disorder: An effectiveness study. J Obsessive Compuls Relat Disord 2016;11:13–21.

[37] Riise EN, Kvale G, Öst L-G, et al. Concentrated exposure and response prevention for adolescents with obsessive-compulsive disorder: A replication study. J Obsessive Compuls Relat Disord 2018;19:15–22.

[38] Havnen A, Hansen B, Haug ET, et al. Intensive group treatment of obsessive-compulsive disorder: A pilot study. Clin Neuropsychiatry J Treat Eval 2013;10(3): 48–55.

[39] Havnen A, Hansen B, Öst L-G, et al. Concentrated ERP delivered in a group setting: An effectiveness study. J Obsessive Compuls Relat Disord 2014;3(4):319–24.

[40] Havnen A, Hansen B, Öst L-G, et al. Concentrated ERP delivered in a group setting: A replication study. Behav Cogn Psychotherapy 2017;45(5):530–6.

[41] Kvale G, Hansen B, Björgvinsson T, et al. Successfully treating 90 patients with obsessive compulsive disorder in eight days: the Bergen 4-day treatment. BMC Psychiatry 2018;18(1). https://doi.org/10.1186/s12888-018-1887-4.

[42] Hansen B, Hagen K, Öst L-G, et al. The Bergen 4-day OCD treatment delivered in a group setting: 12-month follow-up. Front Psychol 2018;9. https://doi.org/10.3389/fpsyg.2018.00639.

[43] Hansen B, Kvale G, Hagen K, et al. The Bergen 4-day treatment for OCD: Four years follow-up of concentrated

ERP in a clinical mental health setting. Cogn Behav Ther 2019;48(2):89–105.

[44] Launes G, Hagen K, Sunde T, et al. A randomized controlled trial of concentrated ERP, self-help and waiting list for obsessive-compulsive disorder: The Bergen 4-day treatment. Front Psychol 2019;10. https://doi.org/10.3389/fpsyg.2019.02500.

[45] Kazdin A. Research design in clinical psychology. New York, NY: Pearson; 2003.

[46] Craske MG, Kircanski K, Zelikowsky M, et al. Optimizing inhibitory learning during exposure therapy. Behav Res Ther 2008;46(1):5–27.

[47] Jacoby RJ, Abramowitz JS. Inhibitory learning approaches to exposure therapy: A critical review and translation to obsessive-compulsive disorder. Clin Psychol Rev 2016;49:28–40.

[48] Abramowitz JS, Blakey SM, Reuman L, et al. New directions in the cognitive-behavioral treatment of OCD: Theory, research, and practice. Behav Ther 2018;49(3): 311–22.

[49] Bouton ME. Context, time, and memory retrieval in the interference paradigms of Pavlovian learning. Psychol Bull 1993;114(1):80–99.

[50] Bouton ME, King DA. Contextual control of the extinction of conditioned fear: Tests for the associative value of the context. J Exp Psychol Anim Behav Process 1983; 9(3):248–65.

[51] Arch JJ, Abramowitz JS. Exposure therapy for obsessive-compulsive disorder: An optimizing inhibitory learning approach. J Obsessive Compuls Relat Disord 2015;6: 174–82.

[52] McGuire JF, Storch EA. An inhibitory learning approach to cognitive-behavioral therapy for children and adolescents. Cogn Behav Pract 2019;26(1):214–24.

[53] Tolin DF. Inhibitory learning for anxiety-related disorders. Cogn Behav Pract 2019;26(1):225–36.

[54] Abramowitz JS, Arch JJ. Strategies for improving long-term outcomes in cognitive behavioral therapy for obsessive-compulsive disorder: Insights from learning theory. Cogn Behav Pract 2014;21(1):20–31.

[55] Mineka S, Mystkowski JL, Hladek D, et al. The effects of changing contexts on return of fear following exposure therapy for spider fear. J Consulting Clin Psychol 1999; 67(4):599–604.

[56] Bouton ME. Context, ambiguity, and unlearning: Sources of relapse after behavioral extinction. Biological Psychiatry 2002;52(10):976–86.

[57] Vansteenwegen D, Vervliet B, Iberico C, et al. The repeated confrontation with videotapes of spiders in multiple contexts attenuates renewal of fear in spider-anxious students. Behav Res Ther 2007;45(6):1169–79.

[58] Craske MG, Treanor M, Conway CC, et al. Maximizing exposure therapy: an inhibitory learning approach. Behav Res Ther 2014;58:10–23.

[59] Gunther LM, Denniston JC, Miller RR. Conducting exposure treatment in multiple contexts can prevent relapse. Behav Res Ther 1998;36(1):75–91.

[60] Bjork RA, Bjork EL. A new theory of disuse and an old theory of stimulus fluctuation. In: Healy A, Kosslyn S, Shiffrin R, editors. From learning processes to cognitive processes: Essays in honor of William K. Estes. Mahwah (NJ): Lawrence Erlbaum Associates, Inc; 1992. p. 35–67.

[61] Bjork RA, Bjork EL. Optimizing treatment and instruction: Implications of a new theory of disuse. In: Nilsson L-G, Ohta N, editors. Memory and society: psychological perspectives. Hove (UK): Psychology Press; 2006. p. 116–40.

[62] Rowe MK, Craske MG. Effects of an expanding-spaced vs massed exposure schedule on fear reduction and return of fear. Behav Res Ther 1998;36(7–8):701–17.

[63] Tsao JCI, Craske MG. Timing of treatment and return of fear: Effects of massed, uniform-, and expanding-spaced exposure schedules. Behav Ther 2000;31(3):479–97.

[64] Rescorla RA. Deepened extinction from compound stimulus presentation. J Exp Psychol Anim Behav Process 2006;32(2):135–44.

[65] Bouton ME, Woods AM, Pineño O. Occasional reinforced trials during extinction can slow the rate of rapid reacquisition. Learn Motiv 2004;35(4):371–90.

Advances in Psychiatry and Behavioral Health 1 (2021) 37–51

ADVANCES IN PSYCHIATRY AND BEHAVIORAL HEALTH

Third-Wave Cognitive Behavioral Therapy for Obsessive Compulsive Disorder?

A Promising Approach if It Includes Exposure

Erika S. Trent, MA[a], Andrew G. Guzick, PhD[b,*], Andres G. Viana, PhD, ABPP[a,c], Eric A. Storch, PhD[b]

[a]Department of Psychology, University of Houston, Health and Biomedical Sciences Building 1, 4849 Calhoun Road, Houston, TX 77204, USA; [b]Department of Psychiatry & Behavioral Sciences, Baylor College of Medicine, 1977 Butler Boulevard, Houston, TX 77030, USA; [c]Texas Institute of Measurement, Evaluation, and Statistics, University of Houston, 4849 Calhoun Road, Houston, TX 77204, USA

KEYWORDS

- Acceptance and commitment therapy • Metacognitive therapy • Mindfulness • Third-wave treatments
- Randomized controlled trials • Exposure and response prevention • Exposure therapy

INTRODUCTION/BACKGROUND

Exposure and response prevention (ERP) is an evidence-based, gold standard form of cognitive behavioral therapy (CBT) for individuals with obsessive compulsive disorder (OCD). This treatment has shown strong efficacy relative to active controls as well as psychopharmacological monotherapy [1,2]. In ERP, therapists assist patients to challenge obsessive fears through facing obsession-provoking situations ("exposure") while reducing or eliminating compensatory compulsions and avoidance ("response prevention") [3,4].

Despite its strong efficacy, a common critique of ERP is that 30% to 35% of patients are estimated to be "non-responders" [1,2]. Critics have noted that because ERP requires sustained contact with anxiety-provoking situations, many patients may drop out, refuse treatment, or not engage fully in therapy (although it is worth noting dropout rates are at least as high in other treatments) [5,6]. Furthermore, most individuals with OCD meet criteria for at least one comorbid disorder, particularly anxiety and depressive disorders [7], and some clinicians express concern that ERP focuses on OCD symptoms and neglects other areas that cause distress or impairment. While these concerns are mitigated by evidence that anxiety and depressive symptoms improve after ERP [8], such secondary symptoms likely complicate the course of treatment.

ERP, which takes a problem-focused approach to helping patients change discrete thoughts and behaviors, was developed in the "second wave" of CBT [9,10]. Building on the first wave of CBT, which focused on changing observable behaviors, the second wave incorporates cognitive principles [11]. The "third wave" of CBT extends the first two waves by emphasizing the function of thoughts beyond their content, contextual conceptualization and experiential exercises in addition to didactic approaches, and the development of transdiagnostic skills (eg, mindfulness, acceptance, values-based action) that can be applied flexibly to various problem areas or diagnoses [11]. It also integrates theoretic knowledge from diverse behavioral and cognitive traditions.

*Corresponding author, *E-mail address:* andrew.guzick@bcm.edu

https://doi.org/10.1016/j.ypsc.2021.05.004
2667-3827/21/

Therapies that fit under this third-wave umbrella include acceptance and commitment therapy (ACT), dialectical behavior therapy, mindfulness-based cognitive therapy, and metacognitive therapy, among others, and have accumulated a strong evidence base for broad forms of psychopathology [12]. In some cases, these contemporary CBT approaches may be more beneficial than traditional CBT; for example, in one randomized comparison trial between ACT and CBT for adults with anxiety disorders, ACT outperformed CBT in terms of long-term outcomes [13] and short-term outcomes among individuals with comorbid depressive disorders [14]. Similarly, a recent randomized trial comparing metacognitive therapy and CBT for adults with depression found a recovery rate of 74% in metacognitive therapy relative to 52% in CBT [15]. Likewise, some argue that using third-wave CBT frameworks may enhance treatment engagement, reduce dropout, and promote better outcomes in terms of both OCD severity and co-occurring symptoms for individuals with OCD [16].

As third-wave therapies have gained empirical support for diverse problem areas, clinicians have increasingly turned to them in their routine practice, including for children and adults with OCD. For example, when searching for OCD specialists on the International OCD Foundation's website within 200 miles of New York City, 202 of the 461 (44%) listed providers or clinics offer ACT, including 114 who treat children, 172 who treat adolescents, and 197 who treat adults [17].

Accordingly, clinical investigators have begun developing and testing third-wave approaches among individuals with OCD [18,19]. While traditional ERP emphasizes extinction learning and expectancy disconfirmation during exposure, ACT emphasizes acceptance of emotional discomfort and exposures that help patients live consistently with their values [16]. Some have argued that the theoretic rationale of ACT could improve patient buy-in and enhance outcomes, as processes such as acceptance decrease distress related to intrusive thoughts [20] and mindfulness increases emotional engagement during exposure [21]. Mindfulness and acceptance also lead to greater exposure therapy participation [22,23]. Thus, it may be that an ACT rationale leads to lower drop out and greater engagement during ERP [16,18]. This has led proponents of the third wave to propose integrating ACT or other third-wave therapies into ERP to improve outcomes, in addition to testing third-wave therapies as standalone treatments [16,18].

Several core "treatment kernels" that emerged in the third wave, including mindfulness and focusing on values, have popularity and scientific support in treating broad forms of psychopathology [12]. Although this theoretic framework is appealing to many clinicians, it is unclear if its evidence base matches its popularity in the treatment of individuals with OCD [24]. To this end, the goal of this article was to evaluate the evidence for third-wave therapies for individuals with OCD, focusing on ACT but also incorporating other third-wave therapies that have been tested, and to provide recommendations for future research in this area. A prior review with a similar aim concluded that there was a dearth of studies comparing ACT with traditional ERP [24]. Since that review, several randomized trials have been published and may have implications for the role of third-wave treatment and research in OCD. In addition to improvement in OCD symptom severity, co-occurring anxiety and depression was also examined, in light of the hypothesis that an emphasis on transdiagnostic skills in third-wave therapies results in superior outcomes for problems that fall outside the primary diagnostic category [14].

RATIONALE

The theoretic bases of third-wave therapies include the ACT model of OCD [25] and the metacognitive model of OCD [26]. The ACT framework, which is based in functional contextualism and the relational frame theory [27], conceptualizes OCD as a disorder of rigid, rule-governed behavior [25]. Patients with OCD exhibit negative evaluations of inner experiences as dangerous and believe they must suppress these inner experiences. ACT targets the cognitive system that reinforces obsessive thoughts (ie, decrease experiential avoidance and increase acceptance) and the behavioral pattern of responding to obsessions in ways that are incongruent with one's values [25]. The ACT model of OCD is empirically supported, as ACT constructs (eg, low acceptance, psychological inflexibility) are associated with OCD symptom severity [28]. Multiple case studies, case series, open trials, and randomized controlled trials (RCTs) have supported the effectiveness of ACT for reducing OCD symptoms [29–31]. Furthermore, a subset of these studies identified ACT-relevant mechanisms of change, such as improvements in psychological flexibility and mindfulness [32–34].

The metacognitive model of OCD argues that OCD is maintained through two processes. Patients misinterpret obsessions as more dangerous and consequential than they are because of fusion beliefs (ie, the belief that thoughts can cause actions, lead to events, or be passed on to objects) and perform rituals because of metacognitive beliefs that such rituals are needed to reduce the perceived threat [35]. Metacognitive therapy targets these beliefs about the power of intrusive thoughts and the necessity to perform rituals. Metacognitive therapy differs from cognitive therapy in that it does not challenge the content of the thoughts, but rather the appraisal and management of these thoughts. Empirically, metacognitions are strong longitudinal predictors of OCD symptoms after controlling for age, sex, and depressive symptoms [36]. Several case studies, case series, open trials, and RCTs have found that metacognitive therapy may be an efficacious treatment for OCD [37–39].

APPROACH

A literature search was conducted on PsycInfo and PubMed. Search criteria included the following descriptors located within the abstract: (1) "obsessive compulsive disorder"; (2) "acceptance and commitment therapy" or "dialectical behavior therapy" or "mindfulness" or "metacognitive" or "third-wave"; and (3) "cognitive behavioral" or "exposure and response prevention." The search included all years up to September 2020. This search was complemented with manual searches of references within the selected articles, as well as manual searches on Google Scholar. Articles were included if they met the following inclusion criteria: (1) sample consists of patients with a diagnosis of OCD; (2) examines the outcomes of a third-wave CBT treatment on OCD symptoms; (3) uses an RCT design; (4) presents original, quantitative data; (5) published in a peer-reviewed journal; and (6) written in English. Twelve articles met inclusion criteria and thus were included in the narrative review.[a] For each measure of OCD symptoms, depressive symptoms, or anxiety symptoms reported, Cohen's *d* was calculated to compare posttreatment scores between third-wave CBT treatments and other treatments. Table 1 provides an abbreviated summary of each study and corresponding effect sizes (see Supplemental Table for a detailed summary).

[a]Vakili and colleagues's [41] 2013 report was chosen over their 2015 report of the same data set because it included more outcomes of interest (OCD, depressive, and anxiety outcomes). Moritz and colleagues's [47] online RCT consisted of participants who reported that they received an OCD diagnosis from a mental health professional. Moritz and colleagues present data from past investigations demonstrating this method has adequate diagnostic validity; thus, the study was included in the present review. Ong and colleagues's secondary analysis [33] examining moderators in Twohig and colleagues's [19] RCT was not included in Table 1 as it did not contain unique data. However, it was included in the narrative review to contextualize Twohig and colleagues's findings.

CURRENT EVIDENCE

Acceptance and Commitment Therapy

Primary outcomes comparing acceptance and commitment therapy to control or non-cognitive-behavioral therapy treatments

Four studies tested the efficacy of ACT against control groups or non-CBT treatments for OCD. Twohig and colleagues [32] examined the efficacy of eight sessions of ACT ($n = 41$) versus progressive relaxation training (ie, an active control; $n = 48$) without in-session exposure among adults with OCD. ACT yielded significantly lower OCD symptoms after treatment than progressive relaxation training ($d = 0.82$). ACT was also more likely to induce clinically significant change in OCD severity at both posttreatment and 3-month follow-up. Esfahani and colleagues [40] examined the efficacy of ACT and two non-CBT treatments—time perspective therapy and narrative therapy—as compared to a waitlist control (total $N = 60$). ACT and narrative therapy, but not time perspective therapy, yielded improvements in OCD symptoms at posttreatment and 2-month follow-up, compared with the waitlist control. The authors report statistically significant differences between groups. Descriptively, Yale-Brown Obsessive Compulsive Scale (Y-BOCS) scores in the ACT group ($M = 13.73$) were lower than those in the time perspective therapy, narrative therapy, or waitlist control groups (*Ms* = 28.13, 18.26, and 27.73, respectively); however, insufficient information was reported to statistically compare between-group differences.

Two studies investigated the efficacy of combinations of ACT and selective serotonin reuptake inhibitors (SSRIs). Vakili and colleagues [41] found that patients who received ACT ($n = 10$; $d = 1.41$) or a combination of ACT and one of two SSRIs (sertraline or fluoxetine; $n = 11$; $d = 1.61$) showed greater improvement in OCD symptom severity than patients who received SSRIs alone ($n = 11$). No significant differences emerged between patients who received ACT alone or the ACT + SSRI combination, although it is worth noting limited power to detect between-group differences in this study and mixed use of antidepressants. These findings are partially consistent with those of Rohani and colleagues [42], who randomized SSRI-medicated patients to either receive group ACT while continuing to take heterogeneous SSRIs ($n = 23$) or only continue taking SSRIs ($n = 23$). Both groups showed significant decreases in OCD symptom severity at posttreatment and follow-up. No group differences were present at posttreatment, but at follow-up, the ACT + SSRI group showed lower OCD symptom severity than the SSRI-only group ($d = 1.93$).

TABLE 1
Summary of Randomized Controlled Trials Included in the Narrative Review

Study	Intervention (n)	Comparison (n)	Sample Characteristics: % fem.	Sample Characteristics: Ave. age (y)	Sample Characteristics: % White[b]	Dropout Rates (%): Inter-vention	Dropout Rates (%): Compar-ison(s)	Treatment Length	Follow-up Period	Measure	Intervention vs Comparison Scores at Posttreatment[c]	Summary[d]
Acceptance and commitment therapies (ACT)												
Twohig et al, [32] 2010	ACT ($n = 41$)	Progressive relaxation training (PRT) ($n = 38$)	66	37	89	9.8	13.2	8 sessions	3 mo	Y-BOCS	$d = 0.82$	ACT>PRT at post-treatment and follow-up
										BDI-II	$d = 0.50$ among all patients	ACT>PRT among patients who reported at least mild depression (BDI≥13)
Esfahani et al, [40] 2015	ACT (subgroup *n*s not reported; total $N = 60$)	Time persp-ective therapy (TPT) Narrative therapy (NT) Waitlist	N/R	N/R (range 6–20)	N/R (Iran)	N/R	N/R	ACT: 10 sessions TPT: 6 sessions NT: 8 sessions Waitlist: 5-h educational workshop	2 mo.	Y-BOCS	Not reported; insufficient information to calculate	ACT>control NT>control TPT = control Statistically significant group differences in OCD symptoms from pretreatment to posttreatment and from posttreatment to follow-up are reported. No follow-up tests reported.
Vakili et al, [41] 2013	ACT ($n = 10$)	ACT + SSRI ($n = 11$) SSRI only ($n = 11$)	44[e]	27[e]	N/R (Iran)	10.0	ACT + SSRI: 9.1 SSRI: 27.3	8 sessions across 10 wk	N/A	Y-BOCS	ACT vs ACT + SSRI: $d = -.05$ ACT vs SSRI: $d = 1.41$ ACT + SSRI vs SSRI: $d = 1.61$	ACT = ACT + SSRI > SSRI

										BDI-II	ACT vs ACT + SSRI: d = 0.14 ACT vs SSRI: d = 0.14 ACT + SSRI vs SSRI: d = .008	ACT = ACT + SSRI = SSRI Patients in all conditions showed significant decreases in BDI-II scores. No significant group differences.
										BAI	ACT vs ACT + SSRI: d = .05 ACT vs SSRI: d = .43 ACT + SSRI vs SSRI: d = .36	ACT = ACT + SSRI = SSRI Patients in all conditions showed significant decreases in BAI scores. No s ignificant group differences.
Rohani et al, [42] 2018	Group ACT + continued SSRI (n = 23)	Continued SSRI only (n = 23)	100	28	0	0	0	16 wk	N/R	Y-BOCS-SR	d = 0.82 at posttreatment (ns) d = 1.93 at follow-up	ACT + SSRI = SSRI at posttreatment ACT + SSRI>SSRI at follow-up
										BDI-II	d = 0.21 at posttreatment (ns) d = 0.48 at follow-up	ACT + SSRI = SSRI at posttreatment ACT + SSRI>SSRI at follow-up
[a]Shabani et al, [43] 2019	Group ACT + continued SSRI (n = 22)	Group CBT + continued SSRI (n = 22) Continued SSRI only (n = 25)	44.9	15	0	9.1	CBT + SSRI: 13.6 SSRI: 0	ACT + SSRI: 10 sessions CBT + SSRI: 12 sessions	3 mo	Y-BOCS	ACT + SSRI vs CBT + SSRI: d = -0.12 *(ns)* CBT + SSRI vs SSRI: d = 1.37 ACT + SSRI vs SSRI: d = 1.02	ACT + SSRI = CBT + SSRI > SSRI at post-treatment and follow-up

(*continued on next page*)

TABLE 1
(continued)

Study	Intervention (*n*)	Comparison (*n*)	Sample Characteristics: % fem.	Sample Characteristics: Ave. age (y)	Sample Characteristics: % White[b]	Dropout Rates (%): Inter-vention	Dropout Rates (%): Compar-ison(s)	Treatment Length	Follow-up Period	Measure	Intervention vs Comparison Scores at Posttreatment[c]	Summary[d]
										CDI	ACT + SSRI vs CBT + SSRI: *d* = 0.03 (*ns*) CBT + SSRI vs SSRI: *d* = 0.68 ACT + SSRI vs SSRI: *d* = 0.67	ACT + SSRI = CBT + SSRI = SSRI at posttreatment and follow-up
[a]Twohig et al, [18] 2018	ACT + ERP (*n* = 28)	ERP (*n* = 30)	68.0	27	80	17.9	17.0	16 sessions across 8 wk	6 mo	Y-BOCS	*d* = 0.04 (ns)	ACT + ERP = ERP at posttreatment and follow-up
										DOCS	*d* = 0.20 (ns)	ACT + ERP = ERP at posttreatment and follow-up
										BDI-II	*d* = 0.25 (ns)	ACT + ERP = ERP at posttreatment and follow-up
Mindfulness-based therapies												
Cludius et al, [44] 2015	Mindfulness-based training (*n* = 49)	Progressive relaxation (PR) (*n* = 38)	66.7	MB: 40 PR: 41	N/R	46.9	39.5	6 wk	N/A	OCI-Total	*d* = 0.32 (ns)	OCD symptom severity did not significantly improve in either condition.
										CES-D	*d* = 0.53 (ns)	Depressive symptom severity did not significantly improve in either condition.

Key et al, [45] 2017	Group mindfulness-based cognitive therapy (MBCT) ($n = 18$)	Waitlist control ($n = 18$)	47.2	32	100	27.7	16.7	8 weekly 2-h sessions	N/A	Y-BOCS-SR	$d = 0.70$	MBCT>waitlist at posttreatment
										BDI-II	$d = 0.93$	MBCT>waitlist at posttreatment
										BAI	$d = 0.70$	MBCT>waitlist at post-treatment
Kulz et al, [46] 2019	Group MBCT ($n = 61$)	Psycho-education group ($n = 64$)	61.6	39	N/R (Germany)	6.6	9.4	8 weekly two-h sessions, plus a booster session at 3 and 6 mo	6 mo	Y-BOCS	$d = 0.40$ (ns)	MBCT = OCD-EP at posttreatment and follow-up
										OCI-R	$d = 0.33$	MBCT>OCD-EP at posttreatment MBCT = OCD-EP at follow-up
										BDI-II	$d = 0.32$	MBCT>OCD-EP at posttreatment MBCT = OCD-EP at follow-up
[a]Strauss et al, [19] 2018	Group mindfulness-based ERP ($n = 19$)	Group ERP ($n = 18$)	64.9	MB-ERP: 33 ERP: 27	97.3	21.0	5.6	10 two-h sessions	6 mo	Y-BOCS-II	$d = -0.20$	MB-ERP = ERP at posttreatment and follow-up
										BDI-II	$d = -0.41$	MB-ERP = ERP at posttreatment and follow-up
Metacognitive therapies												
Moritz et al, [47] 2016	Full ($n = 32$) or adapted ($n = 28$) meta-cognitive therapy	Waitlist ($n = 29$)	48.3	Full: 25 Adapt: 26 Waitlist: 25	N/R (Russia)	53.0	21.0	6 wk	N/A	Y-BOCS Total	Researchers report $d = 0.62$ ($P = .044$) based on change score	MCT (full and adapted) >waitlist MCT-full = MCT-adapted
										OCI-R Total	Researchers report $d = 0.84$ ($P = .006$) based on change score	MCT (full and adapted)>waitlist MCT-full = MCT-adapted
										BDI-II	Researchers report $d = 0.07$ (ns) based on change score	MCT (full and adapted) = waitlist

(continued on next page)

TABLE 1
(*continued*)

Study	Intervention (*n*)	Comparison (*n*)	Sample Characteristics: % fem.	Sample Characteristics: Ave. age (y)	Sample Characteristics: % White[b]	Dropout Rates (%): Inter-vention	Dropout Rates (%): Compar-ison(s)	Treatment Length	Follow-up Period	Measure	Intervention vs Comparison Scores at Posttreatment[c]	Summary[d]
[a]Simons et al, [48] 2006	Metacognitive therapy ($n = 6$)	ERP ($n = 5$)	36.4[e]	MCT: 15 ERP: 13[e]	N/R (Germany)	16.7	0	MCT: ave. 9 sessions ERP: ave. 13 sessions (up to 20 offered)	3 mo 2 y	CY-BOCS	Not reported; insufficient information to calculate	OCD symptom severity improved significantly after treatment, and these improvements were retained at both follow-ups, in both groups. Between-group differences were not analyzed because of small sample size.
										CDI	Not reported; insufficient information to calculate	Depressive symptoms declined, but failed to reach statistical significance because of small sample size and low baseline depressive symptoms.
[a]Rupp et al, [49] 2019	Detached mindfulness (DM) ($n = 21$)	Cognitive re-structuring (CR) ($n = 22$)	58.1	DM: 21 CR: 31	N/R	5.0	9.1	Four 100-mn sessions across 2 wk	4 wk	Y-BOCS	$d = 0.06$ (ns)	DM = CR at post-treatment and follow-up
										BDI-II	$d = 0.16$ (ns)	DM = CR at posttreatment and follow-up

Abbreviations: BAI, Beck Anxiety Inventory; BDI-II, Beck Depression Inventory-II; CES-D, Center for Epidemiologic Studies Depression Scale; CDI, Children's Depression Inventory; DOCS, Dimensional Obsessive-Compulsive Scale; fem., female; MB-ERP, mindfulness-based ERP; MCT, metacognitive therapy; N/A, not applicable; N/R, not reported; ns, nonsignificant; OCI-R, Obsessive Compulsive Inventory–Revised; Y-BOCS-SR, Y-BOCS-Self Report.

[a] Randomized controlled trials that compared third-wave CBT to traditional CBT.

[b] For trials that did not report racial composition of the sample, the country where the trial took place (if reported) is noted.

[c] Cohen's *d* comparing posttreatment scores across treatment group was calculated using mean scores, standard deviations, and sample size at posttreatment among the treatment group and comparison group. Positive *d*s indicate that the third-wave CBT group had lower scores (ie, better outcomes) than the comparison condition. Sizes of *d*s may differ from those reported in the original trials.

[d] ">" indicates that one treatment performed better (ie, lower symptom severity scores) than the other treatment; " = " indicates that differences between two treatments were not statistically significant.

[e] Vakili et al. [41] and Simons et al. [48] reported demographic data on final sample of completers only, rather than the full intent-to-treat sample.

Primary outcomes comparing acceptance and commitment therapy to traditional cognitive-behavioral therapy

Two head-to-head trials compared ACT to traditional CBT. Twohig and colleagues [18] compared a combination of ACT and ERP (which focused on exposure to obsession-provoking situations but provided an ACT framework by incorporating acceptance and values; $n = 28$) to an ERP condition (which provided a "second-wave" rationale for ERP; $n = 30$). Both the ACT + ERP and ERP groups showed significant reductions in OCD symptom severity from pretreatment to posttreatment, and these reductions were maintained at 6-month follow-up. No group differences emerged. Contrary to their predictions, Twohig and colleagues [32] noted comparable changes in obsessive beliefs (ie, an ERP target) and psychological inflexibility (ie, an ACT target), as well as comparable dropout rates (9.8%–13.2%), across the ACT + ERP and ERP groups.

The RCT by Shabani and colleagues [43] is one of the few testing third-wave CBT for adolescents with OCD. SSRI-medicated adolescents ($M_{age} = 15$ years) were randomized to 10 sessions of individual ACT with continued SSRIs ($n = 22$), 12 sessions of individual CBT with continued SSRIs ($n = 22$), or continued SSRIs only ($n = 25$). Adolescents in the ACT + SSRI or CBT + SSRI conditions showed greater reductions in OCD symptom severity at posttreatment than those in the SSRI-only condition ($ds = 1.02$ and 1.37, respectively), and these reductions were maintained at 3-month follow-up. Improvements in OCD symptom severity did not significantly differ between ACT + SSRI and CBT + SSRI conditions at posttreatment or follow-up. Regarding ACT targets, ACT + SSRI youth showed statistically significant improvements in psychological flexibility, mindfulness, and valued living compared with youth in CBT + SSRI or SSRI-only conditions. Youth in the SSRI-only condition did not show statistically significant improvements in any ACT targets. These findings suggest that changes in psychological flexibility, mindfulness, and valued living are processes of change in ACT for OCD.

Secondary outcomes

ACT led to improvements in depression compared with an active control, but only among patients who reported depressive symptoms in the mild range or above at pretreatment [32]. Regardless of treatment condition (third-wave CBT or traditional CBT), patients generally showed significant reductions in depressive symptoms at posttreatment that were maintained at follow-up [18,41,43]. It appears both third-wave CBT and traditional CBT decrease secondary depressive symptoms, and these reductions may not differ across treatment.

Moderators

A secondary analysis of the RCT by Twohig and colleagues [18] examined empirically and theoretically relevant moderators: anxiety symptom severity, depressive symptom severity (due to high comorbidity between internalizing symptoms and OCD), psychological inflexibility (which maintains OCD symptoms from an ACT framework), and interpretation of intrusions (which maintains OCD symptoms from an ERP framework) [33]. Patients with fewer dysfunctional appraisals at pretreatment showed greater OCD symptom improvements in ERP than in ACT + ERP, suggesting that ERP may be a better fit for patients with stronger catastrophic interpretations of intrusive thoughts. Comorbid anxiety, depression, and psychological inflexibility at pretreatment did not moderate treatment outcomes.

Mindfulness-Based Therapies

Primary outcomes comparing mindfulness-based therapies to non-cognitive-behavioral therapy treatments

Cludius and colleagues [44] compared the effects of self-administered mindfulness-based training ($n = 49$) and progressive muscle relaxation ($n = 38$). No statistically significant improvements were observed in either group ($ds = 0.01$ and -0.03, respectively). Key and colleagues [45] tested the efficacy of clinician-delivered group mindfulness-based cognitive therapy ($n = 18$) versus waitlist control ($n = 18$). Patients in group mindfulness-based cognitive therapy showed statistically significant improvements in OCD symptom severity at posttreatment, compared with waitlist ($d = 0.70$). Külz and colleagues [46] compared the outcomes of group mindfulness-based cognitive therapy ($n = 61$) with those of a psychoeducation group (ie, active control; $n = 64$). At posttreatment, mindfulness-based cognitive therapy patients self-reported significantly lower OCD symptom severity than psychoeducation patients ($d = 0.33$), but clinician reports of OCD symptoms did not significantly differ across groups. Moreover, differences in patient self-reports were no longer significant at 6-month follow-up.

Primary outcomes comparing mindfulness-based therapies to traditional cognitive-behavioral therapy

Strauss and colleagues [19] compared outcomes of group mindfulness-based ERP (n = 19) to group traditional ERP (n = 18). As expected, patients undergoing mindfulness-based ERP showed significant improvements in mindfulness (ie, the targeted process of change) compared with those undergoing traditional ERP (d = 0.20). However, although both mindfulness-based ERP and traditional ERP patients showed improvements in OCD symptoms, there were no statistically significant group differences at posttreatment or 6-month follow-up. Strauss and colleagues concluded that mindfulness-based ERP may be unlikely to lead to greater clinically significant improvements than traditional ERP alone [19].

Secondary outcomes

Depressive symptoms typically decreased in treatment conditions compared with control conditions, but did not significantly differ between third-wave CBT and traditional CBT [45,46]. Similarly, mindfulness-based cognitive therapy decreased co-occurring anxiety compared with waitlist [45]. However, no RCTs to date comparing third-wave CBT to traditional CBT have examined anxiety outcomes.

Metacognitive Therapy

Primary outcomes comparing metacognitive therapy to non-cognitive-behavioral therapy treatments

Moritz and colleagues [47] compared the effects of the full version of a self-administered metacognitive therapy manual (n = 32), an "individually adapted" version of the same manual (n = 28), and a waitlist (n = 29). At pretreatment, participants completed 14 yes/no questions that each corresponded to a article in the manual. Participants in the "individually adapted" condition received only the introductory article and articles corresponding to the problems they endorsed. The researchers posited that participants who received the "individually adapted" manual would show greater improvements in OCD symptoms than those who received the full manual because of the focus on more personally relevant domains. Contrary to expectation, OCD symptom improvement did not differ between the full and adapted versions of the manual. Patients who received the manual (whether the full or adapted version) showed improved OCD symptoms compared with waitlist (d = 0.62).

Primary outcomes comparing metacognitive therapy to traditional cognitive-behavioral therapy

In a randomized-allocation case series [48], Simons and colleagues randomly assigned youths aged 8 to 17 years to receive up to 20 weekly sessions of either individual metacognitive therapy (n = 6, of which one patient dropped out; M_{age} = 14.5 years) or individual ERP (n = 5; M_{age} = 13.4 years). All ten youths who completed treatment showed an improvement of over 30% on the child Y-BOCS (CY-BOCS) at posttreatment, and thus were considered responders. While between-group differences were not analyzed because of small sample size, corrected effect sizes of 2.9 for metacognitive therapy patients (average CY-BOCS score decrease from 26 to 6 from pretreatment to posttreatment) and 2.2 for ERP patients (average CY-BOCS score decrease from 20 to 1 from pretreatment to posttreatment) were reported. Moreover, youths in both groups maintained improvements at 3-month and 2-year follow-ups. Descriptively, however, youth who received metacognitive therapy showed a wider spread in follow-up scores (ie, ranges of 0–23 and 0–12 at 3-month and 2-year follow-up, respectively) than youth who received ERP (ie, ranges of 0–3 at both 3-month and 2-year follow-up, respectively). Although this trial suggests that metacognitive therapy may be a viable alternative to traditional CBT for youth with OCD, its methodological limitations and small sample prohibit between-group analyses and thus necessitate replication.

Rupp and colleagues [49] compared the effects of detached mindfulness (a third-wave technique) and cognitive restructuring (a second-wave technique). Detached mindfulness is a metacognitive technique used to develop awareness of one's thoughts as "mental events" that can be observed without acting on them. Cognitive restructuring involves identifying "automatic thoughts" and guiding patients in considering alternative interpretations of a situation that provokes those thoughts. Patients were randomized to eight sessions of detached mindfulness treatment (n = 21) or cognitive restructuring treatment (n = 22); 21 of these patients (10 from the detached mindfulness group and 11 from the cognitive restructuring group) were placed on a 2-week waitlist before beginning treatment. Both detached mindfulness and cognitive restructuring led to improvements in OCD symptoms at posttreatment and 4-week follow-up, compared with the waitlist (ds = 1.55 and 1.67, respectively), but no group differences emerged. Of note, an RCT by Melchior and colleagues [50] comparing metacognitive therapy to ERP in a sample of 100 adults in the Netherlands is currently underway.

Secondary outcomes

Both detached mindfulness and cognitive restructuring led to slight improvements in depressive symptoms at posttreatment and follow-up, with no between-group differences [49]. Similarly, youths' depressive symptoms declined from pretreatment to posttreatment after receiving metacognitive therapy or ERP, but these improvements did not reach statistical significance in the small sample of 10 youths [48]. Finally, patients who self-administered metacognitive therapy showed no changes in depressive symptoms [47].

DISCUSSION

Based on the twelve RCTs reviewed, several findings emerge. First, in comparison to control conditions or non-CBT treatments, third-wave CBT may be effective in treating OCD symptoms, including ACT (eg, ACT vs progressive muscle relaxation [32]; ACT alone or in combination with SSRIs vs SSRIs alone [41]; group ACT + SSRIs vs SSRIs [42]), mindfulness-based therapies (eg, group mindfulness-based cognitive therapy vs waitlist [19]), and metacognitive therapies (eg, metacognitive therapy vs waitlist [47]). However, the evidence is mixed, particularly for interventions that do not incorporate exposure; self-administered mindfulness-based training was not effective [44], and group mindfulness-based cognitive therapy was no more effective than a psychoeducation group [46].

Second, third-wave CBT treatments *which incorporate exposure* are sometimes comparable to, but not more effective than, traditional CBT treatments in treating OCD symptoms. OCD symptom outcomes of traditional ERP/CBT did not statistically differ from ACT (eg, group ACT + SSRI vs group CBT + SSRI [43]), mindfulness-based ERP (eg, group mindfulness-based ERP vs group traditional ERP [19]), and metacognitive therapies (eg, detached mindfulness vs cognitive restructuring [49]). This, of course, begs the question of the active therapeutic elements. Of note, studies that found no lasting improvements in OCD symptoms did not involve explicit exposure (eg, mindfulness-based training vs progressive relaxation [44]; group mindfulness-based cognitive therapy vs psychoeducation group [46]). On the other hand, studies that showed comparable, lasting effects between third-wave CBT and traditional CBT included exposure (eg, ACT + ERP vs traditional ERP [18]; group mindfulness-based ERP vs group traditional ERP [19]). This suggests that ERP is the "active ingredient" of effective OCD treatments. Of note, Twohig and colleagues [33] found similar improvements in ACT targets (psychological flexibility) and traditional ERP targets (obsessional beliefs), suggesting overlapping mechanisms in the two treatments. Together, findings suggest that clinicians should use tried-and-true exposure methods when treating OCD.

Third, improvements in co-occurring depressive symptoms generally did not differ between third-wave CBT and traditional CBT. This challenges previous arguments that third-wave CBT may better treat co-occurring symptoms than traditional CBT [16]. Findings regarding co-occurring anxiety symptoms were reported in only two studies and thus are inconclusive. It is recommended that future RCTs include assessments of co-occurring anxiety and depressive symptoms.

Fourth, the three RCTs testing combinations of ACT and SSRIs yielded similar patterns of findings to prior studies testing combinations of traditional CBT and SSRIs for OCD. Collectively, these RCTs found that ACT + SSRIs outperformed SSRIs alone in the short- and long-term [42,43] and that ACT performed comparably to ACT + SSRIs [41]. However, it is important to note that these studies suffered from significant methodological concerns including small sample size (eg, *ns* = 10–11 per treatment group), unclear rationale (eg, including two types of SSRIs for only 10 wk), absence of follow-up, or a female-only sample [41,42]. In larger and more rigorous RCTs testing combinations of ERP and SSRIs, ERP outperformed first-line medication in head-to-head trials with children and adults with OCD, and the combination of ERP and antidepressants was no different from ERP plus placebo in two of three trials [51–53]. To evaluate the efficacy of combinations of third-wave CBT and SSRIs compared with combinations of ERP and SSRIs, replication through rigorous RCTs is required.

Recommendations

While ACT has shown some promise, the strength of the literature on third-wave CBT for OCD is still in its early stages and does not justify departure from CBT/ERP models as a first-line treatment. First, only a small number of RCTs have evaluated third-wave CBT for OCD, and even fewer of those have compared third-wave CBT to traditional CBT/ERP. Second, many of these RCTs have poor methodological rigor and are based on unclear rationale. Third, many of these RCTs have been conducted by expert groups with biases toward third-wave treatments. Considering Chambless and Hollon's definition of empirically supported treatments [54] and Tolin and colleagues's more recent update [55], only ACT-based ERP meets criteria for a "possibly efficacious" treatment.

Although preliminary research supporting ACT and mindfulness could lead clinicians to use broad ACT or mindfulness skills in place of exposure, the current evidence base does not justify this shift in practice. We suggest that CBT/ERP should remain the gold standard in adult OCD treatment as recommended in current guidelines,[56], with a newer appreciation of data that preliminarily support more flexibility in conceptualizing this treatment from different theoretic frameworks (ie, that ACT-based ERP may be considered "possibly efficacious"). A positive outcome of this new understanding is that it could engender participation in ERP from clinicians from more diverse theoretic backgrounds and a better ability to tailor treatment to the individual.

Future Directions

Future research is needed in this area. First, rigorous dismantling studies are required to ascertain the "active ingredients" in OCD treatment. Second, sufficiently powered moderator analyses in the context of large, head-to-head RCTs comparing third-wave CBT and traditional CBT are needed to predict who responds better to which treatment. The presence of treatment moderators [33] highlights a need for personally tailored intervention. If individual-level moderators (eg, symptom severity, rate of change, presence of co-occurring symptoms, patient preferences) predict improved response to one treatment over another, we may need to better *personalize* treatment for individual patients, rather than develop new treatments that universally outperform traditional CBT. From a biopsychosocial perspective, including biological (eg, brain circuits, genetic factors), psychological (eg, cognitive beliefs, psychological flexibility), and social variables (eg, family accommodation, social environment) in RCTs may help us identify additional moderators or predictors of treatment outcomes in third-wave CBT and traditional CBT. Third, considering the growing popularity of ACT for children and adolescents, more studies of third-wave CBT for youth with OCD are warranted as well, as only two of the studies identified in this review included youth. These studies were limited by small sample sizes prohibiting between-group comparisons, wide age ranges, differing lengths of CBT and ACT treatments or differing lengths of treatment between patients, and variations in SSRIs between patients.

SUMMARY

This narrative review set out to evaluate the evidence for third-wave CBT for individuals with OCD. Using a systematic approach, we identified twelve RCTs testing third-wave CBTs for OCD patients. Studies varied in terms of methodological rigor, treatment components, sample characteristics, and rationale. Third-wave CBTs were generally effective in treating OCD symptoms compared with control or non-CBT treatments, although two studies found no effect (both of which did not include exposure). Third-wave CBT treatments incorporating exposure were often comparable to, but no more effective than, traditional ERP. Co-occurring depressive symptoms tended to improve in conjunction with OCD symptoms; evidence on co-occurring anxiety symptoms is lacking. In summary, third-wave CBT treatments are increasingly used to treat individuals with OCD, yet the evidence for this treatment modality is nascent. Indeed, the popularity of third-wave CBT treatments for OCD has in some ways outpaced the evidence. While CBT/ERP should be the first-line psychotherapeutic treatment, clinicians may consider third-wave CBTs such as ACT for patients who do not respond to traditional CBT, as long as exposure remains an essential component of treatment. Future research should examine active ingredients and moderators that contribute to treatment outcomes.

CLINICS CARE POINTS

- A review of twelve randomized controlled trials revealed that third-wave cognitive behavioral therapy (CBT) that incorporates exposure is sometimes comparable to traditional CBT for individuals with obsessive compulsive disorder, whereas third-wave CBT without exposure is less effective.
- While acceptance and commitment therapy show some promise, the strength of the literature is still in its infancy and does not justify departure from CBT/exposure and response prevention (ERP) as first-line treatment.
- While traditional CBT/ERP should be the first-line psychotherapeutic treatment, clinicians may consider third-wave CBTs with exposure for patients who do not respond to traditional CBT.
- Future research requires dismantling studies and moderator analyses in the context of large and rigorous randomized controlled trials comparing third-wave and traditional CBT.

DISCLOSURE

The authors have no conflicts of interests to disclose.

SUPPLEMENTARY DATA

Supplementary data related to this article can be found online at https://doi.org/10.1016/j.ypsc.2021.05.004.

REFERENCES

[1] Öst L-G, Havnen A, Hansen B, et al. Cognitive behavioral treatments of obsessive–compulsive disorder. A systematic review and meta-analysis of studies published 1993–2014. Clin Psychol Rev 2015;40:156–69.

[2] McGuire JF, Piacentini J, Lewin AB, et al. A meta-analysis of cognitive behavior therapy and medication for child obsessive-compulsive disorder: Moderators of treatment efficacy, response, and remission. Depress Anxiety 2015;32(8):580–93.

[3] Storch EA, McGuire JF, McKay D. The clinician's guide to cognitive-behavioral therapy for childhood obsessive-compulsive disorder. Cambridge (MA): Academic Press; 2017.

[4] Foa EB, Yadin E, Lichner TK. Exposure and response (ritual) prevention for obsessive compulsive disorder: therapist guide. New York, NY: Oxford University Press; 2012.

[5] Johnco C, McGuire JF, Roper T, et al. A meta-analysis of dropout rates from exposure with response prevention and pharmacological treatment for youth with obsessive compulsive disorder. Depress Anxiety 2020;37(5):407–17.

[6] Ong CW, Clyde JW, Bluett EJ, et al. Dropout rates in exposure with response prevention for obsessive-compulsive disorder: What do the data really say? J Anxiety Disord 2016;40:8–17.

[7] Rector NA, Wilde JL, Richter MA. Obsessive compulsive disorder and comorbidity: rates, models, and treatment approaches. In: Abramowitz JS, McKay D, Storch EA, editors. The Wiley Handbook of Obsessive-Compulsive Disorders. vol. 2. Chichester, UK: John Wiley & Sons; 2017. p. 697–725.

[8] Rosa-Alcázar AI, Sánchez-Meca J, Gómez-Conesa A, et al. Psychological treatment of obsessive-compulsive disorder: A meta-analysis. Clin Psychol Rev 2008;28(8):1310–25.

[9] Meyer V. Modification of expectations in cases with obsessional rituals. Behav Res Ther 1966;4(4):273–80.

[10] Foa EB, Goldstein A. Continuous exposure and complete response prevention in the treatment of obsessive-compulsive neurosis. Behav Ther 1978;9(5):821–9.

[11] Hayes SC. Acceptance and commitment therapy, relational frame theory, and the third wave of behavioral and cognitive therapies. Behav Ther 2004;35(4):639–65.

[12] Dimidjian S, Arch JJ, Schneider RL, et al. Considering Meta-Analysis, Meaning, and Metaphor: A Systematic Review and Critical Examination of "Third Wave" Cognitive and Behavioral Therapies. Behav Ther 2016;47(6):886–905.

[13] Arch JJ, Eifert GH, Davies C, et al. Randomized clinical trial of cognitive behavioral therapy (CBT) versus acceptance and commitment therapy (ACT) for mixed anxiety disorders. J Consult Clin Psychol 2012;80(5):750–65.

[14] Wolitzky-Taylor KB, Arch JJ, Rosenfield D, et al. Moderators and non-specific predictors of treatment outcome for anxiety disorders: A comparison of cognitive behavioral therapy to acceptance and commitment therapy. J Consult Clin Psychol 2012;80(5):786–99.

[15] Callesen P, Reeves D, Heal C, et al. Metacognitive therapy versus cognitive Behaviour therapy in Adults with Major Depression: A parallel Single-Blind Randomised trial. Scientific Rep 2020;10(1):1–10.

[16] Twohig MP, Abramowitz JS, Bluett EJ, et al. Exposure therapy for OCD from an acceptance and commitment therapy (ACT) framework. J Obsessive-Compulsive Relat Disord 2015;6:167–73.

[17] International Obsessive-Compulsive Disorder Foundation. Find Help. 2020. Available at: https://iocdf.org/?s=new%2Byork%2Bcity&post_type%5B0%5D=iocdf_provider&post_type%5B1%5D=iocdf_clinic&search-type=provider&filterObj%5B0%5D=language%7Cen&filterObj%5B1%5D=iocdf_tax_provider_strategy%7Cact-2&distance-filter=200mi. Accessed October 11, 2020.

[18] Twohig MP, Abramowitz JS, Smith BM, et al. Adding acceptance and commitment therapy to exposure and response prevention for obsessive-compulsive disorder: A randomized controlled trial. Behav Res Ther 2018;108:1–9.

[19] Strauss C, Lea L, Hayward M, et al. Mindfulness-based exposure and response prevention for obsessive compulsive disorder: Findings from a pilot randomised controlled trial. J Anxiety Disord 2018;57:39–47.

[20] Marcks BA, Woods DW. A comparison of thought suppression to an acceptance-based technique in the management of personal intrusive thoughts: a controlled evaluation. Behav Res Ther 2005;43(4):433–45.

[21] Alex Brake C, Sauer-Zavala S, Boswell JF, et al. Mindfulness-Based Exposure Strategies as a Transdiagnostic Mechanism of Change: An Exploratory Alternating Treatment Design. Behav Ther 2016;47(2):225–38.

[22] Curreri AJ, Farchione TJ, Sauer-Zavala S, et al. Mindful Emotion Awareness Facilitates Engagement with Exposure Therapy: An Idiographic Exploration Using Single Case Experimental Design. Behav Modification 2020. https://doi.org/10.1177/0145445520947662.

[23] Levitt JT, Brown TA, Orsillo SM, et al. The effects of acceptance versus suppression of emotion on subjective and psychophysiological response to carbon dioxide challenge in patients with panic disorder. Behav Ther 2004;35(4):747–66.

[24] Külz A, Barton B, Voderholzer U. Third wave therapies of cognitive behavioral therapy for obsessive compulsive disorder: a reasonable add-on therapy for CBT? State of the art. Psychother Psychosom Med Psychol 2016;66(03/04):106–11.

[25] Twohig MP. The Application of Acceptance and Commitment Therapy to Obsessive-Compulsive Disorder. Cogn Behav Pract 2009;16(1):18–28.

[26] Wells A, Papageorgiou C. Relationships between worry, obsessive-compulsive symptoms and meta-cognitive beliefs. Behav Res Ther 1998;36:899–913.

[27] Hayes SC, Barnes-Holmes D, Roche B. Relational frame theory: a post-skinnerian account of human language and cognition. New York: Springer Science & Business Media; 2001.

[28] Bluett EJ, Homan KJ, Morrison KL, et al. Acceptance and commitment therapy for anxiety and OCD spectrum disorders: An empirical review. J Anxiety Disord 2014; 28(6):612–24.

[29] Twohig MP, Smith BM. Targeting the function of inner experiences in obsessive compulsive and related disorders. Curr Opin Psychol 2015;2:32–7.

[30] Ponniah K, Magiati I, Hollon SD. An update on the efficacy of psychological treatments for obsessive-compulsive disorder in adults. J Obsessive-Compulsive Relat Disord 2013;2(2):207–18.

[31] Öst LG. The efficacy of Acceptance and Commitment Therapy: An updated systematic review and meta-analysis. Behav Res Ther 2014;61:105–21.

[32] Twohig MP, Hayes SC, Plumb JC, et al. A randomized clinical trial of acceptance and commitment therapy versus progressive relaxation training for obsessive-compulsive disorder. J Consult Clin Psychol 2010; 78(5):705–16.

[33] Ong CW, Blakey SM, Smith BM, et al. Moderators and processes of change in traditional exposure and response prevention (ERP) versus acceptance and commitment therapy-informed ERP for obsessive-compulsive disorder. J Obsessive-Compulsive Relat Disord 2020;24:1–11.

[34] Fairfax M, Easey K, Fletcher S, et al. Does mindfulness help in the treatment of obsessive compulsive disorder (OCD)? An audit of client experience of an OCD group. Counselling Psychol Rev 2014;29(3):17–27.

[35] Wells A. Emotional disorders and metacognition: innovative cognitive therapy. Chichester (UK): John Wiley & Sons; 2002.

[36] Mather A, Cartwright-Hatton S. Cognitive predictors of obsessive-compulsive symptoms in adolescence: A preliminary investigation. J Clin Child Adolesc Psychol 2004;33(4):743–9.

[37] Fisher PL, Wells A. Metacognitive therapy for obsessive-compulsive disorder: A case series. J Behav Ther Exp Psychiatry 2008;39(2):117–32.

[38] Melchior K, Franken IHA, van der Heiden C. Metacognitive Therapy for Obsessive-Compulsive Disorder: A Case Report. Bull Menninger Clin 2018;82: 375–89.

[39] Miegel F, Cludius B, Hottenrott B, et al. Session-specific effects of the Metacognitive Training for Obsessive-Compulsive Disorder (MCT-OCD). Psychotherapy Res 2019;30(4):474–86.

[40] Esfahani M, Kjbaf MB, Abedi MR. Evaluation and Comparison of the Effects of Time Perspective Therapy, Acceptance and Commitment Therapy and Narrative Therapy on Severity of Symptoms of Obsessive-Compulsive Disorder. J Indian Acad Appl Psychol 2015;41(3):148–55.

[41] Vakili Y, Gharraee B, Habibi M, et al. The Comparison of Acceptance and Commitment Therapy with Selective Serotonin Reuptake Inhibitors in the Treatment of Obsessive-Compulsive Disorder. Zahedan J Res Med Sci J 2013;16(Suppl 1):10–4.

[42] Rohani F, Rasouli-Azad M, Twohig MP, et al. Preliminary test of group acceptance and commitment therapy on obsessive-compulsive disorder for patients on optimal dose of selective serotonin reuptake inhibitors. J Obsessive-Compulsive Relat Disord 2018;16:8–13.

[43] Shabani MJ, Mohsenabadi H, Omidi A, et al. An Iranian study of group acceptance and commitment therapy versus group cognitive behavioral therapy for adolescents with obsessive-compulsive disorder on an optimal dose of selective serotonin reuptake inhibitors. J Obsessive-Compulsive Relat Disord 2019;22. https://doi.org/10.1016/j.jocrd.2019.04.003.

[44] Cludius B, Hottenrott B, Alsleben H, et al. Mindfulness for OCD? No evidence for a direct effect of a self-help treatment approach. J Obsessive-Compulsive Relat Disord 2015;6:59–65.

[45] Key BL, Rowa K, Bieling P, et al. Mindfulness-based cognitive therapy as an augmentation treatment for obsessive–compulsive disorder. Clin Psychol Psychotherapy 2017;24(5):1109–20.

[46] Külz AK, Landmann S, Cludius B, et al. Mindfulness-based cognitive therapy (MBCT) in patients with obsessive–compulsive disorder (OCD) and residual symptoms after cognitive behavioral therapy (CBT): a randomized controlled trial. Eur Arch Psychiatry Clin Neurosci 2019;269(2):223–33.

[47] Moritz S, Stepulovs O, Schröder J, et al. Is the whole less than the sum of its parts? Full versus individually adapted metacognitive self-help for obsessive-compulsive disorder: A randomized controlled trial. J Obsessive-Compulsive Relat Disord 2016;9:107–15.

[48] Simons M, Schneider S, Herpertz-Dahlmann B. Metacognitive therapy versus exposure and response prevention for pediatric obsessive-compulsive disorder: A case series with randomized allocation. Psychother Psychosom 2006;75(4):257–64.

[49] Rupp C, Jürgens C, Doebler P, et al. A randomized waitlist-controlled trial comparing detached mindfulness and cognitive restructuring in obsessive-compulsive disorder. PLoS ONE 2019;14(3). https://doi.org/10.1371/journal.pone.0213895.

[50] Melchior K, Franken I, Deen M, et al. Metacognitive therapy versus exposure and response prevention for obsessive-compulsive disorder: Study protocol for a randomized controlled trial. Trials 2019;20(1). https://doi.org/10.1186/s13063-019-3381-9.

[51] Foa EB, Liebowitz MR, Kozak MJ, et al. Randomized, Placebo-Controlled Trial of Exposure and Ritual Prevention, Clomipramine, and Their Combination in the

Treatment of Obsessive-Compulsive Disorder. Am J Psychiatry 2005;162:151–61.

[52] Storch EA, Bussing R, Small B, et al. Randomized, placebo-controlled trial of cognitive-behavioral therapy alone or combined with sertraline in the treatment of pediatric obsessive-compulsive disorder. Behav Res Ther 2013;51(12):823–9.

[53] The Pediatric OCD Treatment Study (POTS) Team. Cognitive-behavior therapy, sertraline, and their combination for children and adolescents with obsessive-compulsive disorder. JAMA 2004;292(16):1969–76.

[54] Chambless DL, Hollon SD. Defining empirically supported therapies. J Consult Clin Psychol 1998;66(1): 7–18.

[55] Tolin DF, McKay D, Forman EM, et al. Empirically supported treatment: Recommendations for a new model. Clin Psychol Sci Pract 2015;22(4):317–38.

[56] American Psychiatric Association. Practice guideline for the treatment of patients with obsessive-compulsive disorder. Arlington, VA: American Psychiatric Association; 2007. Available at: https://www.psych.org/psych_pract/treatg/pg/prac_guide.cfm. Accessed November 9, 2020.

Suicide Research

Advances in Psychiatry and Behavioral Health 1 (2021) 53–65
ADVANCES IN PSYCHIATRY AND BEHAVIORAL HEALTH

Digital Technology for Suicide Prevention

Jordan M. Braciszewski, PhD
Center for Health Policy & Health Services Research, Henry Ford Health System, One Ford Place, Suite 3A, Detroit, MI 48202, USA

KEYWORDS
• mHealth • eHealth • Technology • Suicide • Mobile

KEY POINTS

- Digital technologies have immense potential to advance our understanding of and robust response to suicide risk.
- Key limitations in these approaches have stalled their widespread implementation.
- While digital approaches as standalone interventions are likely insufficient, and clinicians should be critical curators of available apps, there is strong promise in using technology to augment ongoing clinical care.
- Large, randomized trials, the involvement of those with lived experience, and attention to ethical and legal considerations should assist in advancing digital health care.

INTRODUCTION

Suicide is the 10th-leading cause of death and #1 cause of injury-related death for adults in the United States, accounting for 45,000 deaths per year [1]. Among adolescents, suicide is the second-leading cause of mortality, accounting for more than 1 in 10 deaths [1]. Unfortunately, suicide rates have not improved over time despite numerous initiatives [2–5]. In fact, data indicate that national suicide rates have increased by nearly 25% over the last 15 years [6,7], making it the only top-10 cause of death with an increasing rate during that period. National concern prompted the National Action Alliance for Suicide Prevention and the Surgeon General to publish the *National Strategy for Suicide Prevention* [8], which focuses on suicide prevention as a core aspect of health care services.

Digital technologies have flourished in the mental health space over the past decade, offering strong potential to improve access to care through tailored, personalized interventions. Given the burgeoning landscape of technology-based approaches to suicide prevention and current limitations of the field, practitioners need a strong resource that details the current state of available approaches to risk assessment and intervention tools. The proliferation of mental health–related technologies available to patients and providers *without* a strong evidence base has the potential to result in harmful experiences for users [9]. As such, this comprehensive review provides an overview of technology-based approaches to suicide prevention with a focus on the quality of the evidence supporting adoption that will serve as a guide for clinicians and researchers working with individuals who endorse suicidal ideation.

Gaps in Current Approaches to Identification and Treatment

Psychological autopsy studies suggest that over 90% of individuals at risk for suicide meet criteria for a psychiatric condition prior to death [10]; as such, it appears natural to intervene primarily with individuals who have these conditions and to do so within behavioral health care settings. However, the modifiable suicide

E-mail address: jbracis1@hfhs.org
Twitter: @jmbrockphd (J.M.B.)

https://doi.org/10.1016/j.ypsc.2021.05.008
2667-3827/21/

risk through specialty behavioral health is quite small because so few patients with suicidal intent are seen there. Recent data indicate that while more than 80% of those who die by suicide make a health care visit in the year before their death, more than 50% do not have a mental health diagnosis [11]. Few of these patients (fewer than 40%) receive behavioral health services prior to their death. In contrast, the vast majority of visits occur in outpatient primary care or general medical specialty settings [11]. Thus, suicide prevention directed only toward individuals with a mental health diagnosis within behavioral health settings (the group with whom most interventions are currently focused) will reach less than half of all healthcare patients before their death.

Over the past several decades, more attention has been paid to suicide-specific approaches to intervention. Several evidence-based treatment protocols have emerged, including dialectical behavior therapy (DBT) [12], cognitive behavioral therapy (CBT) [13], and collaborative assessment and management of suicidality [14], all of which have shown strong efficacy. However, while instrumental in reducing suicide behaviors, these approaches are often time-intensive and labor-intensive interventions. Each requires extensive training, ongoing supervision to maintain fidelity, adjustments to clinic workflow, and extended time and effort to deliver, all of which limit scalable uptake. Streamlined interventions with broad appeal are therefore paramount to meeting the needs of patients and health care policy while preventing increased labor costs and major disruptions to clinical workflow.

Leveraging Digital Technologies to Address a Major Public Health Problem

The National Institute of Mental Health (NIMH) published *A Prioritized Research Agenda for Suicide Prevention* [15], wherein it aims to "reduce suicide attempt and death outcomes through multiple, synergistic components of quality improvement within and across responsible systems." [15,16] According to NIMH's Suicide Prevention Research Prioritization Task Force, technological enhancements to facilitate help-seeking could catalyze progress across multiple suicide prevention priority areas [15]. Technology-based interventions (eg, computer, cell phone, or tablet) have demonstrated efficacy for mental [17–19] and physical [20,21] health issues, smoking [22,23], and substance use [24,25]. These approaches offer significant advantages, including perfect reproducibility of intervention content and improved access for those unable to engage in traditional services. Technology can also increase the likelihood of honest reporting on sensitive topics [26–28], including suicidal ideation [29]. Mobile phones in particular are nearly ubiquitous, as more than 96% of US adults own a mobile phone [30]. New technologies allow for a high degree of tailoring and personalization, increasing intervention acceptability and effectiveness [31]. Treatment engagement can also be improved, with a recent study noting that mobile health (mHealth) strategies promoted higher engagement (90% vs 58%) and retention (56% vs 40%) in treatment compared with clinic-based care for individuals with severe mental illness [32]. Screening and intervention can be completed in any setting, which may improve scalability and reduce significant delays between problem development and treatment initiation. Such screening may result in an increased likelihood of seeking traditional care [33]. Following the COVID-19 pandemic, health systems and other providers have moved toward technology-based delivery of care (eg, telehealth), with many believing this modality will continue beyond the crisis and become a new standard of treatment across health care settings [34]. One survey estimated that 81% of behavioral health providers began using telehealth for the first time during the pandemic, while 70% plan to continue into the future [35].

Technology-based approaches may be well suited for suicide prevention, as mobile phone apps and other devices can offer immediate support and connection to important resources, including family/friends, care providers, and crisis services. Given that suicide risk can change rapidly, mHealth resources have the strong potential to literally save lives [36]. Patients appear amenable to such approaches, as 80% of psychiatry outpatients aged 45 or younger reported a desire to use a mobile app to track their mental health [37]. Those who endorse suicidal ideation, specifically, may prefer these approaches as well [38], particularly given the lack of formal treatment engagement among this population [39,40]. Researchers and policymakers have specifically noted the impact that technology can have on widespread safety plan implementation. Several states now recommend technology-based platforms for accessing suicide safety plans to increase uptake [41,42]. That said, the NIMH Agenda encourages multiple synergistic components [15]; many technology-based approaches to behavioral health are standalone and may not fully leverage the potential of complementary care (ie, tech as an adjunct to treatment). As detailed below, the research literature is growing substantially, though significant work remains to be completed.

CURRENT EVIDENCE

Technology-Based Screening

Suicide prevention begins with the identification of suicidal thoughts, previous attempts, and intentions to engage in suicidal behavior. Systematic Web-based screening of suicidal ideation and behavior may increase identification at the population level as well as assist in rapidly facilitating further evaluation and engagement in treatment. Large-scale programs have been implemented in university settings [33,43], emergency departments [44], and primary care [45,46] with much success. For example, through e-mail, college students were asked to complete a comprehensive suicide and mental health screening questionnaire developed by the American Foundation for Suicide Prevention (AFSP) that categorized respondents into tiers of risk [33]. Those in the high-risk and moderate-risk tiers received personalized feedback from a university counselor that could be viewed on the Web as well as an invitation to a follow-up with the provider online or in person. Almost 90% of respondents returned to view their postscreening assessments, while 19% of moderate-risk to high-risk participants sought an in-person evaluation with the counselor. Students who sought online conversations with the counselor were more likely to initiate treatment than those who did not (38% vs 12%). An additional test of the AFSP model showed similar findings among students, residents, and faculty of a medical school [47]. While improvement could be made in engagement with this model, raising awareness and willingness to talk with a counselor among nearly 1 in 5 students based on e-mailed feedback alone may be a promising low-cost, high-yield strategy. The vast majority of screening-based studies, however, have lacked control group comparisons, limiting their impact on the field.

Within busy primary care and emergency department settings, Web-based screening tools allow clinical staff to collect important data, triage patients, and provide appropriate referrals to services while minimizing the impact on clinical workflow and maximizing important quality metrics like standardization, reliability, efficiency, and validity [48]. Computer-adapted approaches, with branching logic that can tailor screening and assessment to severity, can collect a great deal of clinical information with fewer questions, further increasing efficiency and impact. Integrating such screenings with electronic health records can assist researchers and clinical providers in developing machine learning algorithms that can better predict which patients are at greatest risk of harming themselves [49,50]. Such integration is essential so that providers are not burdened by the need to interact with multiple systems to provide clinical care.

Self-Guided Internet-Based Approaches

Internet-based platforms are various and can include research-driven therapy protocols, support groups, message boards, automated chatbots, e-mail-based support, and others. A circumscribed and recent review of Internet-based self-help interventions for suicidal ideation and behavior found strong support for these approaches [51]. This systematic review and meta-analyses focused exclusively on randomized controlled trials of self-help, Internet-based platforms designed to target suicidal ideation and behavior. Collectively, the interventions in these trials used CBT and DBT concepts, including emotional regulation, worry scheduling, identifying and modifying automatic thoughts, relapse prevention, behavioral activation/activity scheduling, cognitive restructuring, and problem-solving. The meta-analysis indicated a significant effect for reductions in suicidal ideation among intervention participants over controls following intervention for all studies and 6 months later for 4 of the studies. However, 2 studies reported no differences between intervention and control groups on suicide attempts [52,53].

The majority of review articles and meta-analyses on self-help, Internet-based approaches, however, have concluded that while there are likely benefits from using these strategies, the overall quality of the literature is poor [54–57]. Specifically, the current literature has been noted to suffer from small sample sizes, significant attrition, a focus on broader constructs such as depression rather than suicide specifically, heterogeneous methodologies (eg, randomized trials, cross-sectional studies, qualitative research, pre–post designs), and predominately self-report outcomes, resulting in insufficient evidence to accurately assess the utility of Web-based approaches [58]. While few randomized trials in this area have been undertaken, 2 that focused on individuals with depression suggested that suicidal ideation was reduced for both intervention and control participants [59,60]. This observation parallels outcomes from studies on in-person approaches [61,62] that highlight the importance of using strategies that focus directly on mitigating suicide rather than targeting depression with the hope of indirectly impacting suicide outcomes [56].

Mobile Applications

The ubiquitous nature of smartphone ownership makes the delivery of health care through mobile devices an area that has skyrocketed over the last 10 years. Indeed, recent data indicate that 81% of Americans own a smartphone; a substantial increase from 35% in 2011 [30]. These data further indicate that although smartphone ownership decreases with age, 79% of individuals age 50–64 and 53% of those age 65+ own 1 of these devices. In addition, nearly two-thirds of smartphone owners have used their devices to look up information about a health condition [63], and these devices may be helping to bridge the digital divide experienced by racial and ethnic minorities [64].

This digital boom has resulted in over 10,000 mental health-related apps in the Google and Android stores [65], very few of which have been evaluated systemically, calling into question their efficacy at helping individuals cope with suicidal thoughts. As such, app-based approaches to suicide prevention are in their infancy, with the vast majority providing data only on development, feasibility, and acceptability [66–73] or single-arm/open trials [74–77]. Among 6 randomized trials of app-based suicide prevention tools, only 1 suggested group differences in changes over time in nonsuicidal self-injury, suicide plans, and suicide-related behavior, though these effects were not maintained at follow-up [78]. The remaining studies reported that compared with controls, those using a suicide prevention app were not significantly different on measures of suicidal ideation or behavior [79–83].

On a positive note, these approaches—which have been developed and tested almost exclusively in academic-based settings—tend to feature empirically supported components or theories (for a thorough review and clinical guidance of apps, see [84]). For example, the Virtual Hope Box [72] is based in DBT [85] and designed to provide support, comfort, distraction, and relaxation to users through the creation of a virtual representation of the user's reasons for living (eg, reminders of life successes, positive life experiences, loved ones, and existing coping resources). CALMA [83] is also grounded in DBT approaches, whereas LifeApp'tite [79] adheres to a collaborative assessment and management of suicidality-based approach [14]. A recent text messaging study [71] used self-determination theory [86] and motivational interviewing [87], which have received more attention in the suicide literature of late [88–91]. The overwhelming majority of app-based approaches use some form of the widely used safety planning intervention (SPI) [92], a standalone intervention for increasing self-help behaviors among individuals who are unable to readily engage with mental health services. Safety plans are efficacious in reducing suicide-related behaviors [93–95] as well as increasing suicide-related coping [68,91] and treatment engagement [93,96]. Given its strong empirical support and brevity, it is no surprise that the SPI translates well to a digital approach and is widely used in app-based tools [75,97–101]. Finally, BackUp [66] and Be Safe [67] are rare among app-based approaches in that they use a combination of empirically supported approaches in 1 tool, integrating safety planning, a "hope box," crisis support linkages, local resources, scripts to help users access support, and coping skill strategies that may serve as a more robust standalone tool.

Many of the apps reported in the scientific literature, however, are not available publicly [102], do not contain a breadth of empirically supported material, and are not seamlessly integrated into clinical care. App repositories are the "Wild West," containing any conceivable content that could be attractive to someone seeking resources for suicidal ideation. In a more pragmatic review, Larsen and colleagues [36] conducted a review of "active" (ie, those that require active involvement from the user) suicide prevention apps found within the Australian Google Play and iTunes stores. The authors found 49 apps that contained at least 1 notable suicide prevention feature (eg, self-screening, safety planning, crisis support, means restriction), 49% of which were focused exclusively on suicide. Most apps (41%) were developed by academic/health care institutions or commercial organizations, while others were privately created or the source was unknown; this development share is notably higher than for bipolar disorder [103] and depression [104] apps, only 4% of which were developed by academicians or health care professionals. Only 1 suicide-specific app provided the source (eg, treatment manual) of the content being delivered, leaving questions about who developed the material and whether it stems from an evidence-based source. Among the prevention strategies used by the 24 suicide-specific apps, peer support and safety planning were the most common (67% and 54%, respectively), followed by noncrisis support (42%), crisis support/helpline (42%), and means restriction (25%); ongoing contact was the least common (4%). Most apps, unfortunately, only featured 1 evidence-based suicide prevention strategy, and none offered education on psychotherapy as an additional service option that individuals could seek.

A more recent review assessed adherence to evidence-based clinical guidelines among depression and suicide prevention apps in the Google Play and iTunes stores worldwide [105]. Among 46 suicide prevention-focused apps, 9 featured password protection, and 4 included all 6 of the empirically supported suicide prevention guidelines identified by the authors. Taken together, mobile apps are the most widespread approach to digital health options within suicide prevention, though very few involve both empirically supported content and have been subjected to robust evaluation via randomized trials. In addition, the paucity of suicide-specific approaches (and overwhelming focus on depression-related material) contained within each app limits their use as standalone interventions, which may be coveted by individuals seeking anonymity.

Data-Driven Approaches to Identification

As noted earlier, accurate identification of those at greatest risk for suicide is a crucial endeavor in suicide prevention. The most prevalent methods of identification, however, are poor [106,107], ranging from moderate sensitivity at best [108,109] to no better than chance, at worst [110]. As suicidal ideation has been found to be dynamic over time [111,112], digital technologies have the strong potential to more precisely measure that process through ecological momentary assessment (EMA) of active (eg, questionnaires) and passive (eg, Apple Health Kit, pedometers, sleep recordings, other wearables) data. Active EMA methods involve individuals responding to brief questions in real time while operating in their natural environment and during regular daily activities, thus capturing the dynamics between factors of interest with greater ecological validity.

Such methods have been useful to disentangle complex processes involved in alcohol use [113,114], polysubstance use [115,116], and depression [117]. These methods appear to be feasible within the field of suicide risk [118–120] and can be leveraged to enhance accurate identification and provide just-in-time adaptive interventions personalized to each individual, as has been done for smoking cessation [22,121,122], alcohol use [123], and other mental health issues [124–126]. A recent survey of experts in the field of suicide prevention indicated that leveraging digital technologies to more accurately understand the dynamic interplay between ideation and attempts was the top-rated exciting new development in the field [127]. Through the use of machine learning and predictive modeling, mobile devices could employ algorithms to better detect the points of highest risk for individuals, notifying them or their providers of that threat, and delivering an evidenced-based strategy (eg, safety plan, caring contacts, crisis supports) to prevent escalation to an attempt. Continued advances in identification would be welcome, as several robust risk factors appear to predict suicidal *ideation*, but not the transition from ideation to suicide attempt [128]. This approach also shows the most promise concerning NIMH's call for synergy between technology and clinical care, providing clinicians with direct information on patient safety and risk.

ADOPTION OF DIGITAL STRATEGIES

As noted previously, digital approaches to suicide prevention have the strong potential to increase reach, improve access to traditional health care, and augment existing systems of care through streamlined clinical workflows and leveraging myriad data points for predictive modeling. However, several challenges continue to prevent widespread adoption of digital suicide prevention and should be addressed.

First, clinicians have voiced concern about the role of the therapeutic alliance, comprehensive assessment, and the ability to rapidly respond to patients at risk of suicide [129]. Naturally, any risks that providers perceive with regard to digital health strategies will hold back the proliferation of these approaches. Given a constant influx of mood monitoring data, providers are naturally mindful of their patients' safety [130,131]. The COVID-19 pandemic has forced some providers into using telehealth approaches by necessity [34], possibly enhancing positive attitudes toward digital approaches, though this remains to be seen. Although at face value, Web-based and mobile-based programs may seem limited in their ability to engender the therapeutic alliance, several studies have indicated that the development of rapport and alliance with digital tools is possible [132–136]. The extent of therapeutic alliance is certainly an important area of future study, given that patients may quickly disengage with digital platforms with which they do not feel connected and engaged [137], and clinicians may not endorse such approaches if they feel uncomfortable about their ability to successfully monitor their patients over time.

Indeed, ongoing and rapid crisis intervention is also a significant challenge, as in-person risk assessment can be easily followed by protocol-driven responses to patient severity (eg, more comprehensive assessment, initiating inpatient treatment). While digital approaches to mental health intervention continue to progress by offering adaptive assessment and intervention [126], robust safety protocols are likely needed before health systems and providers are fully comfortable with automating suicide prevention. To date, the literature is limited with regard to whether and how to intervene with trained professionals once patients identify as high risk using digital platforms [138,139].

A recent review [138] has examined safety protocol strategies within suicide-related EMA studies for youth, finding that while most studies addressed safety at study onset, only half continued throughout the course of the investigation. The authors note that while preliminary data indicate no harm associated with repeated assessment of suicidal ideation and behavior in both youth and adults, this area of research is relatively new and requires further study. As such, they encourage the development and testing of robust safety protocols within EMA and other approaches that consistently require patients to self-monitor.

Safety aside, researchers have noted declines in adherence to repeated assessment over study periods [140], further impacting the implications of this approach. Another review of safety protocols in digital health solutions for suicide prevention indicated that while most studies acknowledged the use of safety protocols, few directly indicated what took place, limiting the ability of clinicians and researchers to determine what safety monitoring approaches would work best [139]. Ironically, the benefit of anonymity that is so often championed with regard to Web-based and mobile-based interventions conflicts with these goals [139]; that is, study participants are required to provide contact information to evaluate the intervention, possibly introducing selection bias into the study and limiting its external validity. However, without such assurances of safety, digital platforms are unlikely to see widespread implementation.

FUTURE DIRECTIONS

Although digital applications hold much promise in preventing suicide, most available digital interventions do not have sufficient support to be considered standalone services while also lacking integration with current health care delivery (eg, electronic health records). First, and perhaps most importantly, interventions that target suicide prevention should be designed with suicide-specific strategies and content. A sizable proportion of the research literature on digital health for suicide relies on protocols designed for depression, with few to no effects on suicide outcomes [51,56,141]. These findings mirror evidence from large trials of in-person approaches, where protocols for depression or other mental health difficulties related to depression are mostly ineffective toward changes in suicidal ideation and behavior [61,62,142]. More recent approaches (predominately digital apps) have been guided by evidence-based, suicide-specific protocols to directly target ideation and behavior, showing initial promise [74,75,78].

Second, multiple reviews indicate poor adherence to Web-based and mobile phone–based interventions. A recent review noted that nearly two-thirds of studies reported that participants completed less than 50% of the treatment modules [141], with others noting similar rates [57]. If we hope that providers will recommend these tools to patients and that health systems will implement them as regular clinical care, a stronger evidence base is needed and begins with user engagement. Indeed, researchers have noted that evidence does not yet exist to support the "prescription" of standalone digital interventions for suicide prevention [143]. Personalization, user-based design methods, machine learning algorithms, gamification, and dynamic approaches—such as just-in-time adaptive interventions—should be explored to meet the needs of specific individuals [51,141,143]. Interventions that use these attractive options would serve patients by offering a robust delivery system that could meet the goals of standalone interventions, or perhaps more powerfully, adjuncts to traditional care.

While researchers may advocate for and have experience with involving research ethics committees to improve their digital interventions for suicide prevention, a minority of the literature base has focused on the voice of those with lived experience [139], those who have had personal experience with suicidal thoughts, behavior, or have supported a loved one through a suicidal crisis. A recent review of all suicide prevention research (ie, not just digital approaches) from 2010 to 2019 produced only 11 studies that involved individuals with lived experience in developing interventions [144]. Individuals with lived experience can help identify gaps in clinical care that are not evident to practitioners, enhancing the efficacy and validity of intervention content and process [144]. Indeed, patient stakeholders—particularly youth—can develop innovative solutions that improve engagement with digital tools [130], thereby addressing the major weakness of adherence noted throughout this review.

Many current digital approaches rely on a single suicide prevention strategy rather than integrating these within a platform [36,143], leaving individuals to download multiple apps or engage with separate media to get their needs met. Given the relative ease with which digital platforms can handle multiple processes, it would appear natural for robust interventions to include crisis supports, regular self-monitoring, a safety plan, psychotherapy modules, links to peer support, and connection to treatment or emergency services, such as the National Suicide Prevention Lifeline. Relatedly, although mHealth tools can effectively deliver suicide prevention best practices, efforts have focused on technology-based services (ie, standalone interventions) rather than technology-enabled interventions. While the former select components that may be helpful in isolation (eg, safety plans), a technology-enabled approach focuses on the service being provided and how technology can enhance that service [145]. Using this strategy, researchers can take an empirically supported approach, enhance its full delivery through a rigorous mHealth conduit, and augment effects seen in standalone interventions. Such an approach would likely ease concerns noted by providers and increase the likelihood of widespread dissemination.

As noted throughout this review, the current literature base remains heterogeneous and in its infancy. Although fully powered trials will offer important insight into digital interventions for suicide prevention [146], the vast majority of studies with any signal suffer from nonrandom assignment and small sample sizes [56,57,137]. Studies also often use different outcome measures, making aggregation across the literature very challenging [143]. Among app-based approaches that have been tested against control groups, improvement on suicidal ideation or behaviors has largely not been found [79–83]. Finally, despite the widespread use of safety planning in digital approaches to care, the safety plan is a clinical process whereby listening to, empathizing with, and engaging patients is most effective for developing the safety plan and the likelihood of its use [92]. Without the guidance of a collaborator, effectiveness may be reduced.

Finally, a significant number of ethical and legal issues remain. The promise of machine learning, artificial intelligence, and advanced modeling of millions of data points to more accurately identify suicide risk and intervene to prevent suicidal behaviors is outstanding. However, with such great power comes equal levels of responsibility, both legally and ethically. While these early data models will likely engender trust due to their novelty and impressive nature, they will, ultimately, have inaccuracies. Indeed, researchers have noted their limited predictive power and therefore limited clinical utility [147–149]. Apps and other digital devices will label individuals as at risk for suicide before ever indicating intent, while others will be identified as low risk and eventually engage in self-harm. Questions about informed consent, privacy protections, and data sharing will and should be asked as the field moves forward [150]. Indeed, institution-sponsored predictive modeling through digital data collection may result in ethical questions around fair and equitable use of resources and privacy, as well as legal questions should false positives and negatives resulted in inappropriate consequences (eg, involuntary hospitalization, death after low risk categorization) [148,149].

Overall, however, there is still great promise for technology-based suicide prevention approaches. As research continues to focus on the abovementioned shortcomings, integration of standalone interventions with clinical care has strong potential to augment outcomes for patients. Indeed, the most traditional forms of treatment would involve weekly sessions for 45 to 60 minutes, whereas the remainder of the week consists of 167 other hours in which patients may need support. Synergy between digital interventions and traditional care may more rapidly reduce symptoms and improve quality of life while leaving room for the therapy hour to be more focused and efficient.

SUMMARY AND RECOMMENDATIONS FOR PRACTITIONERS

Given the wealth of digital options available to patients, providers are likely to encounter questions about the efficacy of these approaches to suicide prevention, whether from colleagues or patients themselves. In particular, clinicians are most likely to receive questions about the efficacy of mobile apps due to their overwhelming share of the digital technology market. Torous and colleagues [150] offer several important clinical considerations surrounding this burgeoning field. The authors first note that privacy is paramount and that such mobile applications should not sell private, personal data to third parties. Studies have indicated the lack of privacy statements, secure data, and requirements for a username and password on available apps [36], and without such protections, patients can be at serious risk of their data falling into the hands of those to whom they did not provide informed consent. Second, the authors suggest that providers educate patients on the overall lack of evidence in this arena. While there are very exciting possibilities ahead, the literature is very limited and new; thus, patients should not expect robust results from the use of digital technologies, especially standalone tools. Torous and colleagues add that perhaps providers should introduce these approaches as "off label," as they could provide benefit to any given individual, yet the empirical evidence has not yet accumulated for a wholesale recommendation. In addition to improved usability, they argue that app data should be shared with the clinician. It is most likely that apps and other digital technologies will meet their true potential by being informed by those with lived experience and delivered in combination with clinical expertise, which can also alleviate concerns about ongoing symptom tracking without clinical support.

CLINICS CARE POINTS

- Standalone digital interventions are likely insufficient.
- Clinicians should be aware of what data digital interventions are collecting before recommending them to patients.
- Digital interventions that serve as adjuncts to care will likely be more beneficial to patients.
- Evidence to support digital interventions for suicide preventions is in its infancy.

DISCLOSURE

The author has nothing to disclose.

REFERENCES

[1] Centers for Disease Control and Prevention. WISQARS leading causes of death reports, 1981–2016 2017. Available at: https://webappa.cdc.gov/sasweb/ncipc/leadcause.html. Accessed December 15, 2020.

[2] Crosby AE, Ortega L, Stevens MR. Suicides - United States, 1999-2007. MMWR Suppl 2011;60(Suppl):56–9.

[3] Holinger PC, Klemen EH. Violent deaths in the United States, 1900-1975. Relationships between suicide, homicide and accidental deaths. Soc Sci Med 1982;16(22):1929–38.

[4] Mann JJ, Apter A, Bertolote J, et al. Suicide prevention strategies: a systematic review. JAMA 2005;294(16):2064–74.

[5] Kessler RC, Berglund P, Borges G, et al. Trends in suicide ideation, plans, gestures, and attempts in the United States, 1990-1992 to 2001-2003. JAMA 2005;293(20):2487–95.

[6] Centers for Disease Control and Prevention. Suicide among adults aged 35-64 years - United States, 1999-2010. MMWR Morb Mortal Wkly Rep 2013;62(17):321–5.

[7] Curtin SC, Warner M, Hedegaard H. Increase in suicide in the United States, 1999–2014. Hyattsville, MD: National Center for Health Statistics, Centers for Disease Control and Prevention; 2016.

[8] U.S. Department of Health and Human Services Office of the Surgeon General and National Action Alliance for Suicide Prevention. 2012 national strategy for suicide prevention: goals and objectives for action. Washington, DC: US Department of Health and Human Services; 2012.

[9] Baumel A, Torous J, Edan S, et al. There is a non-evidence-based app for that: a systematic review and mixed methods analysis of depression-and anxiety-related apps that incorporate unrecognized techniques. J Affect Disord 2020;273:410–21.

[10] Cavanagh JT, Carson AJ, Sharpe M, et al. Psychological autopsy studies of suicide: a systematic review. Psychol Med 2003;33(3):395–405.

[11] Ahmedani BK, Simon GE, Stewart C, et al. Health care contacts in the year before suicide death. J Gen Intern Med 2014;29(6):870–7.

[12] Linehan MM, Comtois KA, Murray AM, et al. Two-year randomized controlled trial and follow-up of dialectical behavior therapy vs therapy by experts for suicidal behaviors and borderline personality disorder. Arch Gen Psychiatry 2006;63(7):757–66.

[13] Brown GK, Ten Have T, Henriques GR, et al. Cognitive therapy for the prevention of suicide attempts: a randomized controlled trial. JAMA 2005;294(5):563–70.

[14] Jobes DA. The Collaborative Assessment and Management of Suicidality (CAMS): an evolving evidence-based clinical approach to suicidal risk. Suicide Life Threat Behav 2012;42(6):640–53.

[15] National Action Alliance for Suicide Prevention Research Prioritization Task Force. A prioritized research agenda for suicide prevention: an action plan to save lives. Rockville, MD: National Institute of Mental Health and the Research Prioritization Task Force; 2014.

[16] Pringle B, Colpe LJ, Heinssen RK, et al. A strategic approach for prioritizing research and action to prevent suicide. Psychiatr Serv 2013;64(1):71–5.

[17] Ebert DD, Zarski A-C, Christensen H, et al. Internet and computer-based cognitive behavioral therapy for anxiety and depression in youth: a meta-analysis of randomized controlled outcome trials. PLoS One 2015;10(3):e0119895.

[18] Proudfoot J, Clarke J, Birch M-R, et al. Impact of a mobile phone and web program on symptom and functional outcomes for people with mild-to-moderate depression, anxiety and stress: a randomised controlled trial. BMC Psychiatry 2013;13(1):312.

[19] Richards D, Richardson T. Computer-based psychological treatments for depression: a systematic review and meta-analysis. Clin Psychol Rev 2012;32(4):329–42.

[20] Fanning J, Mullen SP, McAuley E. Increasing physical activity with mobile devices: a meta-analysis. J Med Internet Res 2012;14(6):e161.

[21] Pal K, Eastwood SV, Michie S, et al. Computer-based interventions to improve self-management in adults with type 2 diabetes: a systematic review and meta-analysis. Diabetes Care 2014;37(6):1759–66.

[22] Bock BC, Heron KE, Jennings EG, et al. A text message delivered smoking cessation intervention: the initial

trial of TXT-2-QUIT, a randomized, controlled trial. JMIR Mhealth Uhealth 2013;1(2):e17.
[23] Whittaker R, McRobbie H, Bullen C, et al. Mobile phone-based interventions for smoking cessation. Cochrane Database Syst Rev 2016;(4):CD006611.
[24] Mason M, Ola B, Zaharakis N, et al. Text messaging interventions for adolescent and young adult substance use: a meta-analysis. Prev Sci 2015;16(2):181–8.
[25] Marsch LA, Carroll KM, Kiluk BD. Technology-based interventions for the treatment and recovery management of substance use disorders: a JSAT special issue. J Subst Abuse Treat 2014;46(1):1–4.
[26] Butler SF, Villapiano A, Malinow A. The effect of computer-mediated administration on self-disclosure of problems on the Addiction Severity Index. J Addict Med 2009;3(4):194–203.
[27] Gnambs T, Kaspar K. Disclosure of sensitive behaviors across self-administered survey modes: a meta-analysis. Behav Res Methods 2015;47(4):1237–59.
[28] Newman JC, Des Jarlais DC, Turner CF, et al. The differential effects of face-to-face and computer interview modes. Am J Public Health 2002;92(2):294–7.
[29] Torous J, Staples P, Shanahan M, et al. Utilizing a personal smartphone custom app to assess the patient health questionnaire-9 (PHQ-9) depressive symptoms in patients with major depressive disorder. JMIR Ment Health 2015;2(1):e8.
[30] Mobile fact sheet. 2019. Available at: http://www.pewinternet.org/fact-sheet/mobile/. Accessed December 2, 2020.
[31] Ondersma SJ, Chase SK, Svikis DS, et al. Computer-based brief motivational intervention for perinatal drug use. J Subst Abuse Treat 2005;28(4):305–12.
[32] Ben-Zeev D, Brian RM, Jonathan G, et al. Mobile health (mHealth) versus clinic-based group intervention for people with serious mental illness: a randomized controlled trial. Psychiatr Serv 2018;69(9):978–85.
[33] Haas A, Koestner B, Rosenberg J, et al. An interactive web-based method of outreach to college students at risk for suicide. J Am Coll Health 2008;57(1):15–22.
[34] Wosik J, Fudim M, Cameron B, et al. Telehealth transformation: COVID-19 and the rise of virtual care. J Am Med Inform Assoc 2020;27(6):957–62.
[35] Telemental health survey reveals 70 percent of behavioral health providers will continue offering telehealth options post-COVID-19. Available at: https://tridiuum.com/in-the-news-telemental-health-survey-reveals-70-percent-of-behavioral-health-providers-will-continue-offering-telehealth-options-post-covid-19/. Accessed December 14, 2020.
[36] Larsen ME, Nicholas J, Christensen H. A systematic assessment of smartphone tools for suicide prevention. PLoS One 2016;11(4):e0152285.
[37] Torous J, Friedman R, Keshavan M. Smartphone ownership and interest in mobile applications to monitor symptoms of mental health conditions. JMIR Mhealth Uhealth 2014;2(1):e2.
[38] Wilks CR, Coyle TN, Krek M, et al. Suicide ideation and acceptability toward online help-seeking. Suicide Life Threat Behav 2018;48(4):379–85.
[39] Bruffaerts R, Demyttenaere K, Hwang I, et al. Treatment of suicidal people around the world. Br J Psychiatry 2011;199(1):64–70.
[40] Michelmore L, Hindley P. Help-seeking for suicidal thoughts and self-harm in young people: a systematic review. Suicide Life Threat Behav 2012;42(5):507–24.
[41] Washington State Department of Health. Washington state suicide prevention plan. Olympia (WA): Author; 2016.
[42] Suicide Prevention Resource Center. Safety plan mobile app. Available at: https://zerosuicide.edc.org/resources/safety-plan-mobile-app. Accessed May 23, 2020.
[43] Garlow SJ, Rosenberg J, Moore JD, et al. Depression, desperation, and suicidal ideation in college students: results from the American Foundation for Suicide Prevention College Screening Project at Emory University. Depress Anxiety 2008;25(6):482–8.
[44] Fein JA, Pailler ME, Barg FK, et al. Feasibility and effects of a Web-based adolescent psychiatric assessment administered by clinical staff in the pediatric emergency department. Arch Pediatr Adolesc Med 2010;164(12):1112–7.
[45] Gadomski AM, Fothergill KE, Larson S, et al. Integrating mental health into adolescent annual visits: impact of previsit comprehensive screening on within-visit processes. J Adolesc Health 2015;56(3):267–73.
[46] Lawrence ST, Willig JH, Crane HM, et al. Routine, self-administered, touch-screen, computer-based suicidal ideation assessment linked to automated response team notification in an HIV primary care setting. Clin Infect Dis 2010;50(8):1165–73.
[47] Moutier C, Norcross W, Jong P, et al. The suicide prevention and depression awareness program at the University of California, San Diego School of Medicine. Acad Med 2012;87(3):320–6.
[48] Boudreaux ED, Horowitz LM. Suicide risk screening and assessment: designing instruments with dissemination in mind. Am J Prev Med 2014;47(3):S163–9.
[49] Simon GE, Johnson E, Lawrence JM, et al. Predicting suicide attempts and suicide deaths following outpatient visits using electronic health records. Am J Psychiatry 2018;175(10):951–60.
[50] Kessler RC, Warner CH, Ivany C, et al. Predicting suicides after psychiatric hospitalization in US Army soldiers: the Army Study to Assess Risk and Resilience in Servicemembers (Army STARRS). JAMA Psychiatry 2015;72(1):49–57.
[51] Büscher R, Torok M, Terhorst Y, et al. Internet-based cognitive behavioral therapy to reduce suicidal ideation: a systematic review and meta-analysis. JAMA Netw Open 2020;3(4):e203933.
[52] Hetrick SE, Yuen HP, Bailey E, et al. Internet-based cognitive behavioural therapy for young people with suicide-

related behaviour (Reframe-IT): a randomised controlled trial. Evid Based Ment Health 2017;20(3):76–82.
[53] Van Spijker BA, Werner-Seidler A, Batterham PJ, et al. Effectiveness of a web-based self-help program for suicidal thinking in an Australian community sample: randomized controlled trial. J Med Internet Res 2018;20(2):e15.
[54] Lai MH, Maniam T, Chan LF, et al. Caught in the web: a review of web-based suicide prevention. J Med Internet Res 2014;16(1):e30.
[55] Perry Y, Werner-Seidler A, Calear AL, et al. Web-based and mobile suicide prevention interventions for young people: a systematic review. J Can Acad Child Adolesc Psychiatry 2016;25(2):73.
[56] Christensen H, Batterham PJ, O'Dea B. E-health interventions for suicide prevention. Int J Environ Res Public Health 2014;11(8):8193–212.
[57] Witt K, Spittal MJ, Carter G, et al. Effectiveness of online and mobile telephone applications ('apps') for the self-management of suicidal ideation and self-harm: a systematic review and meta-analysis. BMC Psychiatry 2017;17(1):297.
[58] Leavey K, Hawkins R. Is cognitive behavioural therapy effective in reducing suicidal ideation and behaviour when delivered face-to-face or via e-health? A systematic review and meta-analysis. Cogn Behav Ther 2017; 46(5):353–74.
[59] Christensen H, Farrer L, Batterham PJ, et al. The effect of a web-based depression intervention on suicide ideation: secondary outcome from a randomised controlled trial in a helpline. BMJ Open 2013;3(6):e002886.
[60] Moritz S, Schilling L, Hauschildt M, et al. A randomized controlled trial of internet-based therapy in depression. Behav Res Ther 2012;50(7–8):513–21.
[61] Meerwijk EL, Parekh A, Oquendo MA, et al. Direct versus indirect psychosocial and behavioural interventions to prevent suicide and suicide attempts: a systematic review and meta-analysis. Lancet Psychiatry 2016; 3(6):544–54.
[62] Cuijpers P, de Beurs DP, van Spijker BA, et al. The effects of psychotherapy for adult depression on suicidality and hopelessness: a systematic review and meta-analysis. J Affect Disord 2013;144(3):183–90.
[63] The smartphone difference. Available at: http://www.pewinternet.org/2015/04/01/us-smartphone-use-in-2015/. Accessed December 8, 2020.
[64] Smartphones help blacks, Hispanics bridge some – but not all – digital gaps with whites. Available at: https://www.pewresearch.org/fact-tank/2019/08/20/smartphones-help-blacks-hispanics-bridge-some-but-not-all-digital-gaps-with-whites/. Accessed December 8, 2020.
[65] Torous J, Roberts LW. Needed innovation in digital health and smartphone applications for mental health: transparency and trust. JAMA Psychiatry 2017;74(5):437–8.
[66] Pauwels K, Aerts S, Muijzers E, et al. BackUp: Development and evaluation of a smart-phone application for coping with suicidal crises. PLoS One 2017;12(6): e0178144.
[67] Gregory JM, Sukhera J, Taylor-Gates M. Integrating smartphone technology at the time of discharge from a child and adolescent inpatient psychiatry unit. J Can Acad Child Adolesc Psychiatry 2017;26(1):45.
[68] Melvin GA, Gresham D, Beaton S, et al. Evaluating the feasibility and effectiveness of an Australian safety planning smartphone application: a pilot study within a tertiary mental health service. Suicide Life Threat Behav 2019;49(3):846–58.
[69] Muscara F, Ng O, Crossley L, et al. The feasibility of using smartphone apps to manage self-harm and suicidal acts in adolescents admitted to an inpatient mental health ward. Digital Health 2020;6:2055207620975315.
[70] Grist R, Porter J, Stallard P. Acceptability, use, and safety of a mobile phone app (BlueIce) for young people who self-harm: qualitative study of service users' experience. JMIR Ment Health 2018;5(1):e16.
[71] Czyz EK, Arango A, Healy N, et al. Augmenting safety planning with text messaging support for adolescents at elevated suicide risk: development and acceptability study. JMIR Ment Health 2020;7(5):e17345.
[72] Bush NE, Dobscha SK, Crumpton R, et al. A virtual hope box smartphone app as an accessory to therapy: proof-of-concept in a clinical sample of veterans. Suicide Life Threat Behav 2015;45(1):1–9.
[73] O'Brien KHM, Wyman Battalen A, Sellers CM, et al. An mHealth approach to extend a brief intervention for adolescent alcohol use and suicidal behavior: qualitative analyses of adolescent and parent feedback. J Technol Hum Serv 2019;37(4):255–85.
[74] Stallard P, Porter J, Grist R. A smartphone app (BlueIce) for young people who self-harm: open phase 1 pre-post trial. JMIR Mhealth Uhealth 2018;6(1):e32.
[75] Boudreaux ED, Brown GK, Stanley B, et al. Computer administered safety planning for individuals at risk for suicide: development and usability testing. J Med Internet Res 2017;19(5):e149.
[76] Dickter B, Bunge EL, Brown LM, et al. Impact of an online depression prevention intervention on suicide risk factors for adolescents and young adults. Mhealth 2019; 5:11.
[77] Rizvi SL, Hughes CD, Thomas MC. The DBT Coach mobile application as an adjunct to treatment for suicidal and self-injuring individuals with borderline personality disorder: a preliminary evaluation and challenges to client utilization. Psychol Serv 2016; 13(4):380.
[78] Franklin JC, Fox KR, Franklin CR, et al. A brief mobile app reduces nonsuicidal and suicidal self-injury: evidence from three randomized controlled trials. J Consult Clin Psychol 2016;84(6):544.
[79] O'Toole MS, Arendt MB, Pedersen CM. Testing an app-assisted treatment for suicide prevention in a randomized controlled trial: effects on suicide risk and depression. Behav Ther 2019;50(2):421–9.
[80] Kennard BD, Goldstein T, Foxwell AA, et al. As Safe as Possible (ASAP): a brief app-supported inpatient

intervention to prevent postdischarge suicidal behavior in hospitalized, suicidal adolescents. Am J Psychiatry 2018;175(9):864–72.

[81] Tighe J, Shand F, Ridani R, et al. Ibobbly mobile health intervention for suicide prevention in Australian Indigenous youth: a pilot randomised controlled trial. BMJ Open 2017;7(1):e013518.

[82] Bush NE, Smolenski DJ, Denneson LM, et al. A virtual hope box: randomized controlled trial of a smartphone app for emotional regulation and coping with distress. Psychiatr Serv 2017;68(4):330–6.

[83] Rodante DE, Kaplan MI, Olivera Fedi R, et al. CALMA, a mobile health application, as an accessory to therapy for reduction of suicidal and non-suicidal self-injured behaviors: a pilot cluster randomized controlled trial. Arch Suicide Res 2020;1–18.

[84] Luxton DD, June JD, Chalker SA. Mobile health technologies for suicide prevention: feature review and recommendations for use in clinical care. Curr Treat Options Psychiatry 2015;2(4):349–62.

[85] Linehan MM. Dialectical behavior therapy for borderline personality disorder: theory and method. Bull Menninger Clin 1987;51(3):261.

[86] Deci EL, Ryan RM. Overview of self-determination theory: an organismic dialectical perspective. Handbook of self-determination research. 2002. p. 3–33.

[87] Miller WR, Rollnick S, editors. Motivational interviewing: helping people change. New York: The Guilford Press; 2013.

[88] Britton PC, Conner KR, Chapman BP, et al. Motivational interviewing to address suicidal ideation: a randomized controlled trial in veterans. Suicide Life Threat Behav 2020;50(1):233–48.

[89] Britton PC, Patrick H, Wenzel A, et al. Integrating motivational interviewing and self-determination theory with cognitive behavioral therapy to prevent suicide. Cogn Behav Pract 2011;18(1):16–27.

[90] Britton PC, Williams GC, Conner KR. Self-determination theory, motivational interviewing, and the treatment of clients with acute suicidal ideation. J Clin Psychol 2008;64(1):52–66.

[91] Czyz E, King C, Biermann B. Motivational interviewing-enhanced safety planning for adolescents at high suicide risk: a pilot randomized controlled trial. J Clin Child Adolesc Psychol 2019;48(2):250–62.

[92] Stanley B, Brown GK. Safety planning intervention: a brief intervention to mitigate suicide risk. Cogn Behav Pract 2012;19(2):256–64.

[93] Stanley B, Brown GK, Brenner LA, et al. Comparison of the safety planning intervention with follow-up vs usual care of suicidal patients treated in the emergency department. JAMA Psychiatry 2018;75(9):894–900.

[94] Bryan CJ, Mintz J, Clemans TA, et al. Effect of crisis response planning vs. contracts for safety on suicide risk in US Army soldiers: a randomized clinical trial. J Affect Disord 2017;212:64–72.

[95] Brodsky BS, Spruch-Feiner A, Stanley B. The Zero suicide Model: applying evidence-based suicide prevention practices to clinical care. Front Psychiatry 2018;9:33.

[96] Stanley B, Brown GK, Currier GW, et al. Brief intervention and follow-up for suicidal patients with repeat emergency department visits enhances treatment engagement. Am J Public Health 2015;105(8):1570–2.

[97] Hill RM, Dodd CG, Gomez M, et al. The safety planning assistant: feasibility and acceptability of a web-based suicide safety planning tool for at-risk adolescents and their parents. Evidence-based practice in child and adolescent mental health. 2020:5(2);1-9

[98] Nuij C, van Ballegooijen W, Ruwaard J, et al. Smartphone-based safety planning and self-monitoring for suicidal patients: rationale and study protocol of the CASPAR (Continuous Assessment for Suicide Prevention And Research) study. Internet Interv 2018;13:16–23.

[99] O'Grady C, Melia R, Bogue J, et al. A mobile health approach for improving outcomes in suicide prevention (SafePlan). J Med Internet Res 2020;22(7):e17481.

[100] Larsen JLS, Frandsen H, Erlangsen A. MYPLAN–A mobile phone application for supporting people at risk of suicide. Crisis 2016;37(3):236–40.

[101] Spangler DA, Muñoz RF, Chu J, et al. Perceived utility of the Internet-based safety plan in a sample of internet users screening positive for suicidality. Crisis 2019; 41(2):146–9.

[102] Donker T, Petrie K, Proudfoot J, et al. Smartphones for smarter delivery of mental health programs: a systematic review. J Med Internet Res 2013;15(11):e247.

[103] Nicholas J, Larsen ME, Proudfoot J, et al. Mobile apps for bipolar disorder: a systematic review of features and content quality. J Med Internet Res 2015;17(8):e198.

[104] Shen N, Levitan M-J, Johnson A, et al. Finding a depression app: a review and content analysis of the depression app marketplace. JMIR Mhealth Uhealth 2015; 3(1):e16.

[105] Martinengo L, Van Galen L, Lum E, et al. Suicide prevention and depression apps' suicide risk assessment and management: a systematic assessment of adherence to clinical guidelines. BMC Med 2019;17(1):1–12.

[106] O'Connor RC, Nock MK. The psychology of suicidal behaviour. Lancet Psychiatry 2014;1(1):73–85.

[107] De Beurs D, Kirtley O, Kerkhof A, Portzky G, O'Connor RC. The role of mobile phone technology in understanding and preventing suicidal behavior. *Crisis* 2015;36(2):79–82.

[108] Simon GE, Coleman KJ, Rossom RC, et al. Risk of suicide attempt and suicide death following completion of the Patient Health Questionnaire depression module in community practice. J Clin Psychiatry 2016;77(2):221.

[109] Louzon SA, Bossarte R, McCarthy JF, et al. Does suicidal ideation as measured by the PHQ-9 predict suicide among VA patients? Psychiatr Serv 2016;67(5):517–22.

[110] Franklin JC, Ribeiro JD, Fox KR, et al. Risk factors for suicidal thoughts and behaviors: a meta-analysis of 50 years of research. Psychol Bull 2017;143(2):187.

[111] Joiner TE Jr, Rudd MD. Intensity and duration of suicidal crises vary as a function of previous suicide attempts and negative life events. J Consult Clin Psychol 2000;68(5):909.
[112] Zisook S, Trivedi MH, Warden D, et al. Clinical correlates of the worsening or emergence of suicidal ideation during SSRI treatment of depression: an examination of citalopram in the STAR* D study. J Affect Disord 2009; 117(1–2):63–73.
[113] Merrill JE, Boyle HK, Jackson KM, et al. Event-level correlates of drinking events characterized by alcohol-induced blackouts. Alcohol Clin Exp Res 2019;43(12): 2599–606.
[114] Wray TB, Merrill JE, Monti PM. Using ecological momentary assessment (EMA) to assess situation-level predictors of alcohol use and alcohol-related consequences. Alcohol Res Curr Rev 2014;36(1):19.
[115] Shiffman S. Ecological momentary assessment (EMA) in studies of substance use. Psychol Assess 2009; 21(4):486.
[116] Sokolovsky AW, Gunn RL, Micalizzi L, et al. Alcohol and marijuana co-use: consequences, subjective intoxication, and the operationalization of simultaneous use. Drug Alcohol Depend 2020;212:107986.
[117] Armey MF, Schatten HT, Haradhvala N, et al. Ecological momentary assessment (EMA) of depression-related phenomena. Curr Opin Psychol 2015;4:21–5.
[118] Husky M, Olié E, Guillaume S, et al. Feasibility and validity of ecological momentary assessment in the investigation of suicide risk. Psychiatry Res 2014;220(1–2): 564–70.
[119] Kleiman EM, Turner BJ, Fedor S, et al. Examination of real-time fluctuations in suicidal ideation and its risk factors: results from two ecological momentary assessment studies. J Abnorm Psychol 2017; 126(6):726.
[120] Haines A, Chahal G, Bruen AJ, et al. Testing out suicide risk prediction algorithms using phone measurements with patients in acute mental health settings: a feasibility study. JMIR Mhealth Uhealth 2020;8(6):e15901.
[121] Rodgers A, Corbett T, Bramley D, et al. Do u smoke after txt? Results of a randomised trial of smoking cessation using mobile phone text messaging. Tob Control 2005;14(4):255–61.
[122] Businelle MS, Ma P, Kendzor DE, et al. An ecological momentary intervention for smoking cessation: evaluation of feasibility and effectiveness. J Med Internet Res 2016;18(12):e321.
[123] Wright C, Dietze PM, Agius PA, et al. Mobile phone-based ecological momentary intervention to reduce young adults' alcohol use in the event: a three-armed randomized controlled trial. JMIR Mhealth Uhealth 2018;6(7):e149.
[124] Newman MG, Przeworski A, Consoli AJ, et al. A randomized controlled trial of ecological momentary intervention plus brief group therapy for generalized anxiety disorder. Psychotherapy 2014;51(2):198.
[125] Depp CA, Ceglowski J, Wang VC, et al. Augmenting psychoeducation with a mobile intervention for bipolar disorder: a randomized controlled trial. J Affect Disord 2015;174:23–30.
[126] Myin-Germeys I, Klippel A, Steinhart H, et al. Ecological momentary interventions in psychiatry. Curr Opin Psychiatry 2016;29(4):258–63.
[127] O'Connor RC, Portzky G. Looking to the future: a synthesis of new developments and challenges in suicide research and prevention. Front Psychol 2018;9:2139.
[128] Nock MK, Kessler RC, Franklin JC. Risk factors for suicide ideation differ from those for the transition to suicide attempt: the importance of creativity, rigor, and urgency in suicide research. Clin Psychol Sci Pract 2016;23(1):31–4.
[129] Gilmore AK, Ward-Ciesielski EF. Perceived risks and use of psychotherapy via telemedicine for patients at risk for suicide. J Telemed Telecare 2019;25(1):59–63.
[130] Hetrick SE, Robinson J, Burge E, et al. Youth codesign of a mobile phone app to facilitate self-monitoring and management of mood symptoms in young people with major depression, suicidal ideation, and self-harm. JMIR Ment Health 2018;5(1):e9.
[131] Sundram F, Hawken SJ, Stasiak K, et al. Tips and traps: lessons from codesigning a clinician e-monitoring tool for computerized cognitive behavioral therapy. JMIR Ment Health 2017;4(1):e3.
[132] Loree AM, Yonkers KA, Ondersma SJ, et al. Comparing satisfaction, alliance and intervention components in electronically delivered and in-person brief interventions for substance use among childbearing-aged women. J Subst Abuse Treat 2019;99:1–7.
[133] Ondersma SJ, Martin J, Fortson B, et al. Technology to augment early home visitation for child maltreatment prevention: a pragmatic randomized trial. Child Maltreat 2017;22(4):334–43.
[134] Braciszewski JM, Tzilos Wernette GK, Moore RS, et al. A pilot randomized controlled trial of a technology-based substance use intervention for youth exiting foster care. Child Youth Serv Rev 2018;94:466–76.
[135] Braciszewski JM, Tran TB, Moore RS, et al. Feeling heard and not judged: Perspectives on substance use services among youth formerly in foster care. Child Maltreat 2018;23(1):85–95.
[136] Braciszewski JM, Tzilos Wernette GK, Moore RS, et al. Developing a tailored substance use intervention for youth exiting foster care. Child Abuse Neglect 2018;77:211–21.
[137] Arshad U, Gauntlett J, Husain N, et al. A systematic review of the evidence supporting mobile-and internet-based psychological interventions for self-harm. Suicide Life Threat Behav 2020;50(1):151–79.
[138] Bai S, Babeva KN, Kim MI, et al. Future directions for optimizing clinical science & safety: ecological momentary assessments in suicide/self-harm research. J Clin Child Adolesc Psychol 2020;50(1):141–53.
[139] Bailey E, Mühlmann C, Rice S, et al. Ethical issues and practical barriers in internet-based suicide prevention

research: a review and investigator survey. BMC Med Ethics 2020;21:1–16.
[140] Czyz EK, King CA, Nahum-Shani I. Ecological assessment of daily suicidal thoughts and attempts among suicidal teens after psychiatric hospitalization: lessons about feasibility and acceptability. Psychiatry Res 2018;267:566–74.
[141] Torok M, Han J, Baker S, et al. Suicide prevention using self-guided digital interventions: a systematic review and meta-analysis of randomised controlled trials. Lancet Digital Health 2020;2(1):e25–36.
[142] Mewton L, Andrews G. Cognitive behavioral therapy for suicidal behaviors: improving patient outcomes. Psychol Res Behav Manag 2016;9:21.
[143] Melia R, Francis K, Hickey E, et al. Mobile health technology interventions for suicide prevention: systematic review. JMIR Mhealth Uhealth 2020;8(1):e12516.
[144] Watling D, Preece M, Hawgood J, et al. Developing an intervention for suicide prevention: a rapid review of lived experience involvement. Arch Suicide Res 2020;1–16.
[145] National Institute of Mental Health. Opportunities and challenges of developing information technologies on behavioral and social science clinical research 2017 Bethesda, MD.
[146] Simon GE, Beck A, Rossom R, et al. Population-based outreach versus care as usual to prevent suicide attempt: study protocol for a randomized controlled trial. Trials 2016;17(1):452.
[147] Kessler RC, Bossarte RM, Luedtke A, et al. Suicide prediction models: a critical review of recent research with recommendations for the way forward. Mol Psychiatry 2020;25(1):168–79.
[148] Berman AL, Carter G. Technological advances and the future of suicide prevention: ethical, legal, and empirical challenges. Suicide Life Threat Behav 2020;50(3):643–51.
[149] Berman AL, Silverman MM. Hospital-based suicides: challenging existing myths. Psychiatr Q 2020;1–13.
[150] Torous J, Larsen ME, Depp C, et al. Smartphones, sensors, and machine learning to advance real-time prediction and interventions for suicide prevention: a review of current progress and next steps. Curr Psychiatry Rep 2018;20(7):51.

Advances in Psychiatry and Behavioral Health 1 (2021) 67–76

ADVANCES IN PSYCHIATRY AND BEHAVIORAL HEALTH

Identifying People at Risk for Suicide

Implementation of Screening for the Zero Suicide Initiative in Large Health Systems

Karen J. Coleman, PhD[a,*], Christine C. Stewart, PhD[b], Cambria Bruschke, MSW[c], Jean P. Flores, DrPH[c], Andrea Altschuler, PhD[d], Arne Beck, PhD[e], Frances L. Lynch, PhD, MSPH[f], Ashli A. Owen-Smith, PhD, SM[g], Julie E. Richards, PhD, MPH[b], Rebecca Rossom, MD, MS[h], Gregory E. Simon, MD, MPH[b], Stacy Sterling, DrPH, MSW[d], Brian K. Ahmedani, PhD, LCSW[i]

[a]Department of Research and Evaluation, Kaiser Permanente Southern California, 100 South Los Robles, Pasadena, CA 91101, USA; [b]Kaiser Permanente Washington Health Research Institute, 1730 Minor Suite 1600, Seattle, WA 98101, USA; [c]Care Management Institute, Kaiser Permanente, 1 Kaiser Plaza, 16th Floor, Oakland, CA 94612, USA; [d]Kaiser Permanente Division of Research, Kaiser Permanente Northern California, 2000 Broadway, Oakland, CA 94612, USA; [e]Institute for Health Research, Kaiser Permanente Colorado, 2550 South Parker Road, Aurora, CO 80014-8066, USA; [f]Center for Health Research Kaiser Permanente Northwest, 3800 North Interstate Avenue, Portland, OR 97227, USA; [g]School of Public Health, Georgia State University, 140 Decatur Street Office #434, Atlanta, GA 30303, USA; [h]HealthPartners Institute, 8170 33rd Ave S, MS21112R, Minneapolis, MN 55425, USA; [i]Center for Health Policy & Health Services Research, Henry Ford Health System, 1 Ford Place, Suite 3A, Detroit, MI 48202, USA

KEYWORDS

• Learning healthcare system • Electronic medical records • Zero suicide framework • Suicidal ideation

KEY POINTS

The following six actions are recommended to implement wide-scale screening for suicide risk:

- *Health System "Buy-In".* Align screening for suicide risk with efforts clinical systems have already made in obtaining patient-reported outcomes to assist executive leadership achieve goals in which they are already invested.
- *Cross-Disciplinary Collaboration.* Assemble key decision-makers in a workgroup that is coordinated by staff dedicated to the initiative.
- *Evidence-Based Screening Tools.* Use validated instruments recommended by the Joint Commission.
- *Electronic Health Record–Embedded Clinical Tools.* Automate any screening algorithm and collection of patient-reported outcomes using discrete, abstractable structured formats (eg, questionnaires, flowsheets, and so forth) that can be easily assembled for reporting and quality improvement.
- *Well-Defined Clinical Workflows.* Define clear workflows that outline who is responsible for what aspects of the screening, depending on the algorithms developed and data obtained from the electronic health record–embedded clinical tools.
- *Performance Feedback.* Create and maintain a regular set of metrics with benchmarks for screening from the electronic health record–embedded clinical tools that can be distributed to all clinical partners involved in the work.

Funding: This work was funded by award number #U01MH114087 from the National Institute of Mental Health.

*Corresponding author. Department of Research and Evaluation, Kaiser Permanente Southern California, 100 South Los Robles, Pasadena, CA 91101. *E-mail address:* Karen.J.Coleman@kp.org

https://doi.org/10.1016/j.ypsc.2021.05.016
2667-3827/21/

INTRODUCTION

A recent report from the National Center for Health Statistics at the Centers for Disease Control and Prevention found that death from suicide increased by 35% across U.S. populations from 1999 to 2018 [1]. It is estimated that for every suicide death, there are 25 attempts [2], suggesting multiple opportunities for prevention. Increasing suicide rates have prompted many national organizations to improve identification and intervention strategies for those at highest risk. For example, the Joint Commission released an official National Patient Safety Goal on suicide prevention to be implemented in all hospital settings by July 2020 [3]. In response to multiple agency recommendations regarding suicide prevention, the Suicide Prevention Resource Center was created to address suicide prevention throughout the U.S. [4]. As part of their efforts, in partnership with other collaborating national advocacy groups, they created the Zero Suicide Framework specific to health care settings [5].

The Zero Suicide Framework is a flexible set of evidence-based clinical practices and implementation strategies encompassing seven domains (lead, train, identify, engage, treat, transition, and improve) that are designed to mitigate suicide risk, enhance protective factors, and close gaps in health care that leave at-risk patients vulnerable [5]. The domains are meant to be used as needed, depending on the resources of any one health care system, and are designed as a set of recommendations to improve the quality of suicide-prevention efforts. One of the key clinical practices of this framework is "identify" which includes two components: screening for suicidal ideation and assessment of suicide risk including intent and plans. Without identifying those at risk for suicide, there is no opportunity to enact the clinical practices of the framework: engage, treat, and transition.

Unfortunately, with few exceptions, screening for mental health conditions in general, including suicidal ideation, is not a standard part of care in U.S. health settings. Screening rates for depression in U.S. primary care settings are universally low, less than 5% of patients, generally [6,7], and rates of systematic screening specifically for suicide are even lower. A few health systems, most notably the Veteran's Health Administration (VHA), the Department of Defense, and Henry Ford Health System (HFHS), have implemented robust and systematic suicide-screening and risk-assessment programs [8–12]. As a result, the VHA has achieved a suicide risk screening rate of 94.5% [9], and the U.S. Air Force significantly reduced suicide rates among its members [10]. The "perfect depression care" program at HFHS [11,12] has resulted in some of the lowest rates of suicide in the nation and has been used as a model program for the Zero Suicide Framework.

Identifying people at risk for suicide depends in part on having measures and methods that are accurate determinants of risk. Clinical leaders are often concerned that asking about suicidal ideation will require significant resources. One approach to address this concern is to use a staged screening and risk-assessment approach as recommended for the identify domain of the Zero Suicide Framework. The first stage screens for suicidal ideation, and the second stage determines the level to which the risk is imminent by assessing intent and plans [5]. This staged approach helps to deploy resources to accurately match level of risk with the appropriate evidence-based approach [13].

The first stage can be carried out with specialized screening instruments such as The Ask Suicide-Screening Questions [14]; however most large health care systems are already using tools for depression screening/symptom severity assessment, such as the Patient Health Questionnaire (PHQ9) [15,16] which includes a single question asking about the frequency in the last 2 weeks of a patient having "thoughts that you would be better off dead, or of hurting yourself in some way." In this way, health care systems can meet their national quality metrics for depression screening and care [17] while also identifying patients at risk for suicide. The second stage entails assessing suicide risk severity and intent so that appropriate treatment plans can be enacted. For this stage, the Joint Commission [3] has recommended many processes and measures including the Columbia-Suicide Severity Rating Scale (C-SSRS) [18]. A recent study from Sweden found that using the C-SSRS in emergency departments was a strong predictor of death from suicide especially soon after the visit [19].

In addition to considering the characteristics of and the evidence base for screening and assessment tools, the feasibility of administration and the potential to integrate tools into the current workflows of health care systems are critical to address. One important consideration is how broadly to screen [4,20,21]. Some health care systems take a broad approach and screen everyone in a population regardless of known risk. For example, the U.S. quality metrics for depression screening and care [17] have a universal requirement for annual screening of all patients 12 years and older, and many systems are using the PHQ9 to meet this requirement. Because it can be difficult to get "buy-in" to screen broadly for suicide risk (especially initially), many systems choose to begin with selective screening of groups known to be at higher risk. For instance, they may screen all persons with a depression diagnosis because that is a group known to have higher suicide rate than those without this diagnosis [1]. This approach is consistent with the minimum requirement from the Joint Commission's mandate for screening and assessment [3].

A second major feasibility consideration is the setting in which screening will occur [20,21]. Most experts recommend screening in specialty behavioral health care where a more extensive process can be used to both screen and assess level of risk [3]. This approach is likely to screen those most at risk and comprehensively address both elements of the identify clinical practice of the Zero Suicide Framework. Unfortunately, it is also likely to miss patients because many people who die by suicide are not receiving specialty mental health care at that time or have not been diagnosed with any mental health conditions [22,23]. For this reason, other settings have been proposed for suicide screening such as the emergency department, hospitals, and primary care [3,19]. However, these settings have a number of barriers to screening for mental health conditions and suicide risk including providers who are not well trained or comfortable managing patients with suicide risk and the time and resources it takes to do the work.

The present study presents the rationale and results for the implementation of the screening clinical practice in the identify domain of the Zero Suicide Framework over a period of 2 to 8 years in five regions of a large integrated health care system, serving over 10 million members. Screening involved a two-stage approach with the PHQ9 and the C-SSRS and used a learning health care system partnership which paired clinical leadership with embedded research scientists to work toward the long-term goal of "zero suicides" [24]. These findings can be used as a road map for other large U.S. health care systems that initiate population-based screening for suicide risk.

METHODS

Study Design

The evaluation of the screening clinical practice in the identify domain of the Zero Suicide Framework was designed as a retrospective observational study of a natural experiment implemented over a period of 2 to 8 years in five regions of a large integrated health care system. Data were obtained passively in each quarter of each year of implementation. The implementation and evaluation of the Zero Suicide Framework in these health care settings was also designed *a priori* as a partnership between clinical leadership and embedded research scientists [24].

Settings and Population

Kaiser Permanente (KP) is a large, integrated health care delivery system, composed of eight health care service regions across the U.S., which provides care and insurance and oversees hospitals and medical offices for a defined membership population. Many national clinical initiatives implemented across KP regions are supported by the Care Management Institute [25] which resides in the KP Program Office, located in Oakland, CA. These national clinical initiatives often begin with the assembly of operational leaders and research scientists from each KP region to represent a topic area (eg, suicide risk screening). These leaders are responsible for enacting the goals of the initiative in their respective regions.

Five regions of KP were included in the present study across four states: Washington, Oregon, California, and Colorado. To describe the systems in which screening was implemented, patients with continuous membership in these regions in 2019 were included ($n = 9,948,080$). All regions were participating in the Mental Health Research Network (MHRN), a nationwide consortium of public-domain research centers based in large, not-for-profit health care systems in the U.S. [26]. The institutional review boards for human subjects in each region approved all study procedures. Informed consent was not required because of the retrospective nature and minimal risks of the study.

Zero Suicide Care Improvements

Implementation of the Zero Suicide Framework at KP, led by the Care Management Institute, first began in 2014 and then gained traction in 2016. Many KP regions had already been screening for suicidal ideation; however, there was not a systematic way to track this work in the electronic health record, and it was not governed by a unified approach to address the Zero Suicide Framework. Traction came with a growing awareness of the Zero Suicide Framework and an interest in the significant outcomes in reducing suicide mortality demonstrated by other organizations in the health care industry [9–12].

One of these organizations, HFHS, was asked to partner with the Care Management Institute to guide the implementation of the Zero Suicide Framework across KP regions. In addition to the guidance from HFHS, one KP region began assessing risk for suicide using the C-SSRS and recording it in a discrete structured format in the electronic health record during the second quarter (Q2) 2012, serving as an early adoption mentor for the other regions who followed in 2017 and 2018. To provide a coordinated approach to implementation, an interregional Suicide Prevention Learning Collaborative workgroup was formed which included mental health leaders and champions from each KP region, risk management and patient safety partners, researchers, key external collaborators and field experts such as HFHS, and KP members with lived experience of suicide themselves or in family members.

A two-step screening process, informed by research generated by the MHRN [15,16,22–24] and the Joint Commission recommendations [3], was adopted to identify individuals at risk of suicide attempt. Initially the 9th question from the PHQ9 was completed and then was followed by the C-SSRS. In addition, it was decided that the initiative would target behavioral health and addiction medicine providers because of the expertise in these departments for assessing the level of risk and to provide safety and treatment planning. The PHQ9 and C-SSRS were used starting at 10 years of age given that suicidal ideation could not be reliably detected with commonly available instruments in younger children [27]. The screening practices for children and adolescents also included other measures such as the PHQ for adolescents (PHQA) and the Patient-Reported Outcomes Measurement Information System measures [28] for depression followed by the C-SSRS, and in some cases, a single-step C-SSRS was implemented.

The actual workflows used to administer the PHQ9 and subsequent C-SSRS varied across KP regions. For the most part, mental health specialty providers were already using the PHQ9 to assess depression symptoms, including suicidal ideation because of the national quality metrics for depression screening and care [17]. However, only one region systematically used the C-SSRS to conduct the second screening for suicide risk severity before implementation of the Zero Suicide Framework. In order to facilitate the systematic use of the C-SSRS, the Care Management Institute facilitated the creation of an Epic Systems Corporation (EPIC)-based electronic health record version of the C-SSRS so that all regions could capture this risk information discretely in a structured format for monitoring and quality improvement. The Care Management Institute also developed a standard training for staff on the background and administration of the C-SSRS to increase comfort level with the tool.

Systematic measurement of the efforts to identify patients at risk for suicide was critical to the success of adopting the Zero Suicide Framework. The Care Management Institute worked with the operational leadership and research scientists in each KP region to create a standardized set of metrics and processes to support cross-regional implementation of screening practices. The processes for obtaining and standardizing the data were based on the work previously carried out by research scientists who were part of the KP regional implementation teams [22–24]. A formal agreement was created among the KP regions participating in the Zero Suicide Framework that stipulated what data would be abstracted, how and when they would be processed and shared with the Care Management Institute, in what format they would be shared, and with which stakeholders. Funding for the measurement process was provided by the National Institutes of Mental Health, the Care Management Institute, and the local KP regions.

Data and Sources for Evaluation

All screening and membership data were abstracted from electronic health record sources and other secure databases used to collect patient-reported outcomes in the departments of psychiatry and addiction medicine. Specifically, all responses to the PHQ9 and C-SSRS were obtained between April 01, 2012, and October 31, 2019, and demographics including age, gender, race/ethnicity, insurance status, and neighborhood census-tract-derived education were used from 2019. These data are organized in a virtual data warehouse for all systems to facilitate population-based research [29]. Protected health information remains at each health care system, but sites apply common data definitions and formats to ensure equivalent deidentified data for analysis. Only frequencies are shared between institutions for analyses.

ANALYSES

Screening and membership data are presented as descriptive statistics. Means and standard deviations were used to summarize continuous variables, and frequencies and percentages were used for categorical variables. The rate of C-SSRS administration was the key metric used to assess how each KP region implemented the screening clinical practice of the Zero Suicide Framework identify domain. The rate was defined as a C-SSRS completed within 2 business days of a positive 9th item (at least 1 on a scale of 0–3) of the PHQ9/PHQA among patients 10 years and older seen in specialty behavioral health or addiction medicine departments.

RESULTS

Descriptive statistics for the membership in 2019 across all five participating KP regions (n = 9,948,080) are provided in Table 1. Most KP members were aged between 20 and 64 years (61.5%), female (51.8%), White (53.3%), had commercial insurance (70.7%), and had higher census-track-estimated neighborhood education which was operationalized as the number of people in that census-track with at least a college degree (56.7%). Table 2 presents demographics for the denominator of the C-SSRS administration rate in 2019 (positive response on the 9th item of the PHQ9/PHQA; n = 70,036). Most patients reporting positive suicidal

TABLE 1
Descriptive Characteristics for Patients Who Were Continuously Enrolled Across all Five Kaiser Permanente Regions During 2019 (n = 9,948,080)

Characteristic	N	%
Age (y)		
≤19	2,192,469	22.0%
20–39	2,699,562	27.1%
40–64	3,423,963	34.4%
≥65	1,632,086	16.4%
Sex		
Female	5,152,675	51.8%
Male	4,794,707	48.2%
Other/Unknown	698	0.0%
Race		
White	5,301,995	53.3%
Asian	1,413,685	14.2%
Black	710,677	7.1%
Hawaiian/Pacific Islander	94,883	1.0%
American Indian/ Alaskan Native	66,838	0.7%
Multiple Race/Other	74,509	0.7%
Unknown	2,285,499	23%
Hispanic Ethnicity (% Yes)	2,717,901	27.3%
Insurance		
Commercial	7,035,047	70.7%
Medicare	1,679,763	16.9%
Medicaid	813,214	8.2%
Private	392,885	3.9%
Other	27,171	0.3%
Higher neighborhood education (25% or more with a college degree) (% yes)	5,640,561	56.7%

TABLE 2
Descriptive Statistics for All Patient Health Questionnaires (PHQ9) Completed in Psychiatry and Addiction Medicine in 2019 (n = 70,036) that Indicated a Patient Needed Further Assessment with a Columbia Suicide Severity Rating Scale (C-SSRS)

Characteristic	N	%
Age (y)		
10–17	4940	7.1%
18–64	57,890	82.7%
≥65	7206	10.3%
Sex		
Female	45,569	65.1%
Male	24,436	34.9%
Insurance		
Commercial	46,218	66.0%
Medicare	10,029	14.3%
Medicaid	9206	13.1%
Private	4437	6.3%
Other	181	0.3%
Race/Ethnicity		
Non-Hispanic White	40,137	57.3%
Hispanic	15,230	21.7%
Non-Hispanic Black	5159	7.4%
Asian	4813	6.9%
Hawaiian/Pacific Islander	660	0.9%
American Indian/ Alaskan Native	769	1.1%
Multiple Race/Other	476	0.7%
Unknown	2783	4.0%

Notes: Data are presented in aggregate for 5 Kaiser Permanente (KP) regions. This indication was a response of "some/most/almost all days in the last 2 weeks" to the 9th item of the PHQ9, "How often in the last 2 weeks have you had thoughts that you would be better off dead, or of hurting yourself in some way?" Data are presented as sample size and percentage. The rates of C-SSRS administration by KP region are shown in Fig. 1.

ideation were adults aged 18 to 64 years (82.7%), women (65.1%), had commercial insurance (66.0%), and were non-Hispanic White (57.3%).

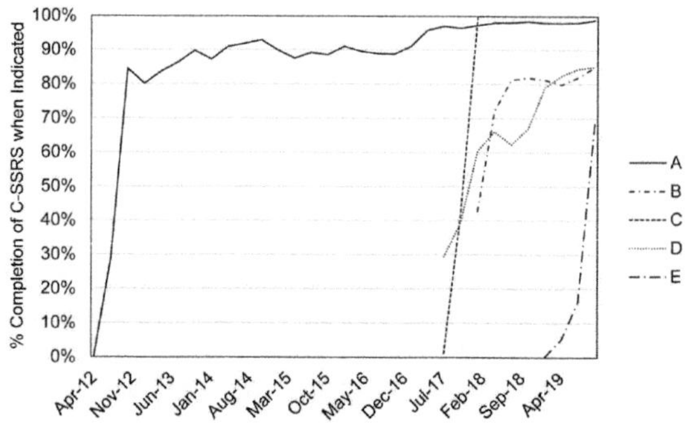

FIG. 1 Rates of Columbia Suicide Severity Rating Scale (C-SSRS) administration in psychiatry and addiction medicine over time (April 2012 – October 2019) for each Kaiser Permanente region (A – E). Rates are calculated for all Patient Health Questionnaires (PHQ9) with a positive response (some/most/almost all days in the last 2 wk) to the 9th item of the PHQ9: "How often in the last 2 weeks have you had thoughts that you would be better off dead, or of hurting yourself in some way?".

Fig. 1 provides the proportion of C-SSRS screenings completed over time starting in 2012 in each of the five KP regions when the PHQ9 item 9 score was at least 1. The pattern of C-SSRS screening rates varied greatly among regions. One region (A) was the early adopter mentioned previously. Two regions switched to administration of the C-SSRS in the electronic medical record in 2017 (C, D) with one achieving 100% administration rates by the end of 2017 (C) and one achieving 85% by December 2018 (D). Finally, the last 2 of the 5 regions to implement the C-SSRS (B, E) began in January 2018 (B) and January 2019 (E) and had rates of 85% (B) and 69% (E) by October 2019.

DISCUSSION

A learning health care system approach [24] to implementing the screening clinical practice of the Zero Suicide Framework identify domain significantly increased systematic suicide screening rates recorded in the electronic health record to an average of 82%, with one region achieving 100%, in less than 3 years across 5 regions of KP serving nearly 10 million patients. Despite this success overall, KP regions varied greatly in the rate with which they implemented the screening clinical practice. Many factors could account for these differences. One is the comparative size and complexity of the regions. The range in annual membership among the 5 KP regions was just over 600,000 to 4.7 million, nearly 1300 to 9400 physicians, and some regions serving entire states. Although each KP region is part of the same entity, each region's organizational culture, structure, labor management partnerships, and competing health system priorities were very different.

Another approach was the implementation of the C-SSRS within the electronic health record. Although an EPIC-based electronic health record version of the C-SSRS was created by the Care Management Institute for all regions to capture this risk information discretely in a structured format for monitoring and quality improvement, local processes were still necessary to activate the C-SSRS locally (EPIC platforms were adopted and modified differently by each KP region.). Another was the creation of specific clinical workflows, acceptability to all parties involved, that would clearly state what was to be done and who would do it when the screening indicated risk for suicide. Although the Care Management Institute could suggest workflows, each KP region had to establish and implement them locally.

Considerations for Implementation

Based on these findings, we believe that there are *six* essential components necessary to successfully implement the screening clinical practice of the Zero Suicide Framework identify domain for specialty behavioral health and addiction medicine. The *first* is to obtain "buy-in" from the clinical systems in which screening will take place. One important component of this process is understanding the investments that clinical systems have already made in obtaining patient-reported outcomes related to suicide prevention such as the PHQ9 for depression screening. The learning health care system approach [24] is particularly important to this step as it embeds researchers in clinical teams which can then help those teams present evidence that will convince executive leaders in these systems to adopt effective practices and implementation strategies. This first step is also critical to the "lead" domain in the Zero Suicide Framework [5].

The *second* is an assembly of all key decision-makers in a workgroup that is coordinated by staff dedicated to the initiative. Key decision-makers should include health technology experts, workflow consultants, clinical experts on screening for and treatment of suicidal ideation such as providers and research scientists, administrators who oversee and train staff, clinical informatics personnel for data reporting, implementation scientists, risk management personnel, and people with lived experience who also have experience with health care system workflows regarding screening for suicide. The *third* is the use of validated instruments for screening [3]. Careful consideration should be made for choosing evidence-based instruments that already align with the health care systems' needs for patient-reported outcome quality metrics [17].

The *fourth* is the automation, whenever possible, of the screening algorithm and reporting using discrete, abstractable structured formats (eg, questionnaires, flowsheets, and so forth) that can be easily assembled for reporting and quality improvement. The PHQ9/PHQA and C-SSRS have already been incorporated into EPIC, the largest electronic health record platform in the U.S. [30]. The *fifth* is the creation of clear workflows that designate responsibility for various clinical responses, depending on the outcome of the scoring algorithm, reported data, and quality-improvement expectations. For example, when a patient indicates clear intent for suicide, to whom does that person speak, what is said in the conversation, when must this conversation take place, and how is this process documented? Even though we only describe the results of the KP efforts to implement the screening clinical practice of the identify domain, in reality, the other domains (lead, train, engage, treat, improve) must also be in place for screening to succeed.

And finally, the *sixth* recommendation is to plan for performance feedback involving a standardized set of metrics created with benchmarks for screening that can be distributed to all clinical partners involved in the work. This performance feedback must be administered with a focus on safety and using opportunity instead of blame-based approaches [31]. A strategy for mitigating poor performance should also be clearly articulated including who will be responsible for the remediation and how it will be done. This will also address the "improve" domain of the Zero Suicide Framework.

Limitations

One of the major limitations of the study was that data were only presented for specialty behavioral health settings. Most experts [3] recommend screening in specialty behavioral health care where a more extensive process can be used to both screen and assess level of risk. Unfortunately, it is also likely to miss patients because many people who die by suicide are not receiving specialty mental health care at that time [22,23]. There are well-documented racial and ethnic disparities in specialty mental health treatment initiation [32–36], and implementation of screening in nonspecialty care settings such as primary care might be better at identifying risk for some groups [23,37]. Rural residents, too, are more likely to have mental health–related office visits with a primary care provider than with a psychiatrist [37]. Because of these important issues, efforts are underway to use the learnings from the roll out of screening in specialty mental health and addiction medicine to screen in KP emergency departments and primary care settings. Recent research highlights a successful approach for increasing culturally and linguistically appropriate depression screening which could be applied to screening and assessment for suicide risk [38].

Another limitation of the study was that other health care organizations were not included, such as Federally Qualified Health Centers, solo practitioner medical offices, or other health care delivery models. Even though these types of health care settings were not included, KP settings were very diverse in their implementation of the Zero Suicide Framework providing good variability for study. In addition, an advantage of KP is that it serves a racially and ethnically diverse population, with some regions being majority Hispanic/non-Hispanic Black. The insurance coverage of the membership is also diverse including high-deductible plans and limited access to specialty mental health care. We believe that as long as any health care setting can meet the requirements for electronic health records as outlined in the Affordable Care Act [39], and they have an infrastructure for creating national quality metrics such as those required by the National Center for Quality Assurance [17], the processes we report in this study could be implemented across a variety of settings.

Future Directions

Expanding suicide screening and assessment within health care settings promises the possibility of saving lives and of greatly reducing the burden of suicide within health care system populations. Some recent studies suggest that health care systems could improve the efficiency of screening and target screening to those most in need [40,41]. For instance, several research teams have developed suicide identification algorithms that use data from electronic health records, pharmacy data, and other health system information to estimate which people are at greater risk of suicide [40]. This approach shows promise, but there are a number of unanswered questions about how to integrate it into health care systems. Other studies have explored whether genetic markers could identify persons at risk [41], but to date, there have not been any strong markers that have emerged.

The changes in care with the advent of coronavirus disease 2019 (COVID-19) have dramatically increased the use of virtual visits, and many health care systems plan to continue this expansion of telehealth. Several studies have tested the use of computerized or remote suicide screening [42–44]. There is some suggestion that this approach could successfully identify persons at risk, but these methods have primarily been used in university settings. Unfortunately, many tools that have been shown to be effective in clinical settings have not been tested in virtual delivery. Finally, little is known about how well persons identified through algorithms, genetics, or virtual screening methods could be effectively linked to needed care. We will likely see continuing expansion of these approaches in the future and additional research to help ensure that they are used effectively.

CLINICS CARE POINTS

- Use validated questionnaires like the Columbia-Suicide Severity Rating Scale (C-SSRS).
- Use questionnaires that can be incorporated into electronic medical records in abstractable formats for tracking.
- Create clear workflows and benchmarks that specify what should happen and how care systems and providers are doing as a result of screening for suicide risk.

DISCLOSURE

None of the authors have any conflicts of interest to disclose.

REFERENCES

[1] National Center for Health Statistics. Increase in Suicide Mortality in the United States, 1999 – 2018. Available at: https://www.cdc.gov/nchs/products/databriefs/db362.htm. Accessed December 1, 2020.

[2] Mann JJ, Currier D. Prevention of suicide. Psych Ann 2007;37:2331–9.

[3] The Joint Commission. Suicide Prevention. Available at: https://www.jointcommission.org/resources/patient-safety-topics/suicide-prevention/. Accessed April 1, 2020.

[4] Suicide Prevention Resource Center. About the Suicide Prevention Resource Center. Available at: https://www.sprc.org/about-sprc. Accessed April 1, 2020.

[5] Education Development Center. A New Way to Explore Zero Suicide. Available at: https://zerosuicide.edc.org/. Accessed April 1, 2020.

[6] Akincigil A, Matthews EB. National rates and patterns of depression screening in primary care: Results from 2012 and 2013. Psychiatr Serv 2017;68:660–6.

[7] Hirschtritt ME, Kline-Simon AH, Kroenke K, et al. Depression screening rates and symptom severity by

alcohol use among primary care adult patients. J Am Board Fam Med 2018;31:724–32.
[8] United States Government U.S. Army. Army Health Promotion, Risk Reduction and Suicide Prevention - Report 2010. Available at: https://www.armyg1.army.mil/hr/suicide/docs/Commanders%20Tool%20Kit/HPRRSP_Report_2010_v00.pdf. Accessed November 15, 2020.
[9] Bahraini N, Brenner LA, Barry C, et al. Assessment of rates of suicide risk screening and prevalence of positive screening results among US Veterans after implementation of the Veterans Affairs Suicide Risk Identification Strategy. JAMA Netw Open 2020;3:e2022531.
[10] Knox KL, Pflanz S, Talcott GW, et al. The US Air Force suicide prevention program: implications for public health policy. Am J Public Health 2010;100:2457–63.
[11] Coffey CE. Building a system of perfect depression care in behavioral health. Jt Comm J Qual Patient Saf 2007;33:193–9.
[12] Coffey CE, Coffey MJ, Ahmedani BK. An update on perfect depression care. Psychiatr Serv 2013;64:396.
[13] Suicide Prevention Resource Center. Suicide screening and assessment. Available at: https://sprc.org/sites/default/files/migrate/library/RS_suicide%20screening_91814%20final.pdf. Accessed November 15, 2020.
[14] Horowitz LM, Bridge JA, Teach SJ, et al. Ask Suicide-Screening Questions (ASQ): A brief instrument for the pediatric emergency department. Arch Pediatr Adolesc Med 2012;166:1170–6.
[15] Rossom RC, Coleman KJ, Ahmedani BK, et al. Suicidal ideation reported on the PHQ9 and risk of suicidal behavior across age groups. J Affect Disord 2017;215:77–84.
[16] Simon GE, Rutter CM, Peterson D, et al. Does response on the PHQ-9 Depression Questionnaire predict subsequent suicide attempt or suicide death? Psychiatr Serv 2013;64:1195–202.
[17] National Center for Quality Assurance. HEDIS Depression Measures Specified for Electronic Clinical Data Systems. Available at: https://www.ncqa.org/hedis/the-future-of-hedis/hedis-depression-measures-specified-for-electronic-clinical-data/. Accessed January 10, 2020.
[18] Bjureberg J, Dahlin M, Carlborg A, et al. Columbia-Suicide Severity Rating Scale Screen Version: initial screening for suicide risk in a psychiatric emergency department. Psychol Med 2021;26:1–9.
[19] Posner K, Brown GK, Stanley B, et al. The Columbia-Suicide Severity Rating Scale: initial validity and internal consistency findings from three multisite studies with adolescents and adults. Am J Psychiatry 2011;168:1266–77.
[20] Pao M, Mournet A, Horowitz LM. Implementation challenges of universal suicide risk screening in adult patients in general medical and surgical settings. Available at: https://www.psychiatrictimes.com/view/implementation-challenges-universal-suicide-risk-screening-adult-patients-general. Accessed August 15, 2020.
[21] Petrik ML, Gutierrez PM, Berlin JS, et al. Barriers and facilitators of suicide risk assessment in emergency departments: a qualitative study of provider perspectives. Gen Hosp Psychiatry 2015;37:581–6.
[22] Ahmedani BK, Simon GE, Stewart C, et al. Health care contacts in the year before suicide death. J Gen Intern Med 2014;29:870–7.
[23] Simon GE, Coleman KJ, Rossom RC, et al. Risk of suicide attempt and suicide death following completion of the Patient Health Questionnaire depression module in community practice. J Clin Psychiatry 2016;77:221–7.
[24] Rossom RC, Simon GE, Beck A, et al. Facilitating Action for Suicide Prevention by Learning Health Care Systems. Psychiatr Serv 2016;67:830–2.
[25] Kaiser Permanente Care Management Institute. Transforming Care Delivery. Available at: https://kpcmi.org/. Accessed December 11, 2020.
[26] Mental Health Research Network. About MHRN. Available at: https://mhresearchnetwork.org/. Accessed December 11, 2020.
[27] Connolly L. Suicidal behavior: Does it exist in pre-school aged children? Ir J Psychol Med 1999;16:72–4.
[28] National Institutes of Health. Patient-Reported Outcomes Measurement Information System. Available at: https://commonfund.nih.gov/promis/index. Accessed April 1, 2021.
[29] Ross TR, Ng D, Brown JS, et al. The HMO Research Network Virtual Data Warehouse: A Public Data Model to Support Collaboration. EGEMS 2014;2:1049.
[30] Johns Hopkins Medicine. Why Epic?. Available at: https://www.hopkinsmedicine.org/epic/why_epic/. Accessed April 1, 2021.
[31] Hardavella G, Aamli-Gaagnat A, Saad N, et al. How to give and receive feedback effectively. Breathe (Sheff). 2017;13(4):327–33.
[32] Coleman KJ, Johnson E, Ahmedani BK, et al. Predicting suicide attempts for racial and ethnic groups of patients during routine clinical care. Suicide Life Threat Behav 2019;49:724–34.
[33] Marrast L, Himmelstein DU, Woolhandler S. Racial and ethnic disparities in mental health care for children and young adults: A national study. Int J Health Serv 2016;46:810–24.
[34] Ahmedani BK, Stewart C, Simon GE, et al. Racial/Ethnic differences in health care visits made before suicide attempt across the United States. Med Care 2015;53:430–5.
[35] Nestor BA, Cheek SM, Liu RT. Ethnic and racial differences in mental health service utilization for suicidal ideation and behavior in a nationally representative sample of adolescents. J Affect Disord 2016;202:197–202.
[36] Alegria M, Alvarez K, Ishikawa RZ, et al. Removing obstacles to eliminating racial and ethnic disparities in behavioral health care. Health Aff 2016;35:991–9.
[37] Cherry D, Albert M, McCaig LF. Mental health-related physician office visits by adults aged 18 and over: United States, 2012-2014. NCHS Data Brief 2018;311:1–8.
[38] Schaeffer AM, Jolles D. Not missing the opportunity: Improving depression screening and follow-up in a

multicultural community. Jt Comm J Qual Patient Saf 2019;45:31–9.
[39] Blumenthal D, Tavenner M. The "meaningful use" regulation for electronic health records. N Engl J Med 2010; 363:501–4.
[40] Belsher BE, Smolenski DJ, Pruitt LD, et al. Prediction models for suicide attempts and deaths: A systematic review and simulation. JAMA Psychiatry 2019;76:642–51.
[41] Lopes FL, McMahon FJ. The promise and limits of suicide genetics. Am J Psychiatry 2019;176:600–2.
[42] Christensen H, Batterham PJ, O'Dea B. E-health interventions for suicide prevention. Int J Environ Res Public Health 2014;11:8193–212.
[43] Gilmore AK, Ward-Ciesielski EF. Perceived risks and use of psychotherapy via telemedicine for patients at risk for suicide. J Telemed Telecare 2019;25:59–63.
[44] King CA, Eisenberg D, Zheng K, et al. Online suicide risk screening and intervention with college students: a pilot randomized controlled trial. J Consult Clin Psychol 2015;83:630–6.

Advances in Psychiatry and Behavioral Health 1 (2021) 77–89

ADVANCES IN PSYCHIATRY AND BEHAVIORAL HEALTH

Lethal Means Safety Approaches for Suicide Prevention

Leslie Barnard, MPH[a,b], Ali Rowhani-Rahbar, MD, MPH, PhD[c,d], Marian E. Betz, MD, MPH[a,e,*]

[a]Department of Emergency Medicine, University of Colorado School of Medicine, 12401 East 17th Avenue, B-215, Aurora, CO 80045, USA; [b]Department of Epidemiology, University of Colorado School of Public Health, 12401 East 17th Avenue, B-215, Aurora, CO 80045, USA; [c]Department of Epidemiology, University of Washington School of Public Health, University of Washington, Box 351619, Seattle, WA 98195, USA; [d]Harborview Injury Prevention and Research Center, University of Washington, Seattle, WA, USA; [e]VA Eastern Colorado Geriatric Research Education and Clinical Center, 12401 East 17th Avenue, B-215, Aurora, CO 80045, USA

KEYWORDS

• Suicide • Lethal means • Firearm • Overdose • Hanging

KEY POINTS

- Lethal means safety (reducing access to highly lethal methods of suicide, like firearms) is a key component of suicide prevention.
- Means safety interventions can be applied at multiple levels, from society (eg, laws), community (eg, partnerships and education), and interpersonal relationships (eg, engaging friends and family) to individuals (eg, changing behavior in storing dangerous items).
- Approaches and challenges vary between geographic regions and cultures depending on the most common methods of suicide as well as political considerations (eg, acceptability of legislation to reduce access to methods such as firearms).

BACKGROUND

Suicide is a global public health problem that affects people across the life span. Across the world, over 800,000 people die by suicide each year. In 2016 suicide was the 18th leading cause of death worldwide, accounting for 1.4% of all deaths. Suicide affects all socioeconomic groups, sexes, and geographic regions [1]. In the United States, nearly 50,000 people die by suicide each year, and suicide is the 10th leading cause of death in 2018 [2]. From 1999 to 2018, suicide rates in the United States increased by 35%, approximately 2% each year between 2006 and 2018 [3]. Suicide was also the second leading cause of death for persons aged 10 to 14, 15 to 19, and 20 to 24 in 2017, with the rate of increase during this time higher than the preceding 5 years [4]. These worsening rates highlight the importance of taking action to prevent suicides and reduce the lethality of attempts.

Suicide prevention is complex from the individual to societal level, and it generally requires a comprehensive, multipronged approach [5]. This approach includes the identification of at-risk individuals, effective care and treatment (including care linkages), response to crisis (for those in crisis, those around them, and postvention interventions after a suicide), and interventions to build resilience, life skills, and connectedness. Another critical component of this comprehensive approach is lethal means safety (previously referred to as "means restriction," a less-preferred term [6]). Means safety approaches are built on studies and conceptual theories showing that suicide attempts can occur after only a short period of deliberation [7–9]. Access to a lethal

*Corresponding author. Department of Emergency Medicine, University of Colorado School of Medicine, 12401 East 17th Avenue, B-215, Aurora, CO 80045. *E-mail address:* Marian.betz@cuanschutz.edu

https://doi.org/10.1016/j.ypsc.2021.05.015

2667-3827/21/

method of suicide during the period of highest risk can increase the likelihood of death should an attempt occur. Thus, means safety approaches work by reducing physical access to methods, thereby delaying an attempt (temporarily or permanently) (Fig. 1). Even if a person substitutes a second method, that method is less likely to be lethal, assuming the most lethal methods (eg, firearms) are the ones to which access has been reduced. Thus, lethal means safety can attenuate or eliminate the role of a critical factor (access to means) during a time of vulnerability and reduce the likelihood of suicide attempts or death [10]. Implementation of means safety approaches varies by setting, from population-based policies to individual-level intervention.

Means safety approaches also vary by method, and the leading methods of suicide attempts (failed or deadly) vary by geographic region. In the United States, firearm suicides are the most common method of suicide death, accounting for nearly half of all suicide deaths with variation among subgroups (eg, approximately 40% among youth and 68% among veterans) [2]. Suffocation (hanging) is the second-leading method of suicide death in the United States, and poisoning or overdose is by far the most common method used in nonfatal suicide attempts. The World Health Organization estimates that internationally, 79% of suicides occur in low-income or middle-income countries, with poisonings from pesticides accounting for 20% of suicides globally [11]. However, the mechanism of suicide varies depending on the country. For example, the leading and second-leading methods of suicide are hanging or burning charcoal in Taiwan [12], hanging or poisoning in the United Kingdom [13], and hanging or jumping in Japan [14].

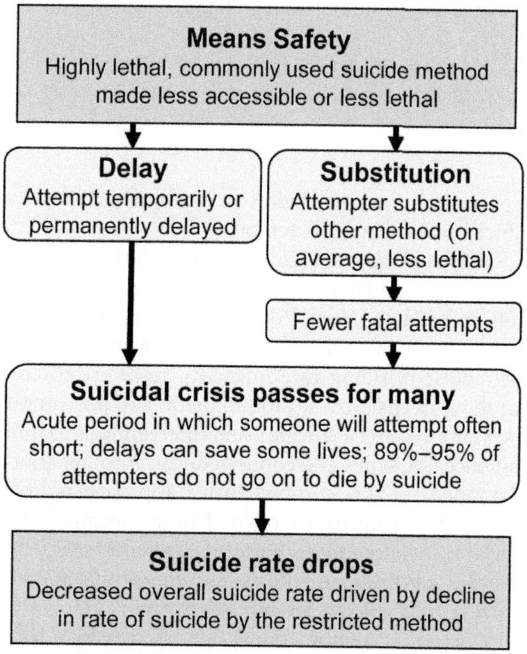

FIG. 1 Conceptual model of how reducing access to a highly lethal and commonly used suicide method saves lives at the population level. (*Adapted from* Barber CW, Miller MJ. Reducing a suicidal person's access to lethal means of suicide: a research agenda. Am J Prev Med. 2014;47(3 Suppl 2):S264-272; with permission.)

FRAMEWORK FOR PREVENTION EFFORTS

One model for organizing means safety suicide prevention strategies is the social-ecological model (SEM) [15]. Understanding how the 4 levels of the SEM (societal, community, relationship, and individual) interact and overlap can inform strategies to address public health issues. This model was previously used with firearm suicide in the United States. [16]. Here we apply it to a broader range of lethal means safety in both mechanism and geography (Table 1). We then discuss the challenges of implementation and evaluation.

Societal

The societal level refers to policies, laws, and culture. There are a plethora of policy studies, both internationally and in the United States, focused on public health approaches to lethal means safety at the societal level.

In the United Kingdom, changing global economics and coal production from 1960 to 1971 reduced the carbon monoxide content of coal. This subsequently led to a significant decrease in overall suicide rates as well as those among age and sex groups [17], as asphyxiation by cooking gas had been a primary method of suicide. The same pattern was observed when barbecue coal was restricted in 1 city in Taiwan but was not regulated in another [18]. Similarly, the regulation and outright ban of sales of certain pesticides in several countries have shown to be an effective method in reducing suicides due to pesticide ingestion [19]. Notably, the pesticide bans were enacted specifically for suicide prevention, while the change in carbon monoxide access in the United Kingdom was a policy unrelated to suicide prevention that had an unexpected, positive benefit through reduced suicide rates.

Regarding firearm suicide, there are some notable examples of means safety approaches at the policy level. In Australia, a 1996 mass shooting prompted a law prohibiting the sale and promoting the buyback of

TABLE 1
Examples of Suicide Prevention Practices at each Level of the Social-Ecological Model

Level	Examples	Sample Resources
Societal	• Consideration of policies reducing access to highly lethal methods of suicide	• Educational Fund to Stop Gun Violence: https://preventfirearmsuicide.efsgv.org/interventions/societal/ • Suicide Prevention on Bridges: https://suicidepreventionlifeline.org/wp-content/uploads/2017/04/Suicide-Bridges-National-Suicide-Prevention-Lifeline-Position-2017-FINAL.pdf
Community	• Collaboration with trusted organizations (eg, "Gun shop projects") • Targeted messaging at higher-risk communities	• Gun Shop Projects: https://www.hsph.harvard.edu/means-matter/gun-shop-project/ • Veterans' PREVENTS: https://www.va.gov/PREVENTS/accomplishments.asp • Utah Firearm Suicide Prevention: https://vimeo.com/175761640 • Gun Storage Maps: o https://coloradofirearmsafetycoalition.org/gun-storage-map/ o https://hiprc.org/firearm/firearm-storage-wa/ o https://mdpgv.org/safestoragemap/ • Trevor Project o https://www.thetrevorproject.org/
Relationship	• Engagement of friends and family in lethal means safety counseling/interventions • Lethal means assessment and counseling by health care providers	• NSSSF/AFSP: https://www.nssf.org/safety/suicide-prevention/suicide-prevention-toolkit/ • Overwatch (Veterans): https://overwatchproject.org/ • BulletPoints project: https://www.bulletpointsproject.org/ • CALM training: https://www.sprc.org/resources-programs/calm-counseling-access-lethal-means
Individual	• Information and tools for individuals about lethal means safety	• Lock to Live: http://lock2live.org/ • Signpost, Assess, Facts, Emotion, Recommend: o https://intheforefront.org/safer-homes-suicide-aware/

semiautomatic and pump-action shotguns and rifles. The observed reduction in firearm suicides following this period was attributed to both cultural changes, such as attitudes on firearm ownership preceding the law, and restriction after the law was enacted [20,21]. A second example comes from Switzerland, where a reduction in army personnel resulted in a reduction in army-issued firearms and led to a statistically significant decrease in suicides by those firearms among this high-risk group [22]. Similarly, in Israel, the Israeli Defense Force (IDF), a population-based army, changed their policy so that IDF soldiers were required to leave their firearms on the army base when they went home; this led to a decreased suicide rate among IDF soldiers of 40%. Notably, the reduction was attributed to a decrease in weekend firearm suicides directly affected by the policy [23]. Some states in the United States implemented policies that enacted background checks in order to purchase a firearm or waiting periods after a firearm purchase. Anestis and colleagues evaluated and concluded that each of these laws was associated with a significantly lower proportion and rate of firearm suicide deaths in those states [24]. Another relatively new intervention in the United States is the use of gun violence restraining orders and extreme risk protection orders, which allow police or family members to petition to have firearms removed temporarily from those who may pose an imminent risk to others or themselves. Evaluation of Connecticut's and Indiana's laws showed a reduction in suicide associated with these laws [25,26]. Another legal approach is child access prevention laws, which impose criminal liability when a child in a home with firearms gains access as a result of poor storage. In states where these laws have been implemented, preliminary evidence indicates that these laws are associated with a reduction in unintentional firearm injuries and suicides among children [27]. Notably, many of these examples at the societal level, such as extreme risk protection orders, rely on community participation—for example, members of the public knowing about and requesting extreme risk protection orders in cases of concern—for their effect to take place. Another example is laws that allow individuals to place themselves on voluntary "do-not-sell" lists to prevent firearm acquisition [28].

Community

Community is the second level of the SEM and refers to the social and physical environment. "Community" exists at various levels depending on the characteristic that unites a group of people; the United States can be seen as a community versus other countries, while the United States also contains myriad communities within it as defined by geographic, demographic, or other subgroupings. Lethal means safety approaches can leverage community ties through physical, cultural, and other approaches.

One example of community-level intervention is physical modification to prevent suicide by jumping, most commonly bridge modifications [29]. The Golden Gate Bridge in San Francisco, California, is a notable example of physical changes made to a historically lethal means of suicide by jumping [30]. Political, financial, and cultural opposition to a physical barrier on the bridge—long a suicide destination—led to initial reliance on hotlines and bridge patrols to thwart suicide attempts. With mixed evidence for the effectiveness of these approaches [31,32], California ultimately passed legislation in 2014 to build a physical barrier, projected to be complete in 2023 [33]. Another community-level example of changing the physical environment is an approach to reduce suicides by hanging from ceiling fans [34]. Lethality would potentially be reduced by adding a weight release or arrester cable/spring to allow for a safe drop. After a cluster of suicides by hanging in dorm rooms, a community in India added this mechanism to their ceiling fans. This pilot program was promising but has yet to be evaluated.

Medication take-back programs are another example of community-based interventions used in the United States and elsewhere. Medication take-back programs are intended to provide safe disposal of unused medications that could otherwise accumulate in the home and thereby increase availability and the likelihood of misuse. Evaluations of these programs have shown them to be highly effective at eliminating excess medications through medication drop-off sites available to members of the public [35]. Local media campaigns relying on community messaging have been shown to increase awareness and the likelihood of community members talking to others about the dangers of prescription drug abuse [36]. Evidence also exists that these programs have low penetration, so expansion may be needed to increase community participation and knowledge [37,38].

There are also several examples of lethal means safety interventions within local geographic communities. With a commitment to nonpolitical approaches, the New Hampshire Firearm Safety Coalition was formed to develop and share firearm suicide prevention education with firearms retailers and ranges [39]. This "Gun Shop Project" model has since expanded to states across the United States, with a key characteristic being local connections and tailoring [40]. Other programs based within local communities include the Colorado Firearm Safety Coalition, which created the first statewide map of voluntary firearms storage locations [41], followed by maps in Washington and Maryland. Another example comes from Utah, which has developed public-facing videos and included suicide prevention information in firearms training courses in Utah [42].

There are several examples of communities at higher risk for suicide that require tailored education and messaging. These communities include specific racial and ethnic minorities, including refugees and indigenous populations. In the United States, there is a concerning trend of increasing suicide rates among Black youth, with a higher proportion of suicides by firearms compared with the youth of other racial/ethnic groups [43,44]. Meyerhoff and colleagues described Bhutanese refugees experience a rate of suicide that is nearly 2 times higher than that of the general population in the United States. A culturally responsive model including preferred, appropriate language, destigmatization of mental health services, and tailored means safety interventions was described as the preferred prevention response [45]. Similarly, indigenous populations in Australia, Canada, the United States, and New Zealand experience disproportionately high rates of suicide. An evaluation of several interventions among this population highlighted the success of community prevention, gatekeeper training, and education. Each of these interventions utilized community and community members with a focus on culturally specific programming in the implementation of empowerment programs; family outreach after suicides; suicide risk screening at community events; community-based education on how to identify and support individuals at high risk of suicide; and educational programs on topics like communication, problem-solving, and alcohol and drug use [46].

Within the LGBTQ community, firearm ownership for self-protection is not uncommon [47]. Especially within the trans community, there are efforts to increase firearm ownership rates for self-protection, given the high rates of hate crimes and violence reported against those identifying as LGBQT [48]. Men identifying as LGBTQ are 4 times more likely to report suicide attempts, and LGBTQ women are 2 times more likely than non-LGBTQ women [49]. This combination may put the LGBTQ firearm-owning community at particularly high risk for firearm suicide. Additionally, LGB and questioning youth report higher rates of suicidal ideation and attempts compared with This should be non-LGB (as is) not non-LGBT as suggested by reviewers youth [50]. One community-level educational resource is the Trevor Project, a national suicide prevention resource center for LGBTQ youth that offers program support services [51], including information on lethal means safety.

Some communities—like those comprised of veterans—stretch across geographic boundaries. In the United States, several programs are designed to address means safety for suicide prevention by leveraging community connections within the veteran community, a community that has a documented higher risk of suicide compared with the nonveteran population [52]. The US Department of Defense (DoD) and its Defense Suicide Prevention Office have developed specific training and educational campaigns related to means safety [53]. The DoD Defense Suicide Prevention Office also convened a Lethal Means Task Force to advise on lethal means safety approaches related to firearms, medications, railways, and other methods of suicide. Similarly, the Department of Veterans Affairs supports lethal means safety counseling by health care providers of veterans with suicide risk [54], a veterans crisis line, and a Center for Suicide Prevention which are well known within the veteran community [55]. The Veteran's Crisis Line has centered on specific reasons why veterans have higher rates of suicide, including having access to lethal means. The Veteran's Crisis Line addresses this elevated risk by including lethal means safety in their counseling and outreach and uses the line to reach people who may not be receiving those messages from the VA [56] or other mental health services. The 2019 PREVENTS [President's Roadmap to Empower Veterans and End a National Tragedy of Suicide] initiative from the White House and the VA includes specific recommendations related to lethal means safety as well [57].

Community approaches to means safety for suicide prevention can also leverage a desire to support and protect other community members. Messaging campaigns encourage reducing access to lethal means during times of crisis, for example, through temporary, voluntary storage of firearms away from the home. This is seen in the Together With Veterans program, which leverages community members who are veterans to take leadership roles in suicide prevention education and training strategies for fellow veterans and those they interact with [58]. This approach is analogous to broad community campaigns like "friends don't let friends drive drunk" to reduce alcohol-impaired driving, motor vehicle crashes, and injuries [59]. Broad campaigns can have the benefit of changing behavioral norms within a community, though such changes are usually slow.

Relationship

Relationship in the SEM refers to interpersonal connections to family, friends, health care providers, or other individuals. Cultural and political challenges can confound people's ability to intervene on behalf of a friend or loved one, especially given the stigma around mental health and the political sensitivity of firearms in the United States. However, targeted strategies, specific messaging, and language for friends/family to help those in crisis exist. Qualitative studies show that preferences for certain words or phrases in addition to group identity may increase the likelihood of message engagement. Culturally specific messaging, including group identity such as rural versus urban, second amendment rights, and knowledge of firearms for firearm owners, increases their likelihood of taking steps to reduce access to firearms during times of crisis [60,61]. The National Shooting Sports Foundation, the trade association for the firearms industry, partnered with the American Foundation for Suicide Prevention to develop suicide prevention educational materials and programming for firearm owners [62] and parents of youth who may be at risk for suicide [63]. Messaging around "have a brave conversation" draws upon core beliefs of strength and responsibility from the firearms community. In areas of Asia with disproportionately higher rates of suicide using pesticides, storage containers were not found to prevent suicide [64], but pesticide vendor education about suicide prevention was promising [65].

Within health care settings, lethal means counseling is recommended for patients at risk of suicide [66].

There is evidence that such counseling can affect behavior, especially when conducted with parents of at-risk adolescents and when combined with the provision of locking devices [67]. The SAFETY study found that an ED-based counseling intervention for parents of youth at risk for suicide appeared to improve home medication storage and firearms storage after the intervention [68]. Individual-level evaluation shows that lethal means safety counseling by providers is an effective tool to reduce subsequent suicide attempts [69]; however, it is infrequently deployed [70]. Training for health care providers exists through Counseling on Access to Lethal Means [71], although studies suggest more work is needed to ensure providers are "culturally competent" in discussing firearms and that assessment and counseling need to be integrated into pathways of care. Multiple medical organizations have developed or are developing resources and guidelines about firearms safety counseling [72,73]. Notably, no current state or federal law in the United States prohibits health care providers from assessing or discussing firearms access among patients at risk of suicide [74]. Additionally, although some health care providers may be untrained or hesitant to discuss firearms out of fear of offending patients, studies have shown that firearm owners are open to questioning and counseling about firearms safety when it occurs in an appropriate context (eg, risk of suicide) [75].

Another opportunity for medical professionals to intervene is with patients with alcohol or substance abuse. While alcohol overdose alone is not necessarily a common suicide method, alcohol intoxication at the time of attempt is highly common across all suicide methods [76]. Alcohol ingestion can contribute to death through cognitive inhibition—thereby potentiating an attempt in a person with ideation—and central nervous system and respiratory depression that can be deadly when combined with a medication overdose [77]. Some studies indicate that those with substance abuse or dependence have higher suicide rates than those with depression [78], and dual treatment programs (treating both substance abuse and concomitant depression or other illnesses) are an important resource. Incorporation of suicide risk screening for patients with identified alcohol or substance may facilitate treatment. Efforts should also leverage other trusted contacts, such as engaging relationships for suicide prevention through counselors and patient/client relationships at substance abuse programs or mental health community programs, by incorporating education about the dangers of alcohol and suicide risk.

Individual

The last level of the SEM is the individual. Suicide risk varies among individuals because of complicated interactions between static and dynamic risk factors (eg, a genetic predisposition for mental illness, relapses in substance abuse, social stressors like divorce or job loss, and bereavement). Behavior change theories explore an individual's beliefs, perceptions, adherence to interventions, and intention to change. Models of behavior change can shed light on why individuals might seek treatment and follow treatment recommendations [79]. Prevention efforts should aim to reach higher-risk groups to encourage action to reduce lethal means access. A recent study showed that brief interventions with firearm owners in community settings (eg, gun shows) effectively encouraged safer home firearms storage [80]. The "Lock to Live" [81] online decision aid was designed to help individuals at risk of suicide (and their friends or family) make decisions about reducing access to firearms, medications, and other suicide methods; in a pilot trial, it had extremely high patient acceptability [82]. The provision of firearms locking devices, whether in clinical or community settings, may help promote individual-level behavior change [83,84].

Individual history, biological factors, and societal constructs affect a person's risk for suicide. Therefore, individual-level interventions should consider the characteristics of an individual that place them in a high-risk group and tailor messaging and educational materials appropriately. For example, targeted language, messaging, and interventions aimed at farmers were used alongside pesticide bans to address high suicide rates by pesticides to affect individual-level action in the purchasing and storing of pesticides [85,86]. Firearm owners may report higher rates of suicidal thoughts and behaviors compared with those who do not own firearms regardless of the primary motivation for firearm ownership [87,88]. However, some evidence supports the idea that firearm owners are not more suicidal than non-firearm owners and that the higher risk of suicide among those living in gun-owning homes is because of the presence of guns, not because they are inherently more suicidal [89,90]. Firearm owners who may be at risk for suicide are more likely to store their firearms unsafely [91,92] and may be less likely to be open to means safety [93]. Men are disproportionately affected by high firearm suicide rates and are also less likely to seek care for depression or mental illness, meaning intervention can be challenging. To affect individual-level change, outreach at gun shows or other community events [80] may be more effective in reaching those in this group, as men may be less likely to interact with mental health services. Education in these settings was reported to be highly valuable, to increase comfort with discussing safe storage, and to increase safe firearm and ammunition storage among participants [84]. To affect individual change, many of these interventions are an example of an approach that spans the SEM levels by using societal, community, and relationship means to affect, enable, or encourage individual behavior and address individual risk factors.

Other individual-level risk factors for suicide include history of depression and other mental illnesses, hopelessness, substance abuse, certain health conditions, previous suicide attempt, violence victimization and perpetration, and genetic and biological determinants [5]. There are prevention strategies that individuals may engage in to reduce their personal risk of suicide. These include engaging in mental health treatment, especially approaches like dialectical behavior therapy or cognitive behavioral therapy that emphasize agency and involvement in the process of changing thought patterns [94,95]. Lethal means safety counseling is a component to address within these therapies, and it is a specific section in the evidence-based intervention of safety planning [96], which also includes coping strategies, problem-solving, and identifying emergency contacts. These individual-level therapies and strategies can be used to reduce suicide risk.

CHALLENGES FOR LETHAL MEANS SAFETY APPROACHES

Challenges to lethal means safety interventions exist across the levels of the SEM. These include challenges related to theoretic considerations, culture, implementation, and evaluation.

First, there is the theoretic question of whether providing information on the lethality of suicide methods could be harmful in that it might alert individuals to which methods are most lethal and thereby prompt them to select those methods. These questions may be particularly relevant in considerations of medications, as the public may not be aware that certain commonly available medications (eg, acetaminophen) are far more toxic than others (eg, ibuprofen). Prescription medications used to treat depression, anxiety, and other conditions that may raise suicide risk can also be problematic; in high doses or in contraindicated combinations, they may be toxic, but reducing access may pose a barrier to effective treatment. For example, there has been an increase in the use of benzodiazepines in combination with opioids in fatal and nonfatal overdoses (some unintentional and some with suicidal intent) recently in the United States and abroad [97,98]. Additional theoretic challenges relate to US laws about firearm transfers, particularly in temporary transfers to an individual or a storage location. These include state-by-state variability in whether a background check is needed as well as questions about liability on the part of the person or location (among both retailers and law enforcement) providing temporary storage [99,100].

In addition to these theoretic challenges, there are also cultural challenges related to methods. In New Zealand, Beautrais and colleagues described hanging and car exhaust as being too widely accessible for lethal means safety approaches to be practical. Additionally, despite evidence supporting regulation of ceiling fan weight releases [34], easy substitutes for hanging may undermine the success of these types of programs [101]. In the United States, firearms pose a particular challenge, given the political sensitivity over the topic and the general cultural divide between researchers and firearm owners. Efforts at using appropriate terminology and engagement of the firearms community in research (both early on and sustained) may help overcome these gaps [102]. Some evidence suggests that affirming cultural values increased safe storage and physician engagement, especially among those who were rural, politically conservative, and gun rights advocates [61,103].

Challenges within the health care setting include those in implementation, at the level of both providers (eg, beliefs and behaviors) and systems. Studies show that many providers are skeptical about the preventability of suicide or may not be comfortable or trained in delivering lethal means counseling [104]. There are also institutional challenges, including limited time and training for medical providers, a lack of existing protocols [105], and where protocols exist, a resistance to change [106] or fear of liability. However, a growing body of evidence supports methods to increase medical setting interventions, such as clinician education to conduct counseling and reminders or prompts in the electronic medical record systems [107].

Lastly, challenges also exist for the evaluation of interventions. Studies show that suicide morbidity and mortality are underreported [108], and without proper universal systematic reporting of suicide death and attempts, accurate evaluation of these programs is impractical. Additionally, many policies are passed without evaluation plans, and the impact is studied through observational designs, limiting our understanding of underlying mechanisms for potential reduction. Differential uptake and versions of recommendations from experts in both policy (eg, extreme risk laws) and medical settings (differential screening tools) make evaluation and generalizability difficult.

FUTURE DIRECTIONS

There are several direct methods to improve means safety within the SEM that require a broad range of stakeholders. In societal-level interventions, political will and the prioritization of suicide prevention are key. These components should include acceptance and uptake of effective recommendations from experts, politicians, physicians, community organizations, and individuals—while this is rare, it should remain a goal. For community-level approaches, partnership and engagement at the international, national, and local levels should reiterate the same messaging and offer complementary programs for means safety. Within the relationship level, cultural change is needed to normalize friends and family to take steps to reduce firearm access when someone is at risk. Similarly, medical provider and institutional cultural change, buy-in and implementation of effective methods of lethal means assessment, and counseling are crucial. Lastly, for individual-level interventions, the application of behavior change science into lethal means safety is key to convincing people to take ownership of their own health. At all 4 of these levels, the stigma associated with suicide needs to be eliminated for effective implementation. While the SEM theoretic framework is well established, many programs do not have strong outcomes research evidence to support their success. More robust research is needed to evaluate means safety within and between each level of the SEM. Interactions of means safety among the 4 levels are unknown, and there may be intersectional benefits or potential negative consequences.

More robust data on suicide globally and in the United States, including methods for nonfatal and fatal suicide, are warranted. The WHO reports that only 80 of 194 member states have data of sufficient quality to directly report suicide rates [11]. Regardless of the country, suicide is more likely to be underreported through misclassification due to religious, legal, and cultural implications of suicide and suicidal behavior [109]. Without accurate reporting at the global and local levels, prevention strategies cannot be properly implemented or evaluated.

Another area of identified research is the evaluation of prevention strategies at the population level rather than in small pilot studies. Many interventions examining safe firearms storage also counsel and provide storage options to their participants [58,59]. Those that provide counseling and safe storage options at no cost to participants (ie, provide a trigger lock or lockbox) are different from those that simply counsel for safe storage and leave the cost burden on the individual—a far more likely scenario. While some evidence exists to show that among those who are at high risk for firearm suicide, counseling is still an effective intervention to increase safe storage [84], more evidence is needed to examine how these interventions can be deployed and evaluated at the population level.

There are also important differences in means safety strategies by suicide method, albeit with a need for a better understanding of the underlying mechanisms. Safe storage lockers and boxes provided to prevent suicide in countries disproportionately affected by pesticide suicide showed that these efforts were not effective [64,110], while there is evidence that this is effective to promote behavior change for safer storage and prevent firearm suicide among youth in the United States. [80,83,84]. Perhaps the more important difference between these 2 suicide methods is that in Asia, where pesticides are a leading cause of suicide, bans at the societal level have been the most effective means of safety [19,64]. In the United States, where firearm suicide is disproportionately high, similar bans are not politically feasible. Therefore, research at the community, relationship, and individual levels should be a more important focus of future research to prevent firearm suicide in the United States.

Culturally appropriate messaging among different groups (politically, geographically, and demographically) needs to be better studied to target prevention of specific means of suicide. Some research has been done to evaluate and encourage culturally sensitive terms to target firearm suicide prevention [60,99,102,107]. Potentially alienating the groups that a prevention strategy is meant to influence can undermine and further isolate and detach those groups, therefore creating more harm. Wherever possible, including members of the community within the design, implementation, and evaluation of suicide-prevention strategies should be prioritized [111]. Messaging and intervention needs may also vary over time. The multiple stressors related to the COVID-19 pandemic have raised concerns about the potential for a coming suicide pandemic. Stay-at-home orders, isolation, and limited access to mental health services contribute to increased anxiety, depression, and suicidal thoughts [112,113], especially among youth [114]. In the United States, the COVID-19 pandemic and social and political unrest fueled gun sales in 2020 [115,116], where an estimated 40% were first-time gun owners [117]. Lethal means safety efforts are doubly important in the United States during a time of increased stress and increased firearms access. A focus on accurate data collection, analysis, and most importantly, sustained prevention [118], is necessary within the volatile climate of this pandemic to mitigate its impact on suicide.

SUMMARY

Overall, means safety is an evidence-based, effective strategy to prevent suicide, but there are challenges within different mechanisms that make its implementation challenging or limited. Therefore, means safety should be used in conjunction with other suicide-prevention strategies within a comprehensive suicide prevention framework and across levels from societal to individual. With coordinated effort, ongoing evaluation, and dissemination of evidence-based practices, means safety approaches offer an opportunity to help prevent suicides in the United States and internationally.

CLINICS CARE POINTS

- Lethal means safety (reducing access to firearms and other highly lethal methods of suicide) is an evidence-based, recommended component of suicide prevention.
- Means safety approaches span from society-level interventions (like laws limiting access) to interventions to encourage individuals to change their own behavior or access.
- Across geographic areas, interventions should be tailored to reflect the most common and most lethal methods of suicide.
- "Culturally competent" approaches to means safety, including collaboration with stakeholders, may help overcome political or cultural objections.

DISCLOSURE

The authors' time was supported by NIH/NIMH Grant Number R61 MH125754. The contents of this work are the authors' sole responsibility and do not necessarily represent official funder views or the views of the Department of Veterans Affairs. The authors report no commercial or financial conflicts of interest.

REFERENCES

[1] Suicide data. In: World Health Organization. 2020. Available at: http://www.who.int/mental_health/prevention/suicide/suicideprevent/en/. Accessed November 6, 2020.

[2] FastStats - Suicide and Self-Inflicted Injury. In: Centers for Disease Control and Prevention. 2020. Available at: https://www.cdc.gov/nchs/fastats/suicide.htm. Accessed September 29, 2020.

[3] Hedegaard H, Curtin SC, Warner M. Increase in Suicide Mortality in the United States, 1999–2018. 2020. In: Centers for Disease Control. Available at: https://www.cdc.gov/nchs/products/databriefs/db362.htm. Accessed November 30, 2020.

[4] Curtin SC, Heron M. Death rates due to suicide and homicide among persons aged 10–24: United States, 2000–2017. NCHS Data Brief, no 352. Hyattsville (MD): National Center for Health Statistics; 2019.

[5] 2012 National Strategy for Suicide Prevention: Goals and Objectives for Action: A Report of the U.S. Surgeon General and of the National Action Alliance for Suicide Prevention. In: US Department of Health & Human Services. Available at: http://www.ncbi.nlm.nih.gov/books/NBK109917/. Accessed November 25, 2020.

[6] Stanley IH, Hom MA, Rogers ML, et al. Discussing firearm ownership and access as part of suicide risk assessment and prevention: "means safety" versus "means restriction. Arch Suicide Res 2017;21(2):237–53.

[7] Victor SE, Klonsky ED. Correlates of suicide attempts among self-injurers: a meta-analysis. Clin Psychol Rev 2014;34(4):282–97.

[8] Burke TA, Alloy LB. Moving Toward an Ideation-to-Action Framework in Suicide Research: A Commentary on. Clin Psychol Publ Div 2016;23(1):26–30.

[9] May AM, Klonsky ED. What distinguishes suicide attempters from suicide ideators? a meta-analysis of potential factors. Clin Psychol Sci Pract 2016;23(1):5–20.

[10] Barber CW, Miller MJ. Reducing a suicidal person's access to lethal means of suicide: a research agenda. Am J Prev Med 2014;47(3 Suppl 2):S264–72.

[11] Suicide. In: World Health Organization. 2020. Available at: https://www.who.int/news-room/fact-sheets/detail/suicide. Accessed November 30, 2020.

[12] Lin J-J, Chang S-S, Lu T-H. The leading methods of suicide in Taiwan, 2002-2008. BMC Public Health 2010;10(1):480.

[13] Suicides in England and Wales - Office for National Statistics. In: Office for National Statistics. 2020. Available at: https://www.ons.gov.uk/peoplepopulationandcommunity/birthsdeathsandmarriages/deaths/bulletins/suicidesintheunitedkingdom/2019registrations. Accessed November 30, 2020.

[14] Ojima T, Nakamura Y, Detels R. Comparative study about methods of suicide between Japan and the United States. J Epidemiol 2004;14(6):187–92.

[15] The Social-Ecological Model: A Framework for Prevention In: Violence Prevention Centers for Disease Control and Prevention. 2020. Available at: https://www.cdc.gov/violenceprevention/publichealthissue/social-ecologicalmodel.html. Accessed November 6, 2020.
[16] Allchin A, Chaplin V, Horwitz J. Limiting access to lethal means: applying the social ecological model for firearm suicide prevention. Inj Prev 2019;25(Suppl 1):i44–8.
[17] Kreitman N. The coal gas story. United Kingdom suicide rates, 1960-71. Br J Prev Soc Med 1976;30(2): 86–93.
[18] Chen Y-Y, Chen F, Chang S-S, et al. Assessing the efficacy of restricting access to barbecue charcoal for suicide prevention in taiwan: a community-based intervention trial. PLoS One 2015;10(8):e0133809.
[19] Gunnell D, Knipe D, Chang S-S, et al. Prevention of suicide with regulations aimed at restricting access to highly hazardous pesticides: a systematic review of the international evidence. Lancet Glob Health 2017; 5(10):e1026–37.
[20] Gilmour S, Wattanakamolkul K, Sugai MK. The Effect of the Australian National Firearms Agreement on Suicide and Homicide Mortality, 1978–2015. Am J Public Health 2018;108(11):1511–6.
[21] Chapman S, Alpers P, Agho K, et al. Australia's 1996 gun law reforms: faster falls in firearm deaths, firearm suicides, and a decade without mass shootings. Inj Prev 2006;12(6):365–72.
[22] Thoeni N, Reisch T, Hemmer A, et al. Suicide by firearm in Switzerland: who uses the army weapon? Results from the national survey between 2000 and 2010. Swiss Med Wkly 2018;148:w14646.
[23] Lubin G, Werbeloff N, Halperin D, et al. Decrease in suicide rates after a change of policy reducing access to firearms in adolescents: a naturalistic epidemiological study. Suicide Life Threat Behav 2010;40(5):421–4.
[24] Anestis MD, Anestis JC. Suicide Rates and State Laws Regulating Access and Exposure to Handguns. Am J Public Health 2015;105(10):2049–58.
[25] Kivisto AJ, Phalen PL. Effects of risk-based firearm seizure laws in connecticut and indiana on suicide rates, 1981-2015. Psychiatr Serv Wash DC 2018;69(8):855–62.
[26] Swanson JW, Easter MM, Alanis-Hirsch K, et al. Criminal justice and suicide outcomes with indiana's risk-based gun seizure law. J Am Acad Psychiatry Law 2019;47(2):188–97.
[27] Kivisto AJ, Kivisto KL, Gurnell E, et al. Adolescent suicide, household firearm ownership, and the effects of child access prevention laws. J Am Acad Child Adolesc Psychiatry 2020. https://doi.org/10.1016/j.jaac.2020.08.442.
[28] Rivara FP, Vars FE, Rowhani-Rahbar A. Three Interventions to Address the Other Pandemic-Firearm Injury and Death. JAMA 2021;325(4):343–4, 206.
[29] Okolie C, Wood S, Hawton K, et al. Means restriction for the prevention of suicide by jumping. Cochrane Database Syst Rev 2020;2:CD013543.
[30] Yeh C, Lester D. Suicides from the Golden Gate Bridge: have they changed over time? Psychol Rep 2010; 107(2):491–2.
[31] Stack S. Crisis phones - suicide prevention versus suggestion/contagion effects. Crisis 2015;36(3):220–4.
[32] Larsen ME, Cummins N, Boonstra TW, et al. The use of technology in Suicide Prevention. Annu Int Conf IEEE Eng Med Biol Soc 2015;2015:7316–9.
[33] Saving Lives at the Golden Gate Bridge. In: Golden Gate Bridge. 2018. Available at: https://www.goldengatebridgenet.org/. Accessed November 25, 2020.
[34] Kariippanon K, Wilson CJ, McCarthy TJ, et al. A call for preventing suicide by hanging from ceiling fans: an interdisciplinary research agenda. Int J Environ Res Public Health 2019;16(15):2708.
[35] Yang CHJ, Doshi M, Mason NA. Analysis of medications returned during a medication take-back event. Pharm J Pharm Educ Pract 2015;3(3):79–88.
[36] Yanovitzky I. The American medicine chest challenge: evaluation of a drug take-back and disposal campaign. J Stud Alcohol Drugs 2016;77(4):549–55.
[37] Egan KL, Gregory E, Sparks M, et al. From dispensed to disposed: evaluating the effectiveness of disposal programs through a comparison with prescription drug monitoring program data. Am J Drug Alcohol Abuse 2017;43(1):69–77.
[38] Kozak MA, Melton JR, Gernant SA, et al. A needs assessment of unused and expired medication disposal practices: A study from the Medication Safety Research Network of Indiana. Res Soc Adm Pharm 2016;12(2): 336–40.
[39] Barber C, Frank E, Demicco R. Reducing suicides through partnerships between health professionals and gun owner groups-beyond docs vs glocks. JAMA Intern Med 2017;177(1):5–6.
[40] Polzer E, Brandspigel S, Kelly T, et al. "Gun shop projects" for suicide prevention in the USA: current state and future directions. Inj Prev 2020;27(2):150–4.
[41] Kelly T, Brandspigel S, Polzer E, et al. Firearm storage maps: a pragmatic approach to reduce firearm suicide during times of risk. Ann Intern Med 2020;172(5): 351–3.
[42] Barber C, Berrigan JW, Sobelson Henn M, et al. Linking public safety and public health data for firearm suicide prevention in Utah. Health Aff Proj Hope 2019;38(10): 1695–701.
[43] Bridge JA, Horowitz LM, Fontanella CA, et al. Age-Related Racial Disparity in Suicide Rates Among US Youths From 2001 Through 2015. JAMA Pediatr 2018;172(7):697–9.
[44] Shain BN. Increases in rates of suicide and suicide attempts among black adolescents. Pediatrics 2019; 144(5):e20191912.
[45] Meyerhoff J, Rohan KJ, Fondacaro KM. Suicide and Suicide-related Behavior among Bhutanese Refugees Resettled in the United States. Asian Am J Psychol 2018; 9(4):270–83.

[46] Clifford AC, Doran CM, Tsey K. A systematic review of suicide prevention interventions targeting indigenous peoples in Australia, United States, Canada and New Zealand. BMC Public Health 2013;13(1):463.

[47] Tomsich EA, Kravitz-Wirtz N, Pallin R, et al. Firearm Ownership Among LGBT Adults in California. Violence Gend 2020;7(3):102–8.

[48] Incidents and Offenses. 2020. In: FBI. Available at: https://ucr.fbi.gov/hate-crime/2019/topic-pages/incidents-and-offenses. Accessed March 23, 2021.

[49] King M, Semlyen J, Tai SS, et al. A systematic review of mental disorder, suicide, and deliberate self harm in lesbian, gay and bisexual people. BMC Psychiatry 2008;8:70.

[50] Ivey Stephenson AZ, Demissie Z, Crosby AE, et al. Suicidal ideation and behaviors among high school students — youth risk behavior survey, United States, 2019. MMWR Suppl 2020;69(1):47–55.

[51] The Trevor Project — Saving Young LGBTQ Lives. 2021. In: The Trevor Project. Available at: https://www.thetrevorproject.org/. Accessed March 23, 2021.

[52] Hoffmire CA, Kemp JE, Bossarte RM. Changes in suicide mortality for veterans and nonveterans by gender and history of VHA Service Use, 2000-2010. Psychiatr Serv Wash DC 2015;66(9):959–65.

[53] Defense Suicide Prevention Office. In: Defense Suicide Prevention Office. 2019. Available at: https://www.dspo.mil/. Accessed October 30, 2020.

[54] Lethal Means Counseling: Recommendations for Providers. In: Department of Veterans Affairs and Department of Defense. 2020. Available at: https://www.healthquality.va.gov/guidelines/MH/srb/LethalMeansProviders20200527508.pdf. Accessed October 30, 2020.

[55] Tsai J, Snitkin M, Trevisan L, et al. Awareness of Suicide Prevention Programs Among U.S. Military Veterans. Adm Policy Ment Health 2020;47(1):115–25.

[56] National Academies of Sciences. Military Service Members and Veterans. 2018. Available at: https://www.ncbi.nlm.nih.gov/books/NBK540132/. Accessed November 6, 2020.

[57] Executive Order 13861 - PREVENTS. In: U.S. Department of Veterans Affairs. 2020. Available at: https://www.va.gov/PREVENTS/EO-13861.asp. Accessed November 6, 2020.

[58] Monteith LL, Wendleton L, Bahraini NH, et al. Together With Veterans: VA National Strategy Alignment and Lessons Learned from Community-Based Suicide Prevention for Rural Veterans. Suicide Life Threat Behav 2020;50(3):588–600.

[59] Flanagan CA, Elek-Fisk E, Gallay LS. Friends don't let friends ...or do they? Developmental and gender differences in intervening in friends' ATOD use. J Drug Educ 2004;34(4):351–71.

[60] Pallin R, Siry B, Azrael D, et al. "Hey, let me hold your guns for a while": A qualitative study of messaging for firearm suicide prevention. Behav Sci Law 2019;37(3):259–69.

[61] Marino E, Wolsko C, Keys S, et al. Addressing the cultural challenges of firearm restriction in suicide prevention: a test of public health messaging to protect those at risk. Arch Suicide Res 2018;22(3):394–404.

[62] Suicide Prevention Toolkit Items. In: NSSF. 2020. Available at: https://nssf.wpengine.com/safety/suicide-prevention/suicide-prevention-toolkit/. Accessed November 25, 2020.

[63] A Guide for Parents: Understanding Youth Mental Health and Preventing Unauthorized Access to Firearms. 2020. Available at: https://www.nssf.org/a-guide-for-parents-understanding-youth-mental-health-and-preventing-unauthorized-access-to-firearms/. Accessed December 16, 2020.

[64] Reifels L, Mishara BL, Dargis L, et al. Outcomes of community-based suicide prevention approaches that involve reducing access to pesticides: a systematic literature review. Suicide Life Threat Behav 2019;49(4):1019–31.

[65] Weerasinghe M, Konradsen F, Eddleston M, et al. Potential interventions for preventing pesticide self-poisoning by restricting access through vendors in Sri Lanka. Crisis 2018;39(6):479–88.

[66] Rowhani-Rahbar A, Simonetti JA, Rivara FP. Effectiveness of interventions to promote safe firearm storage. Epidemiol Rev 2016;38(1):111–24.

[67] Roszko PJD, Ameli J, Carter PM, et al. Clinician Attitudes, Screening Practices, and Interventions to Reduce Firearm-Related Injury. Epidemiol Rev 2016;38(1):87–110.

[68] Miller M, Salhi C, Barber C, et al. Changes in Firearm and Medication Storage Practices in Homes of Youths at Risk for Suicide: Results of the SAFETY Study, a Clustered, Emergency Department-Based, Multisite, Stepped-Wedge Trial. Ann Emerg Med 2020;76(2):194–205.

[69] Boggs JM, Beck A, Ritzwoller DP, et al. A Quasi-Experimental Analysis of Lethal Means Assessment and Risk for Subsequent Suicide Attempts and Deaths. J Gen Intern Med 2020;35(6):1709–14.

[70] Boggs JM, Quintana LM, Powers JD, et al. Frequency of clinicians' assessments for access to lethal means in persons at risk for suicide. Arch Suicide Res 2020;1–10. https://doi.org/10.1080/13811118.2020.1761917.

[71] Mueller KL, Naganathan S, Griffey RT. Counseling on access to lethal means-emergency department (CALM-ED): a quality improvement program for firearm injury prevention. West J Emerg Med 2020;21(5):1123–30.

[72] Talley CL, Campbell BT, Jenkins DH, et al. Recommendations from the American College of Surgeons Committee on Trauma's Firearm Strategy Team (FAST) Workgroup: Chicago Consensus I. J Am Coll Surg 2019;228(2):198–206.

[73] Bulger EM, Kuhls DA, Campbell BT, et al. Proceedings from the Medical Summit on Firearm Injury Prevention: A Public Health Approach to Reduce Death and

Disability in the US. J Am Coll Surg 2019;229(4): 415–30.e12.

[74] Wintemute GJ, Betz ME, Ranney ML. Yes, you can: physicians, patients, and firearms. Ann Intern Med 2016; 165(3):205.

[75] Betz ME, Azrael D, Barber C, et al. Public opinion regarding whether speaking with patients about firearms is appropriate: results of a national survey. Ann Intern Med 2016;165(8):543–50.

[76] James IP. Blood alcohol levels following successful suicide. Q J Stud Alcohol 1966;27(1):23–9.

[77] Pompili M, Serafini G, Innamorati M, et al. Suicidal behavior and alcohol abuse. Int J Environ Res Public Health 2010;7(4):1392–431.

[78] Boggs JM, Beck A, Hubley S, et al. General medical, mental health, and demographic risk factors associated with suicide by firearm compared with other means. Psychiatr Serv 2018;69(6):677–84.

[79] Gipson P, King C. Health behavior theories and research: implications for suicidal individuals' treatment linkage and adherence. Cogn Behav Pract 2012; 19(2):209–17.

[80] Stuber JP, Massey A, Meadows M, et al. SAFER brief community intervention: a primary suicide prevention strategy to improve firearm and medication storage behaviour. Inj Prev 2020. https://doi.org/10.1136/injuryprev-2020-043902.

[81] Lock To Live. In: Lock to Live. 2018. Available at: http://lock2live.org/. Accessed November 25, 2020.

[82] Betz ME, Knoepke CE, Simpson S, et al. An interactive web-based lethal means safety decision aid for suicidal adults (lock to live): pilot randomized controlled trial. J Med Internet Res 2020;22(1):e16253.

[83] Grossman DC, Stafford HA, Koepsell TD, et al. Improving firearm storage in Alaska native villages: a randomized trial of household gun cabinets. Am J Public Health 2012;102(Suppl 2):S291–7.

[84] Simonetti JA, Rowhani-Rahbar A, King C, et al. Evaluation of a community-based safe firearm and ammunition storage intervention. Inj Prev 2018;24(3):218–23.

[85] Cuthbertson C, Brennan A, Shutske J, et al. Developing and implementing farm stress training to address agricultural producer mental health. Health Promot Pract 2020. https://doi.org/10.1177/1524839920931849 1524839920931849.

[86] Kennedy AJ, Brumby SA, Versace VL, et al. The ripple effect: a digital intervention to reduce suicide stigma among farming men. BMC Public Health 2020;20(1): 813.

[87] Bryan CJ, Bryan AO, Anestis MD. Rates of Preparatory Suicidal Behaviors across Subgroups of Protective Firearm Owners. Arch Suicide Res 2020;1–13. https://doi.org/10.1080/13811118.2020.1848672.

[88] Cj B, Ao B, Anestis MD. Associations among exaggerated threat perceptions, suicidal thoughts, and suicidal behaviors in U.S. firearm owners. J Psychiatr Res 2020;131:94–101.

[89] Morgan ER, Gomez A, Rowhani-Rahbar A. Firearm Ownership, Storage Practices, and Suicide Risk Factors in Washington State, 2013-2016. Am J Public Health 2018;108(7):882–8.

[90] Miller M, Swanson SA, Azrael D. Are we missing something pertinent? a bias analysis of unmeasured confounding in the firearm-suicide literature. Epidemiol Rev 2016;38(1):62–9.

[91] Anestis MD, Bandel SL, Butterworth SE, et al. Suicide risk and firearm ownership and storage behavior in a large military sample. Psychiatry Res 2020;291:113277.

[92] Bryan CJ, Bryan AO, Anestis MD, et al. Firearm availability and storage practices among military personnel who have thought about suicide. JAMA Netw open 2019;2(8):e199160.

[93] Butterworth SE, Daruwala SE, Anestis MD. The role of reason for firearm ownership in beliefs about firearms and suicide, openness to means safety, and current firearm storage. Suicide life-threatening Behav 2020; 50(3):617–30.

[94] Buus N, Juel A, Haskelberg H, et al. User Involvement in Developing the MYPLAN Mobile Phone Safety Plan App for People in Suicidal Crisis: Case Study. JMIR Ment Health 2019;6(4):e11965.

[95] Conti EC, Jahn DR, Simons KV, et al. Safety Planning to Manage Suicide Risk with Older Adults: Case Examples and Recommendations. Clin Gerontol 2020;43(1): 104–9.

[96] Stanley B, Brown GK. Safety Planning Intervention: A Brief Intervention to Mitigate Suicide Risk. Cogn Behav Pract 2012;19(2):256–64.

[97] Camidge DR, Wood RJ, Bateman DN. The epidemiology of self-poisoning in the UK. Br J Clin Pharmacol 2003;56(6):613–9.

[98] Gladden RM, O'Donnell J, Mattson CL, et al. Changes in Opioid-Involved Overdose Deaths by Opioid Type and Presence of Benzodiazepines, Cocaine, and Methamphetamine - 25 States, July-December 2017 to January-June 2018. MMWR Morb Mortal Wkly Rep 2019;68(34):737–44.

[99] Pierpoint LA, Tung GJ, Brooks-Russell A, et al. Gun retailers as storage partners for suicide prevention: what barriers need to be overcome? Inj Prev 2019;25(Suppl 1):i5–8.

[100] Brooks-Russell A, Runyan C, Betz ME, et al. Law Enforcement Agencies' Perceptions of the Benefits of and Barriers to Temporary Firearm Storage to Prevent Suicide. Am J Public Health 2019;109(2):285–8.

[101] Gunnell D, Bennewith O, Hawton K, et al. The epidemiology and prevention of suicide by hanging: a systematic review. Int J Epidemiol 2005;34(2):433–42, 8.

[102] Anestis MD, Bond AE, Bryan AO, et al. An examination of preferred messengers on firearm safety for suicide prevention. Prev Med 2021;145:106452.

[103] Wolsko C, Marino E, Keys S. Affirming cultural values for health: The case of firearm restriction in suicide prevention. Soc Sci Med 2020;248:112706.

[104] Betz ME, Miller M, Barber C, et al. Lethal means restriction for suicide prevention: beliefs and behaviors of emergency department providers. Depress Anxiety 2013;30(10):1013–20.

[105] Betz ME, Brooks-Russell A, Brandspigel S, et al. Counseling suicidal patients about access to lethal means: attitudes of emergency nurse leaders. J Emerg Nurs 2018; 44(5):499–504.

[106] Zhou E, DeCou CR, Stuber J, et al. Usual Care for Emergency Department Patients Who Present with Suicide Risk: A Survey of Hospital Procedures in Washington State. Arch Suicide Res 2020;24(3):342–54.

[107] Benjamin Wolk C, Van Pelt AE, Jager-Hyman S, et al. Stakeholder perspectives on implementing a firearm safety intervention in pediatric primary care as a universal suicide prevention strategy: a qualitative study. JAMA Netw Open 2018;1(7):e185309.

[108] Tøllefsen IM, Hem E, Ekeberg Ø. The reliability of suicide statistics: a systematic review. BMC Psychiatry 2012;12:9.

[109] Sainsbury P, Jenkins JS. The accuracy of officially reported suicide statistics for purposes of epidemiological research. J Epidemiol Community Health 1982;36(1): 43–8.

[110] Pearson M, Metcalfe C, Jayamanne S, et al. Effectiveness of household lockable pesticide storage to reduce pesticide self-poisoning in rural Asia: a community-based, cluster-randomised controlled trial. Lancet 2017; 390(10105):1863–72.

[111] Marino E, Wolsko C, Keys SG, et al. A culture gap in the United States: Implications for policy on limiting access to firearms for suicidal persons. J Public Health Policy 2016;37(Suppl 1):110–21.

[112] Gunnell D, Appleby L, Arensman E, et al. Suicide risk and prevention during the COVID-19 pandemic. Lancet Psychiatry 2020;7(6):468–71.

[113] Reger MA, Stanley IH, Joiner TE. Suicide mortality and coronavirus disease 2019-a perfect storm? JAMA Psychiatry 2020;77(11):1093–4.

[114] Zhang L, Zhang D, Fang J, et al. Assessment of mental health of chinese primary school students before and after school closing and opening during the COVID-19 Pandemic. JAMA Netw Open 2020;3(9):e2021482.

[115] Caputi TL, Ayers JW, Dredze M, et al. Collateral Crises of Gun Preparation and the COVID-19 Pandemic: Infodemiology Study. JMIR Public Health Surveill 2020; 6(2):e19369.

[116] Hoops K, Johnson T, Grossman ER, et al. Stay-at-home orders and firearms in the United States during the COVID-19 pandemic. Prev Med 2020;141:106281.

[117] First-Time Gun Buyers Grow to Nearly 5 Million in 2020. In: NSSF. 2020. Available at: https://nssf.wpengine.com/first-time-gun-buyers-grow-to-nearly-5-million-in-2020/. Accessed December 4, 2020.

[118] John A, Pirkis J, Gunnell D, et al. Trends in suicide during the covid-19 pandemic. BMJ 2020;371.

Advances in Psychiatry and Behavioral Health 1 (2021) 91–106

ADVANCES IN PSYCHIATRY AND BEHAVIORAL HEALTH

Treatment of Premenstrual Dysphoric Disorder (PMDD)

Advances and Challenges

Liisa Hantsoo, PhD*, Julia Riddle, MD

Department of Psychiatry and Behavioral Sciences, The Johns Hopkins University School of Medicine, 550 North Broadway Street, Baltimore, MD, USA

KEYWORDS

• Menstrual cycle • Mood disorder • Women • Premenstrual • Selective serotonin reuptake inhibitor
• Hormonal contraceptive • Oophorectomy • Premenstrual dysphoric disorder

KEY POINTS

- PMDD is a severe mood disorder that affects around 5% of reproductive-aged women, but is challenging to diagnose and often underrecognized or misdiagnosed by clinicians.
- Key challenges in diagnosing PMDD are utilizing prospective daily ratings to ensure symptom entrainment to the menstrual cycle, ruling out other psychiatric diagnoses, assessing comorbidities, and ruling out premenstrual worsening of psychiatric diagnoses.
- PMDD treatment options include intermittent or continuous administration of SSRIs, oral contraceptives, cognitive-behavioral treatment, GnRH medications, or hysterectomy-BSO; treatment challenges include appropriate use of intermittent SSRI dosing, nonresponse to SSRIs, managing medications in the context of comorbidities, and managing treatment through reproductive transitions.
- Additional research is needed in nonpharmacologic (third-wave, internet-based interventions), and pharmacologic (nonoral hormonal contraceptives, neuroactive steroid-based medications) management of PMDD, and treatment during reproductive transitions.

INTRODUCTION

Premenstrual dysphoric disorder (PMDD) is an affective disorder characterized by mood symptoms that initiate during the luteal (premenstrual) phase of the menstrual cycle and resolve with menses onset [1,2]. As an affective disorder, primary PMDD symptoms include irritability, depressed mood, anxiety, and mood lability. PMDD may also include physical symptoms (eg, bloating, headache). According to *Diagnostic and Statistical Manual of Mental Disorders* (*DSM-5*) criteria, PMDD requires a premenstrual pattern of at least five mood and/or physical symptoms, including at least one core mood symptom (mood lability, irritability, anxiety, or low mood) [3]. While around one in 20 menstruating women have PMDD [4], the disorder is underrecognized by clinicians and therefore often misdiagnosed or treated suboptimally [5,6]. In this review, we focus on challenges in diagnosing and treating PMDD, and recent treatment developments; for a general overview of PMDD diagnosis and treatment, we refer the reader to other reviews [7–11].

Diagnosis Informs Treatment

Accurate diagnosis of PMDD is the first step toward providing effective treatment. Critically, to meet *DSM-5*

*Corresponding author, *E-mail address:* LHantso1@jhmi.edu

https://doi.org/10.1016/j.ypsc.2021.05.009
2667-3827/21/

diagnostic criteria, symptoms must be confirmed via prospective daily ratings during at least two menstrual cycles and be present for most menstrual cycles in the previous year. There are numerous daily symptom measures to aid in PMDD diagnosis, including the Daily Record of Severity of Problems (DRSP) [12], the Calendar of Premenstrual Experiences (COPE) [13,14], or the Prospective Record of Impact and Severity of Menstrual Symptoms (PRISM) [15]. Prospective daily ratings allow the clinician to confirm that symptoms are entrained to the menstrual cycle, distinguishing PMDD from other cyclic affective disorders such as bipolar disorder or cyclothymia. The clinician should also rule out disorders such as major depressive disorder (MDD); PMDD is distinct from other depressive disorders, as it often presents as mood lability, irritability, and/or anxiety as opposed to low mood [1,16–18]. The clinician should rule out medical causes, such as chronic fatigue syndrome, fibromyalgia, anemia, and migraine disorder.

PMDD should also be distinguished from other menstrual cycle entrained mood symptoms, such as premenstrual syndrome (PMS) or premenstrual exacerbation (PME) of another psychiatric disorder. Importantly, PMS is not a psychiatric disorder per *DSM*; it is a clinical syndrome that can include mild mood symptoms or purely physical symptoms. The American College of Obstetrics and Gynecology (ACOG) defines PMS as one physical or psychological symptom in the 5 days prior to menses [19]. The symptom(s) must occur in three consecutive menstrual cycles, subside within 4 days of menses onset, cause impairment, and be verified by prospective rating. Some women with a psychiatric diagnosis experience PME, a worsening of psychiatric symptoms in the premenstruum. For instance, over 60% of women with MDD reported premenstrual worsening [20–22]. It is crucial to differentiate PMDD from PME when evaluating a patient, as women with PME will likely not respond appropriately to treatments that are indicated for PMDD. Finally, some patients with PMDD meet criteria for a secondary affective disorder. In these cases, the PMDD symptoms are clearly entrained to the menstrual cycle and markedly different from the symptoms of the other psychiatric diagnoses.

PREMENSTRUAL DYSPHORIC DISORDER TREATMENT

For a treatment algorithm for PMDD, we refer the reader to the up-to-date guidelines [23]. The American Academy of Family Physicians [24] also offers PMDD treatment guidelines, while ACOG [19] and the Royal College of Obstetricians and Gynaecologists (RCOG) [25] offer treatment guidelines for PMS. Surprisingly, there are no treatment guidelines from the major psychiatric organizations.

Selective Serotonin Reuptake Inhibitors

The latest up-to-date treatment guidelines [23] recommend pharmacotherapy, particularly selective serotonin reuptake inhibitors (SSRIs), as a first-line treatment for PMDD [19,25]. Clinical trials have examined various SSRIs in treating PMDD or severe PMS, including sertraline [26–37], paroxetine [38–46], citalopram [47], escitalopram [48,49], and fluoxetine [50–55]. Meta-analyses have indicated that SSRIs are effective for PMDD, reducing symptoms significantly more than placebo [56,57], including both mood and physical symptoms [58]. However, in meta-analyses, SSRIs have shown only small to medium effect sizes [59].

Dose ranges

In contrast to MDD, relatively low SSRI doses reduce PMDD symptoms [32]. A 2013 Cochrane meta-analysis summarized dosages used in clinical trials of SSRIs for PMDD, which included low doses (10 mg fluoxetine, 25–50 mg sertraline, 10–12.5 mg paroxetine, 10 mg escitalopram) and moderate doses (20 mg fluoxetine, 100–105 mg sertraline, 20–30 mg paroxetine, 20–50 mg escitalopram, 20–50 mg citalopram) [56]. The meta-analysis concluded that while low doses of SSRIs are effective for PMDD, moderate doses were associated with a larger effect size and higher response rate [56]. Steiner and colleagues, in their 2006 expert treatment guidelines for PMDD and severe PMS, outlined similar low-to-moderate SSRI dose ranges [10]. These relatively low SSRI doses may be effective because SSRIs act as selective brain steroidogenic stimulants at doses that are inactive on serotonergic function, altering the conversion of progesterone to its neuroactive metabolite, allopregnanolone [60].

Intermittent dosing, symptom-onset therapy

SSRIs have a short onset of therapeutic action in PMDD, reducing symptoms within 12 to 36 hours [61,62]. As described above, this is likely due not to serotonergic mechanisms, but via neuroactive steroid mechanisms that occur in a more rapid timeframe [60]. Thus, SSRIs can be administered continuously (taken daily), or intermittently (taken only during the luteal phase) [32,39,63]. Intermittent dosing includes *luteal dosing* and *symptom-onset dosing*. In luteal dosing, a woman takes the SSRI within her luteal phase, starting at ovulation (usually approximated via menstrual cycle tracking). In symptom-onset dosing, she takes the SSRI once her symptoms have initiated, often in the week prior to menses [45,49,62,64]. SSRIs are stopped when menstruation begins, although some women will continue to take the SSRI for the first few days of their cycle if symptoms persist during menses [36]. Both continuous and intermittent SSRI treatments are efficacious for PMDD [56], with meta-analyses showing moderate to large effect sizes for both approaches [57,58]. Intermittent treatment may be most beneficial for irritability and affect lability, with a lesser effect on depressed mood and somatic symptoms [39]. Intermittent treatment may be preferred for patients who experience SSRI side effects, such as nausea, insomnia, headache, or sexual dysfunction [56,58].

Hormonal Contraceptives

While oral contraceptive pills (OCPs) are considered a first-line treatment for PMDD [25], there is mixed evidence for OCPs' efficacy in treating PMDD [65]. The OCP Yaz (drospirenone 3 mg plus ethinyl estradiol 20 μg), which is administered in a 24 to 4 dosing scheme (ie, 24 active hormone pills followed by four hormone-free pills), is the only OCP that is FDA-approved for PMDD treatment. A meta-analysis of combined oral contraceptives found that Yaz reduced severe PMDD symptoms, but there was a large placebo effect [66]. Hormone monotherapy appears less effective than combined hormones. For instance, a Cochrane review meta-analysis of progesterone for PMS did not find strong evidence for progesterone use alone [67]. Regarding monophasic (same dose of hormone daily) versus multiphasic (varying levels of hormones across a 21- or 28-day cycle) OCPs, monophasic pills are generally recommended [23] to avoid fluctuations in hormone levels that may contribute to mood deterioration in PMDD [68]. However, few studies have compared monophasic versus multiphasic OCPs head-to-head [69].

Continuous dosing of oral contraceptives refers to skipping the week of placebo pills, thus avoiding frequent hormonal fluctuations. A randomized, double-blind, placebo-controlled trial with an open-label substudy on continuous dosing of levonorgestrel (90 μg) and ethinyl estradiol (20 μg) showed some improvement of premenstrual symptoms [70]. However, there was a high placebo response rate.

Finally, there have been no rigorous placebo-controlled trials to examine the impact of other hormonal contraceptive formulations, such as patches, vaginal rings, progestin implants or injections, or hormone-containing intrauterine devices (IUDs), on PMDD symptoms [71]. Indeed, progestins in these forms of birth control may exacerbate PMDD symptoms [72].

Psychotherapy

Cognitive-behavioral therapy (CBT) is also a first-line treatment for PMDD, alone or in combination with medication. CBT includes cognitive restructuring and behavioral modification. However, there are no manualized CBT treatments specifically for PMDD.

In meta-analyses, CBT interventions for PMDD produce small to medium effect sizes and are superior to control conditions [59,73]. However, there are few rigorous, high-quality RCTs. A 2009 systematic review of CBT for PMDD found little evidence for CBT effects on premenstrual mood symptoms, largely due to inadequate study design [74]. Those authors recommended more rigorous clinical trials of traditional CBT interventions for PMDD, as well as research on mindfulness or acceptance-based interventions for PMDD. These third-wave interventions may be suited to PMDD. For instance, an 8-week mindfulness group intervention in women with mild to moderate PMS reduced anxiety and depressive symptoms [75]. A similar 8-week mindfulness-based group intervention reduced premenstrual depression, hopelessness, anxiety, mood lability, interpersonal sensitivity, irritability, and conflict with others, compared with a control group [76].

Regarding the combination of psychotherapy and medication, meta-analysis suggests no added benefit from combined treatment [59]. In a study comparing CBT, fluoxetine alone, or fluoxetine plus CBT, all three groups showed similar improvement over 6 months, although fluoxetine improved symptoms more rapidly than CBT [77]. While SSRIs may improve premenstrual affective symptoms, CBT increased the use of adaptive coping strategies and shifted attribution of premenstrual symptoms [59]. CBT also showed better maintenance of treatment effect at follow-up, compared to SSRI [59].

Gonadotropin-Releasing Hormone Medications

Gonadotropin-releasing hormone (GnRH) stimulates the synthesis and secretion of luteinizing hormone (LH) and follicular-stimulating hormone (FSH) via changes in GnRH pulse size and frequency. GnRH pulsatility is essential for the regulation of menstruation. GnRH agonists and antagonists, both of which alter this pulsatility, are a second-line treatment for PMDD, and should only be considered when the patient has failed multiple treatment trials. GnRH medications suppress ovarian function, reducing estradiol and progesterone to postmenopausal levels. In addition to myriad multisystem short-term risks, these medications carry long-term risks even after cessation, including bone density loss, memory changes, insomnia, hypertension, joint pain, weight gain, hot flashes, acne, and decreased libido [78]. This "chemical oophorectomy" may also test how a woman's PMDD symptoms would respond to surgical oophorectomy [79].

Leuprolide acetate (Lupron) is a GnRH agonist that significantly improved PMDD symptoms in several trials [80–83]. Similarly, the low-dose GnRH agonist buserelin significantly reduced premenstrual irritability and depression [84]. Approximately 60% to 70% of women with PMDD respond to GnRH treatment [85], and research suggests that women with fewer acute sharp increases and decreases in mood symptoms and regular cyclic mood changes are more likely to respond to GnRH treatment than women with other symptom dynamics [80,85].

Surgical Oophorectomy

Hysterectomy and bilateral salpingo-oophorectomy (BSO) is a final treatment option for severe PMDD that has not responded to other treatments. In 2013, the International Society for Premenstrual Disorders (ISPMD) included hysterectomy-BSO in its consensus on the management of premenstrual disorders [86]. However, there are few clinical trials on hysterectomy-BSO for PMDD, and sample sizes are small [87–89]. Among women interviewed following hysterectomy-BSO for PMS or PMDD, 96% reported being "satisfied" or "very satisfied" with the treatment, and 93.6% reported complete resolution of their premenstrual symptoms [89].

While existing studies suggest that hysterectomy-BSO is effective in managing PMDD symptoms, the permanent effects of premature menopause, including higher risk of bone loss, heart disease, vaginal dryness, urinary incontinence, and decreased libido, must be weighed against the benefits of relief from PMDD. Because of these lasting effects, confirmation of diagnosis, adequate trials of other treatments, and documented success with medical ovarian suppression (GnRH medications) should be pursued prior to surgical intervention.

TREATMENT CHALLENGES

Medication Nonresponse

While SSRIs are the first-line treatment for PMDD, SSRI response rates tend to be low, ranging from roughly 12% to 60% [90,91]. Many studies do not report response rates, and responder status definition varies among studies (Table 1). A previous review found that when using a 50% reduction in self-reported premenstrual symptoms (measured by visual analogue scale (VAS) [53] or Penn Daily Symptom Report (DSR) [26,27]) to define SSRI response, 51% to 63% of participants responded to SSRI compared with around 28% to 36% of placebo users [92]. When using a Clinical Global Impression (CGI) scale score of very much or much improved to define response, response rates were around 50% to 58% for SSRI and 26% to 47% for placebo [92]. This is similar to SSRI response rates for MDD, which in most studies are around 50% [93]. The CGI is a relatively limited, subjective, clinician-rated measure of treatment response, as opposed to measuring specific symptom response or using a continuous prospective scale such as the DRSP.

It is unclear what clinical characteristics distinguish SSRI responders from nonresponders in PMDD. Duration of premenstrual symptoms, menstrual cycle length, OCP use, age, number of children, and educational level did not predict treatment response [26]. Women diagnosed with severe PMS or PMDD who also experienced some level of symptoms in the follicular phase (specifically days 5–10 of the menstrual cycle) had a poorer response to sertraline; no demographic features, specific symptoms, or symptom clusters predicted treatment response [94]. One study examined citalopram treatment in women with severe PMS who had failed previous SSRI trials [47]. While many of these participants did respond to citalopram, the authors were unable to determine the causes of previous SSRI failure. Additional work needs to be carried out to characterize SSRI responders versus nonresponders in PMDD, as has been examined in postpartum depression [95]. Studies of PMDD treatment response have been limited by the inclusion of women with PMS, and potentially women with PME if this was not carefully screened for. It is possible that there are biological subtypes of PMDD, some of which respond best to SSRIs, while others respond to other agents.

Comorbidities

In some individuals, PMDD is comorbid with other psychiatric illnesses. PMDD may occur with PME or another psychiatric disorder, or PME may occur without PMDD. To distinguish between PME and PMDD symptoms, clinicians should use daily tracking tools, clinical evaluation during luteal and follicular phases, and collateral informants to assess if the symptoms in the premenstruum differ in quality (in the case of PMDD) or merely in quantity/intensity (in the case of PME)

TABLE 1
Rate of Response to SSRI Treatment in PMDD

Trial	Design	Study Groups	Responder Definition	% Responders		N
Steiner 1995	Parallel	Continuous dosing for 6 cycles: 1. Fluoxetine 20 mg 2. Fluoxetine 60 mg 3. Placebo	VAS-tension, irritability, dysphoria mean score improvement/cycle of ≥50% (moderate) or ≥75% (marked)	Moderate: Fluoxetine: 53% Placebo: 28%	Marked: Fluoxetine: 32% Placebo: 14%	277
Yonkers, Halbreirch 1996	Parallel, included PME	Continuous dosing: 1. Sertraline 50–150 mg, 2. Placebo	CGI-I ≤ 2	Sertraline: 68% Placebo: 40%		162
Yonkers, Gullion, 1996	Open, Crossover	Placebo × 1 cycle, then Paroxetine 10–30 mg × 3 cycles, continuous	CGI-I ≤ 2	All participants: 50%		14
Halbreich & Smoller 1997	Crossover	Sertraline 100 mg for all continuous, then responders (n = 11) randomized to crossover study with intermittent dosing	No longer meeting criteria for PMDD/ dysphoric PMS, CGI ≤ 3, HAM-D decrease of ≥50%, and no longer dysphoric during luteal phase	Crossover: Sertraline (9/9): 100% Placebo (2/5): 40%		15
Pearlstein 1997	Parallel	1. Fluoxetine 20 mg 2. Bupropion 100 mg TID, both continuous	CGI-I ≤ 2	Fluoxetine: 100% Bupropion: 33% Placebo: 17%		34
Yonkers & Halbreich 1997	Parallel	Sertraline 50–150 mg x 3 cycles, continuous	CGI-I ≤ 2	Sertraline: 62% Placebo: 34%		243
Steiner 1997	Parallel	1. PMDD + affective disorder or alcoholism – Fluoxetine 20 mg, continuous 2. PMDD alone – Fluoxetine 20 mg, intermittent	> 75% improvement in luteal mood symptoms on PRISM	Continuous dosing comorbid group: 66.7%	Intermittent dosing PMDD only: 75%	48

(continued on next page)

TABLE 1
(continued)

Trial	Design	Study Groups	Responder Definition	% Responders	N
Su[c] 1997	Crossover	Fluoxetine 20–60 mg or placebo × 3 cycles, washout × 2 cycles, crossover, continuous dosing	(a) ≤ 30% increase in negative mood symptoms (VAS) in luteal vs follicular phase vs baseline or (b) ≥ 50% improvement in DRF composite mood and impairment symptom score or (c) ≥ 30% improvement in severity on DRF	**(a)** Fluoxetine: 65% Placebo: 18% **(b)** Fluoxetine: 59% Placebo: 12% **(c)** Fluoxetine: 41% Placebo: 24%	17
Jermain 1999	Crossover	Sertraline 50 mg, then 100 mg, or placebo × 2 cycles, late luteal phase dosing	Not defined, but used COPE: at least a 30% reduction in luteal phase COPE total score after the first cycle	Sertraline: 70% Placebo: 50%	57
Cohen 2002	Parallel	After removing placebo responders (n = 25) in first cycle: 1. Fluoxetine 20 mg 2. Fluoxetine 10 mg Luteal phase dosing 3. Placebo	Responder not defined. Primary efficacy measure defined as statistically significant lower score on Daily Record of Severity of Problems	Fluoxetine 20 mg: 38% Fluoxetine 10 mg: 35% Placebo: 20% Statistically significant difference between fluoxetine 20 mg and placebo, but not fluoxetine 10 mg and placebo	260
Miner 2002	Parallel	After removing placebo responders (n = 27) in first cycle: 1. Fluoxetine 90 mg on 2 luteal days 2. Fluoxetine 90 mg on 1 luteal day (+placebo 2nd day) 3. Placebo	Not defined		257

Halbreich 2002	Parallel	Cycle 1: Placebo Cycle 2–4: Sertraline 50–100 mg vs placebo, intermittent dosing	CGI-I $\leq$ 2	**Cycles 1, 2, 3, 4** Tx: 50%,58%, 63%, Placebo: 26%, 38%, 47%,		228
Cohen 2004	Parallel	1. Paroxetine CR 12.5 mg 2. Paroxetine 25 mg continuous dosing 3. Placebo	(a) $\geq$50% reduction from baseline VAS-Mood (b) CGI-I $\leq$ 2	**(a)** 12.5 mg: 71% 25 mg: 67% Placebo: 49%	**(b)** 12.5 mg: 71% 25 mg: 66% Placebo: 49%	327
Pearlstein 2005	Parallel	1. Paroxetine CR 12.5 2. Paroxetine CR 25 mg continuous dosing	$\geq$50% reduction in VAS-Mood score	Paroxetine 12.5 mg: 67% Paroxetine 25 mg: 76% Placebo: 50%		371
Freeman 2005	Parallel	Intermittent vs Sx onset/5 d prior dosing of Escitalopram 10–20 mg × 3 cycles	Efficacy: DSR score decrease $\geq$ 50% or CGI-I $\leq$ 2	**DSR:** Luteal: 85% Sx onset: 64%	**CGI-I:** Luteal: 77% Sx onset: 64%	27
Steiner 2005	Parallel	1. Paroxetine CR 12.5 mg 2. Paroxetine 25 mg Intermittent dosing	(a) $\geq$ 50% reduction from baseline VAS-Mood scores, (b) mean luteal phase VAS- Mood score of less than or equal to the baseline mean follicular phase VAS-Mood score, (c) CGI-I $\leq$ 2, (d) PGE $\leq$ 2	**(a)** 25 mg: 72% 12.5 mg: 67% Placebo: 49% **(b)** 12.5 mg: 32% 25 mg: 17% Placebo: 7%	**(c)** 25 mg: 68% 12.5 mg: 57% Placebo: 44% **(d)** 25 mg: 48% 12.5 mg: 51% Placebo: 28% a	373
Yonkers 2006	Crossover	Paxil 25 mg or placebo at symptom onset, crossover after 1 cycle, intermittent	CGI-I $\leq$ 2	70% in medication group, 10% in placebo		20
Landen 2007	Parallel	1. Paroxetine, 20 mg, luteal phase dosing, with placebo during follicular phase 2. Paroxetine, 20 mg, continuous doing 3. Placebo, continuous	(a) CGI-I $\leq$ 2 (b) Self-rating as very much improved or much improved on the PGE scale, (c) $\geq$ 50% reduction of irritability and depressed mood on	**(a)** Luteal: 67% Con't: 83% Placebo: 27% **(b)** Luteal: 62% Con't: 85% Placebo: 22%	**(c) VAS, depressed mood** Luteal: 78% Con't: 95% Placebo: 48% **(d)** Luteal: 82%	269

(*continued on next page*)

TABLE 1
(continued)

Trial	Design	Study Groups	Responder Definition	% Responders		N
			VAS (d) no longer meeting the VAS-based inclusion criteria	**(c) VAS Irritability** Luteal: 89% Con't: 91% Placebo: 41%	Con't: 85% Placebo: 34%	
Eriksson 2008	Parallel	Luteal phase dosing: 1. Escitalopram 20 mg 2. Escitalopram 10 mg 3. Placebo	*(a)* $\geq$ 50% reduction in luteal rating total VAS-rated irritability, depression, tension or anxiety, affect lability *(b)* $\geq$ 50% reduction in luteal irritability, *(c)* CGI-I $\leq$ 2 *(d)* PGE $\leq$ 2 Post hoc definitions: (e) $\geq$ 80% reduction in the luteal rating of the sum of the 4 VAS (above) (f) $\geq$ 80% reduction in luteal irritability.	**(a)** 20 mg: 90% 10 mg: 88% Placebo: 72% **(b)** 20 mg: 89% 10 mg: 86% Placebo: 56% **(c)** 20 mg: 88% 10 mg: 67% Placebo: 55%	**(d)** 20 mg: 75% 10 mg: 55% Placebo: 35% **(e)** 20 mg: 87% 10 mg: 56% Placebo: 41% **(f)** 20 mg: 80% 10 mg: 58% Placebo: 30% [b]	151
Steiner 2008	Parallel	1. Paroxetine 20 mg 2. Paroxetine 10 mg Luteal phase dosing 3. Placebo	(a) VAS reduction $\geq$ 50% (b) CGI-I $\leq$ 2	**(a) VAS-Irritability** Paroxetine: 78% Placebo: 48% **(a) VAS - Tension** Paroxetine: 72% Placebo: 46%	**(b)** No statistically significant difference found	99
Wu 2008	Single, then parallel	Paroxetine 20 mg continuous $\times$ 2 cycles, then: 1. Paroxetine 20 mg, continuous dosing $\times$ 4 cycles 2. Paroxetine 20 mg, luteal phase dosing $\times$ 4 cycles	(a) reduction of luteal phase of PRISM $\geq$ 50%; (b) reduction of luteal phase of HAMD $\geq$ 50%; (c) luteal phase HAMD < 8; (d) luteal phase HAMD $\leq$ follicular phase HAMD; and (v) CGI-S $\geq$ 2	**For all outcomes:** Continuous: 50–78.6% Intermittent: 37.5–93.8%		36

Freeman 2009	Parallel, double-blind switch to placebo	1. Short term: Sertraline 50–100 mg × 4 mo, then placebo x 14 mo, luteal phase dosing 2. Long term: Sertraline 50–100 mg × 12 mo, then placebo × 6 mo, luteal phase dosing	DSR < 80 or ≥50% improvement from baseline	72% improved in all participants, no statistically significant difference between groups	174
Yonkers 2015	Parallel	1. Sertraline 50–100 mg during symptomatic interval × 6 cycles 2. Placebo	CGI-I ≤ 2	Sertraline: 67% Placebo: 53%	252

Research into treatment efficacy for PMDD has been limited by differing definitions of treatment response, as well as a high placebo response rate. Studies that identified statistically significant differences in treatment versus placebo groups have been shaded in gray. Unless otherwise specified, the studies used the following criteria for evaluating PMDD: reproductive age women, cycle lengths usually ~23 to 35 d, 2 to 3 cycles of tracking symptoms, confirmation by structured interview of DSM-IV criteria, and the absence of Axis 1 pathology in the prior 6 to 24 mo depending on study.

Abbreviations: CGI-I, Clinical Global Impressions – Improvement; CGI-S, Clinical Global Impression – Severity; COPE, calendar of premenstrual experience; DRF, daily rating form; DSR, Penn daily symptom report; HAM-D, Hamilton depression rating scale; PGE, patient global evaluation; PRISM, prospective record of impact of menstrual symptoms; VAS, visual analog scale.

[a] Estimated from Figure 4 in original publication.
[b] Estimated from Figure 4 in original publication.
[c] Su et al. initially defined participants as PMS, but retrospectively identified them all to meet criteria for PMDD.

from the rest of the menstrual cycle. In a patient with MDD and PMDD, for example, there may be irritability and anger present only in the luteal phase, and dysphoria, guilt, and anhedonia throughout the cycle. These situations present a treatment challenge, particularly in bipolar disorder, where SSRIs may worsen the underlying bipolar illness [96,97]. There is little literature on treatment guidelines for comorbid psychiatric disorders in PMDD. Treatment of PMDD comorbid with another psychiatric disorder and/or PME of an underlying psychiatric disorder can be approached similarly to isolated PMDD, with a focus on optimizing the current treatment regimen and introducing PMDD treatment practices such as luteal phase increases in a continuous SSRI [97]. Finally, we reiterate that diagnosis informs treatment. For instance, while women with PMDD may respond to hormone-based medications such as OCPs, women with PME of major depression typically do not [80,98].

Reproductive Transitions

Preconception, pregnancy, postpartum

The risks of illness vary throughout preconception planning, pregnancy, and the postpartum due to the hormonal changes that occur throughout the peripartum. When planning for pregnancy, many patients will need to change their PMDD regimen, such as stopping birth control, GnRH medications, or, in some cases, changing psychiatric medications and doses. Though there is no current research on PMDD patients during this phase, clinical reasoning would conclude that untreated patients are at high risk of relapse prior to pregnancy. During early pregnancy, without menstrual cycles, patients often experience a remission of symptoms. The third trimester and postpartum period, however, are particularly vulnerable times for patients with PMDD, who have an increased risk for antenatal and postpartum depression (PPD) [99,100]. Weaning from breastfeeding is another time that may present challenges for patients with PMDD and PME due to the hormonal fluctuations following cessation of breastfeeding, although more research is needed in this area.

There are no current guidelines and little published literature on treating PMDD during preconception planning, pregnancy, and the postpartum. Before pregnancy, strategies depend on the previously successful treatment regimen; that is, if hormonal contraception is stopped, for example, then other nonhormonal treatment strategies, such as SSRIs, could be considered. Once pregnant, patients may initially stop SSRI treatment due to cessation of menstrual cycles and thus cessation of symptoms. By the third trimester, however, as marked hormonal fluctuations begin in preparation for delivery, close observation of mood is prudent for potential active or prophylactic treatment of antenatal and postpartum depression. Though little is published about PMDD and breastfeeding, the suppression of menses during breastfeeding may be linked to fewer PMDD symptoms. Nonetheless, close monitoring is also necessary during this time for reemergence of PMDD symptoms and/or PPD.

Perimenopause

The menopausal transition occurs over 2 to 8 years, typically beginning between ages 39 to 51. The menopausal transition includes several stages, including early transition, late transition, and postmenopause [101,102]. During the transition, menstrual cycles undergo change, eventually becoming irregular, and hormonal fluctuations are marked. Some studies suggest that premenstrual mood symptoms lessen with age [103–107], although others have found more severe premenstrual symptoms in older age groups compared with younger groups [108,109]. These studies have been cross-sectional, and prospective longitudinal studies on PMDD symptom course over the menopause transition are lacking. The literature is sparse on treatment of PMDD during perimenopause. Due to the irregular cycles, intermittent SSRI dosing is not ideal and patients may favor continuous daily or symptom-onset dosing instead. Other treatments listed above that do not rely on knowing the timing of menstruation could be viable options during perimenopause, though further research on efficacy and risk is needed. Once menstrual cycles have ceased, PMDD symptoms should resolve and medication can be stopped.

RECENT DEVELOPMENTS IN TREATMENT

Neuroactive Steroid-Based Pharmacotherapy

Neurosteroid-based pharmacotherapies represent an important development in reproductive-related mood disorder treatment. These treatments may be more specific to the pathophysiology underlying reproductive-related mood disorders, particularly targeting the GABA-A receptor, than medications such as SSRIs [110]. In 2018, a groundbreaking study found that brexanolone, an intravenous form of the neuroactive steroid allopregnanolone, rapidly reduced depressive symptoms in women with postpartum depression [111]. Prior to this, SSRIs were considered the first-line treatment for postpartum depression, as they are with PMDD, but they are only effective in a fraction of women [112]. Isoallopregnanolone (UC1010; Sepranolone), a GABA-A receptor modulating steroid antagonist, significantly reduced premenstrual symptoms in women with PMDD, compared with placebo [113]. A later phase IIb study found that Sepranolone similarly reduced PMDD symptoms, but this effect was not statistically significant due to a large placebo response rate [114]. A study published in early 2021 examined ulipristal acetate, a selective progesterone receptor modulator that acts as a progesterone antagonist, in PMDD [115]. Ulipristal acetate reduced total DRSP scores by 41%, compared with 22% in the placebo group, and 85% of the women in the ulipristal group achieved remission or partial remission.

Internet-Based Cognitive-Behavioral Therapy

A recent development in mental health treatment is internet-based cognitive-behavioral therapy (iCBT), which has shown promising results in other female lifespan affective conditions such as postpartum depression [116]. A trial of 174 women with PMDD compared an 8-week therapist-guided iCBT intervention to a waitlist control [117]. Participants in the iCBT condition completed weekly self-guided online modules including psychoeducation (information about PMDD), cognitive strategies (identification, modification of dysfunctional cognitions), and behavioral strategies (eg, balanced diet, relaxation), with weekly email support from a therapist. The iCBT intervention reduced symptom intensity, functional and psychological impairment, and symptom impact on daily function, with effects durable to 6 months posttreatment.

DISCUSSION

While PMDD affects around 5% of reproductive-aged women, this severe mood disorder can be challenging to diagnose, and is underrecognized by clinicians. Thus, PMDD is often misdiagnosed or treated suboptimally. Key challenges in diagnosing PMDD are utilizing prospective daily ratings to ensure symptom entrainment to the menstrual cycle, ruling out other psychiatric diagnoses, assessing comorbidities, and ruling out premenstrual worsening of psychiatric diagnoses. Once a diagnosis of PMDD is established, first-line treatments include SSRIs, oral contraceptives, and cognitive-behavioral treatment. PMDD treatment with SSRIs is unique from other affective disorders, as intermittent dosing and use of lower dosages are possible. If first-line treatments are insufficient, other options include GnRH medications or hysterectomy-BSO, which reduce ovarian hormones to postmenopausal levels and carry significant side-effect risks. Research in PMDD treatment has been limited by different definitions of treatment response (see Table 1), and a high placebo response rate. Treatment challenges include appropriate use of intermittent SSRI dosing, nonresponse to SSRIs, managing medications in the context of comorbidities, and managing treatment through reproductive transitions such as the perinatal and perimenopausal timeframes. Additional research is needed in nonpharmacologic management of PMDD (eg, psychotherapy interventions, hormonal contraceptives beyond oral formulations), characterizing traits of treatment responders versus nonresponders, and in managing PMDD through reproductive transitions. There is also potential in neuroactive steroid-based pharmacotherapies, iCBT, and third-wave psychotherapy interventions, although research is needed in these areas also.

SUMMARY

PMDD is an underrecognized and therefore often suboptimally treated affective disorder. However, with appropriate diagnosis, symptom management can often be achieved. There are numerous treatment options for PMDD, including SSRIs, oral contraceptives, GnRH medications, and hysterectomy-BSO. Despite the challenges in treating this disorder, including comorbidities and reproductive transitions, additional research may provide insight to therapeutic targets and a more personalized approach to PMDD treatment.

CLINICS CARE POINTS

- PMDD is underrecognized by clinicians and is therefore often misdiagnosed or treated suboptimally. Isolating a diagnosis of PMDD requires great care. Prospective daily symptom tracking is vital to define the relationship between symptoms and the luteal phase.
- SSRIs have the largest evidence base for PMDD treatment. There is mixed evidence for oral contraceptives. Evidence is lacking for other hormonal contraceptives such as patches or hormonal intrauterine devices.
- Cognitive-behavioral interventions increase the use of adaptive coping strategies in PMDD, although they reduce symptoms less rapidly than SSRIs.
- GnRH medications are a second-line treatment for PMDD; potential side-effects should be considered.

Hysterectomy-BSO is a last-line treatment for PMDD; as it is an irreversible surgical procedure, risks and benefits should be considered carefully.

- PMDD treatment can be complicated by reproductive transitions. There is little published on treatment during the early stages of conception or during weaning from breastfeeding. The third trimester and postpartum period present an increased risk for postpartum depression; screening and early treatment are critical.

DISCLOSURE

The authors have nothing to disclose. Dr L. Hantsoo's work is supported by NIMH K23MH107831.

REFERENCES

[1] Epperson C, Steiner M, Hartlage SA, et al. Premenstrual dysphoric disorder: evidence for a new category for DSM-5. Am J Psychiatry 2012;169(5):465–75.
[2] Halbreich U. The diagnosis of premenstrual syndromes and premenstrual dysphoric disorder–clinical procedures and research perspectives. Gynecol Endocrinol 2004;19(6):320–34.
[3] American Psychiatric Association. Diagnostic and statistical manual of mental disorders. 5th ed. Arlington, VA: American Psychiatric Publishing; 2013.
[4] Gehlert S, Song IH, Chang C-H, et al. The prevalence of premenstrual dysphoric disorder in a randomly selected group of urban and rural women. Psychol Med 2009; 39(1):129–36.
[5] Craner JR, Sigmon ST, McGillicuddy ML. Does a disconnect occur between research and practice for premenstrual dysphoric disorder (PMDD) diagnostic procedures? Women Health 2014;54(3):232–44.
[6] Weisz G, Knaapen L. Diagnosing and treating premenstrual syndrome in five western nations. Soc Sci Med 2009;68(8):1498–505.
[7] Hantsoo L, Epperson CN. Premenstrual dysphoric disorder: epidemiology and treatment. Curr Psychiatry Rep 2015;17(11):87.
[8] Lanza di Scalea T, Pearlstein T. Premenstrual dysphoric disorder. Med Clin North Am 2019;103(4):613–28.
[9] Reid RL, Soares CN. Premenstrual dysphoric disorder: contemporary diagnosis and management. J Obstet Gynaecol Can 2018;40(2):215–23.
[10] Steiner M, Pearlstein T, Cohen LS, et al. Expert guidelines for the treatment of severe PMS, PMDD, and comorbidities: the role of SSRIs. J Womens Health (Larchmt) 2006;15(1):57–69.
[11] Yonkers KA, Simoni MK. Premenstrual disorders. Am J Obstet Gynecol 2018;218(1):68–74.
[12] Endicott J, Nee J, Harrison W. Daily record of severity of problems (DRSP): reliability and validity. Arch Womens Ment Health 2006;9(1):41–9.
[13] Allen SS, McBride CM, Pirie PL. The shortened premenstrual assessment form. J Reprod Med 1991;36(11): 769–72.
[14] Feuerstein M, Shaw WS. Measurement properties of the calendar of premenstrual experience in patients with premenstrual syndrome. J Reprod Med 2002;47(4): 279–89.
[15] Reid RL. Premenstrual dysphoric disorder (formerly premenstrual syndrome). In: Feingold KR, Anawalt B, Boyce A, et al, editors. Endotext. South Dartmouth, MA: MDText.com, Inc.; 2000.
[16] Angst J, Sellaro R, Merikangas KR, et al. The epidemiology of perimenstrual psychological symptoms. Acta Psychiatr Scand 2001;104(2):110–6.
[17] Freeman EW, Halberstadt SM, Rickels K, et al. Core symptoms that discriminate premenstrual syndrome. J Womens Health (Larchmt) 2011;20(1):29–35.
[18] Landén M, Eriksson E. How does premenstrual dysphoric disorder relate to depression and anxiety disorders? Depress Anxiety 2003;17(3):122–9.
[19] ACOG. ACOG practice bulletin: premenstrual syndrome. Clinical management guidelines for obsetrician-gynecologists. Int J Obstet Gynecol 2001;73: 183–91.
[20] Haley CL, Sung SC, Rush AJ, et al. The clinical relevance of self-reported premenstrual worsening of depressive symptoms in the management of depressed outpatients: a STAR*D report. J Womens Health (Larchmt) 2013;22(3):219–29.
[21] Kornstein SG, Harvey AT, Rush AJ, et al. Self-reported premenstrual exacerbation of depressive symptoms in patients seeking treatment for major depression. Psychol Med 2005;35(5):683–92.
[22] Hartlage, Brandenburg DL, Kravitz HM. Premenstrual exacerbation of depressive disorders in a community-based sample in the United States. Psychosom Med 2004;66(5):698–706.
[23] Casper RF, Yonkers KA. Treatment of premenstrual syndrome and premenstrual dysphoric disorder - UpToDate. 2020. Available at: https://www-uptodate-com.proxy1.library.jhu.edu/contents/treatment-of-premenstrual-syndrome-and-premenstrual-dysphoric-disorder?search="' Treatment%20of%20premenstrual%20syndrome%20and%20premenstrual%20dysphoric%20disorder&source=search_result&selectedTitle=1~150&usage_type=default&display_rank=1. [Accessed 15 June 2020].
[24] Hofmeister S, Bodden S. Premenstrual syndrome and premenstrual dysphoric disorder. AFP 2016;94(3): 236–40.
[25] Premenstrual syndrome, management (Green-top Guideline No. 48). Royal College of Obstetricians & Gynaecologists. 2016. Available at: https://www.rcog.org.uk/en/guidelines-research-services/guidelines/gtg48/. [Accessed 10 October 2018].

[26] Freeman EW, Rickels K, Sondheimer SJ, et al. Differential response to antidepressants in women with premenstrual syndrome/premenstrual dysphoric disorder: a randomized controlled trial. Arch Gen Psychiatry 1999;56(10):932–9.

[27] Freeman EW, Rickels K, Sondheimer SJ, et al. Continuous or intermittent dosing with sertraline for patients with severe premenstrual syndrome or premenstrual dysphoric disorder. Am J Psychiatry 2004;161(2):343–51.

[28] Freeman EW, Rickels K, Sammel MD, et al. Time to relapse after short-term or long-term sertraline treatment for severe premenstrual syndromes. Arch Gen Psychiatry 2009;66(5):537–44.

[29] Halbreich U, Smoller JW. Intermittent luteal phase sertraline treatment of dysphoric premenstrual syndrome. J Clin Psychiatry 1997;58(9):399–402.

[30] Halbreich U, Bergeron R, Yonkers KA, et al. Efficacy of intermittent, luteal phase sertraline treatment of premenstrual dysphoric disorder. Obstet Gynecol 2002;100(6):1219–29.

[31] Jermain DM, Preece CK, Sykes RL, et al. Luteal phase sertraline treatment for premenstrual dysphoric disorder. Results of a double-blind, placebo-controlled, crossover study. Arch Fam Med 1999;8(4):328–32.

[32] Kornstein SG, Pearlstein TB, Fayyad R, et al. Low-dose sertraline in the treatment of moderate-to-severe premenstrual syndrome: efficacy of 3 dosing strategies. J Clin Psychiatry 2006;67(10):1624–32.

[33] Pearlstein TB, Halbreich U, Batzar ED, et al. Psychosocial functioning in women with premenstrual dysphoric disorder before and after treatment with sertraline or placebo. J Clin Psychiatry 2000;61(2):101–9.

[34] Yonkers KA, Halbreich U, Freeman E, et al. Sertraline in the treatment of premenstrual dysphoric disorder. Psychopharmacol Bull 1996;32(1):41–6.

[35] Yonkers KA, Halbreich U, Freeman E, et al. Symptomatic improvement of premenstrual dysphoric disorder with sertraline treatment. A randomized controlled trial. Sertraline Premenstrual Dysphoric Collaborative Study Group. JAMA 1997;278(12):983–8.

[36] Yonkers KA, Kornstein SG, Gueorguieva R, et al. Symptom-onset dosing of sertraline for the treatment of premenstrual dysphoric disorder: a randomized clinical trial. JAMA Psychiatry 2015;72(10):1037–44.

[37] Young SA, Hurt PH, Benedek DM, et al. Treatment of premenstrual dysphoric disorder with sertraline during the luteal phase: a randomized, double-blind, placebo-controlled crossover trial. J Clin Psychiatry 1998;59(2):76–80.

[38] Cohen LS, Soares CN, Yonkers KA, et al. Paroxetine controlled release for premenstrual dysphoric disorder: a double-blind, placebo-controlled trial. Psychosom Med 2004;66(5):707–13.

[39] Landén M, Nissbrandt H, Allgulander C, et al. Placebo-controlled trial comparing intermittent and continuous paroxetine in premenstrual dysphoric disorder. Neuropsychopharmacology 2007;32(1):153–61.

[40] Steiner M, Hirschberg AL, Bergeron R, et al. Luteal phase dosing with paroxetine controlled release (CR) in the treatment of premenstrual dysphoric disorder. Am J Obstet Gynecol 2005;193(2):352–60.

[41] Steiner M, Ravindran AV, LeMelledo J-M, et al. Luteal phase administration of paroxetine for the treatment of premenstrual dysphoric disorder: a randomized, double-blind, placebo-controlled trial in Canadian women. J Clin Psychiatry 2008;69(6):991–8.

[42] Sundblad C, Wikander I, Andersch B, et al. A naturalistic study of paroxetine in premenstrual syndrome: efficacy and side-effects during ten cycles of treatment. Eur Neuropsychopharmacol 1997;7(3):201–6.

[43] Wu K-Y, Liu C-Y, Hsiao M-C. Six-month paroxetine treatment of premenstrual dysphoric disorder: continuous versus intermittent treatment protocols. Psychiatry Clin Neurosci 2008;62(1):109–14.

[44] Yonkers KA, Gullion C, Williams A, et al. Paroxetine as a treatment for premenstrual dysphoric disorder. J Clin Psychopharmacol 1996;16(1):3–8.

[45] Yonkers KA, Holthausen GA, Poschman K, et al. Symptom-onset treatment for women with premenstrual dysphoric disorder. J Clin Psychopharmacol 2006;26(2):198–202.

[46] Pearlstein TB, Bellew KM, Endicott J, et al. Paroxetine controlled release for premenstrual dysphoric disorder: remission analysis following a randomized, double-blind, placebo-controlled trial. Prim Care Companion J Clin Psychiatry 2005;7(2):53–60.

[47] Freeman EW, Jabara S, Sondheimer SJ, et al. Citalopram in PMS patients with prior SSRI treatment failure: a preliminary study. J Womens Health Gend Based Med 2002;11(5):459–64.

[48] Eriksson E, Ekman A, Sinclair S, et al. Escitalopram administered in the luteal phase exerts a marked and dose-dependent effect in premenstrual dysphoric disorder. J Clin Psychopharmacol 2008;28(2):195–202.

[49] Freeman EW, Sondheimer SJ, Sammel MD, et al. A preliminary study of luteal phase versus symptom-onset dosing with escitalopram for premenstrual dysphoric disorder. J Clin Psychiatry 2005;66(6):769–73.

[50] Cohen LS, Miner C, Brown EW, et al. Premenstrual daily fluoxetine for premenstrual dysphoric disorder: a placebo-controlled, clinical trial using computerized diaries. Obstet Gynecol 2002;100(3):435–44.

[51] Miner C, Brown E, McCray S, et al. Weekly luteal-phase dosing with enteric-coated fluoxetine 90 mg in premenstrual dysphoric disorder: a randomized, double-blind, placebo-controlled clinical trial. Clin Ther 2002;24(3):417–33.

[52] Pearlstein TB, Stone AB, Lund SA, et al. Comparison of fluoxetine, bupropion, and placebo in the treatment of premenstrual dysphoric disorder. J Clin Psychopharmacol 1997;17(4):261–6.

[53] Steiner M, Steinberg S, Stewart D, et al. Fluoxetine in the treatment of premenstrual dysphoria. Canadian

Fluoxetine/Premenstrual Dysphoria Collaborative Study Group. N Engl J Med 1995;332(23):1529–34.
[54] Steiner M, Korzekwa M, Lamont J, et al. Intermittent fluoxetine dosing in the treatment of women with premenstrual dysphoria. Psychopharmacol Bull 1997; 33(4):771–4.
[55] Su TP, Schmidt PJ, Danaceau MA, et al. Fluoxetine in the treatment of premenstrual dysphoria. Neuropsychopharmacology 1997;16(5):346–56.
[56] Marjoribanks J, Brown J, O'Brien PMS, et al. Selective serotonin reuptake inhibitors for premenstrual syndrome. Cochrane Database Syst Rev 2013;6:CD001396.
[57] Shah NR, Jones JB, Aperi J, et al. Selective serotonin reuptake inhibitors for premenstrual syndrome and premenstrual dysphoric disorder: a meta-analysis. Obstet Gynecol 2008;111(5):1175–82.
[58] Brown J, O' Brien PMS, Marjoribanks J, et al. Selective serotonin reuptake inhibitors for premenstrual syndrome. Cochrane Database Syst Rev 2009;(2):CD001396.
[59] Kleinstäuber M, Witthöft M, Hiller W. Cognitive-behavioral and pharmacological interventions for premenstrual syndrome or premenstrual dysphoric disorder: a meta-analysis. J Clin Psychol Med Settings 2012; 19(3):308–19.
[60] Pinna G, Costa E, Guidotti A. SSRIs act as selective brain steroidogenic stimulants (SBSSs) at low doses that are inactive on 5-HT reuptake. Curr Opin Pharmacol 2009;9(1):24–30.
[61] Landén M, Thase ME. A model to explain the therapeutic effects of serotonin reuptake inhibitors: the role of 5-HT2 receptors. Psychopharmacol Bull 2006;39(1): 147–66.
[62] Steinberg EM, Cardoso GMP, Martinez PE, et al. Rapid response to fluoxetine in women with premenstrual dysphoric disorder. Depress Anxiety 2012;29(6): 531–40.
[63] Freeman EW. Luteal phase administration of agents for the treatment of premenstrual dysphoric disorder. CNS Drugs 2004;18(7):453–68.
[64] Ravindran LN, Woods S-A, Steiner M, et al. Symptom-onset dosing with citalopram in the treatment of premenstrual dysphoric disorder (PMDD): a case series. Arch Womens Ment Health 2007;10(3):125–7.
[65] Cunningham J, Yonkers KA, O'Brien S, et al. Update on research and treatment of premenstrual dysphoric disorder. Harv Rev Psychiatry 2009;17(2):120–37.
[66] Lopez LM, Kaptein AA, Helmerhorst FM. Oral contraceptives containing drospirenone for premenstrual syndrome. Cochrane Database Syst Rev 2012;2:CD006586.
[67] Ford O, Lethaby A, Roberts H, et al. Progesterone for premenstrual syndrome. Cochrane Database Syst Rev 2012;3:CD003415.
[68] Schmidt PJ, Martinez PE, Nieman LK, et al. Exposure to a change in ovarian steroid levels but not continuous stable levels triggers PMDD symptoms following ovarian suppression. Am J Psychiatry 2017;174(10): 980–9.
[69] Bäckström T, Hansson-Malmström Y, Lindhe BA, et al. Oral contraceptives in premenstrual syndrome: a randomized comparison of triphasic and monophasic preparations. Contraception 1992;46(3):253–68.
[70] Freeman EW, Halbreich U, Grubb GS, et al. An overview of four studies of a continuous oral contraceptive (levonorgestrel 90 mcg/ethinyl estradiol 20 mcg) on premenstrual dysphoric disorder and premenstrual syndrome. Contraception 2012;85(5):437–45.
[71] Rapkin AJ, Korotkaya Y, Taylor KC. Contraception counseling for women with premenstrual dysphoric disorder (PMDD): current perspectives. Open Access J Contracept 2019;10:27–39.
[72] Bäckström T, Andreen L, Birzniece V, et al. The role of hormones and hormonal treatments in premenstrual syndrome. CNS Drugs 2003;17(5):325–42.
[73] Busse JW, Montori VM, Krasnik C, et al. Psychological intervention for premenstrual syndrome: a meta-analysis of randomized controlled trials. Psychother Psychosom 2009;78(1):6–15.
[74] Lustyk MKB, Gerrish WG, Shaver S, et al. Cognitive-behavioral therapy for premenstrual syndrome and premenstrual dysphoric disorder: a systematic review. Arch Womens Ment Health 2009;12(2):85–96.
[75] Panahi F, Faramarzi M. The effects of mindfulness-based cognitive therapy on depression and anxiety in women with premenstrual syndrome. Depress Res Treat 2016;2016:9816481.
[76] Bluth K, Gaylord S, Nguyen K, et al. Mindfulness-based stress reduction as a promising intervention for amelioration of premenstrual dysphoric disorder symptoms. Mindfulness (N Y) 2015;6(6):1292–302.
[77] Hunter MS, Ussher JM, Browne SJ, et al. A randomized comparison of psychological (cognitive behavior therapy), medical (fluoxetine) and combined treatment for women with premenstrual dysphoric disorder. J Psychosom Obstet Gynaecol 2002;23(3):193–9.
[78] Gallagher JS, Missmer SA, Hornstein MD, et al. Long-term effects of gonadotropin-releasing hormone agonists and add-back in adolescent endometriosis. J Pediatr Adolesc Gynecol 2018;31(4):376–81.
[79] Wyatt KM, Dimmock PW, Ismail KMK, et al. The effectiveness of GnRHa with and without "add-back" therapy in treating premenstrual syndrome: a meta analysis. BJOG 2004;111(6):585–93.
[80] Freeman EW, Sondheimer SJ, Rickels K. Gonadotropin-releasing hormone agonist in the treatment of premenstrual symptoms with and without ongoing dysphoria: a controlled study. Psychopharmacol Bull 1997;33(2): 303–9.
[81] Mezrow G, Shoupe D, Spicer D, et al. Depot leuprolide acetate with estrogen and progestin add-back for long-term treatment of premenstrual syndrome. Fertil Steril 1994;62(5):932–7.
[82] Mortola JF, Girton L, Fischer U. Successful treatment of severe premenstrual syndrome by combined use of gonadotropin-releasing hormone agonist and

estrogen/progestin. J Clin Endocrinol Metab 1991; 72(2):252A-252F.
[83] Schmidt PJ, Nieman LK, Danaceau MA, et al. Differential behavioral effects of gonadal steroids in women with and in those without premenstrual syndrome. N Engl J Med 1998;338(4):209–16.
[84] Sundström I, Nyberg S, Bixo M, et al. Treatment of premenstrual syndrome with gonadotropin-releasing hormone agonist in a low dose regimen. Acta Obstet Gynecol Scand 1999;78(10):891–9.
[85] Pincus SM, Alam S, Rubinow DR, et al. Predicting response to leuprolide of women with premenstrual dysphoric disorder by daily mood rating dynamics. J Psychiatr Res 2011;45(3):386–94.
[86] Nevatte T, O'Brien PMS, Bäckström T, et al. ISPMD consensus on the management of premenstrual disorders. Arch Womens Ment Health 2013;16(4):279–91.
[87] Casper RF, Hearn MT. The effect of hysterectomy and bilateral oophorectomy in women with severe premenstrual syndrome. Am J Obstet Gynecol 1990;162(1): 105–9.
[88] Casson P, Hahn PM, Van Vugt DA, et al. Lasting response to ovariectomy in severe intractable premenstrual syndrome. Am J Obstet Gynecol 1990;162(1): 99–105.
[89] Cronje WH, Vashisht A, Studd JWW. Hysterectomy and bilateral oophorectomy for severe premenstrual syndrome. Hum Reprod 2004;19(9):2152–5.
[90] Dimmock PW, Wyatt KM, Jones PW, et al. Efficacy of selective serotonin-reuptake inhibitors in premenstrual syndrome: a systematic review. Lancet 2000; 356(9236):1131–6.
[91] Halbreich U. Selective serotonin reuptake inhibitors and initial oral contraceptives for the treatment of PMDD: effective but not enough. CNS Spectr 2008; 13(7):566–72.
[92] Halbreich U, O'Brien PMS, Eriksson E, et al. Are there differential symptom profiles that improve in response to different pharmacological treatments of premenstrual syndrome/premenstrual dysphoric disorder? CNS Drugs 2006;20(7):523–47.
[93] Biernacka JM, Sangkuhl K, Jenkins G, et al. The International SSRI Pharmacogenomics Consortium (ISPC): a genome-wide association study of antidepressant treatment response. Transl Psychiatry 2015;5(4):e553.
[94] Freeman EW, Sondheimer SJ, Polansky M, et al. Predictors of response to sertraline treatment of severe premenstrual syndromes. J Clin Psychiatry 2000;61(8): 579–84.
[95] Sharma V, Khan M, Baczynski C, et al. Predictors of response to antidepressants in women with postpartum depression: a systematic review. Arch Womens Ment Health 2020;23(5):613–23.
[96] Payne JL, Roy PS, Murphy-Eberenz K, et al. Reproductive cycle-associated mood symptoms in women with major depression and bipolar disorder. J Affect Disord 2007;99(1–3):221–9.
[97] Smith M, Frey BN. Treating comorbid premenstrual dysphoric disorder in women with bipolar disorder. J Psychiatry Neurosci 2016;41(2):E22–3.
[98] Peters W, Freeman MP, Kim S, et al. Treatment of premenstrual breakthrough of depression with adjunctive oral contraceptive pills compared with placebo. J Clin Psychopharmacol 2017;37(5):609–14.
[99] Bloch M, Rotenberg N, Koren D, et al. Risk factors associated with the development of postpartum mood disorders. J Affect Disord 2005;88(1):9–18.
[100] Bloch M, Rotenberg N, Koren D, et al. Risk factors for early postpartum depressive symptoms. Gen Hosp Psychiatry 2006;28(1):3–8.
[101] Dennerstein L, Lehert P, Heinemann K. Global epidemiological study of variation of premenstrual symptoms with age and sociodemographic factors. Menopause Int 2011;17(3):96–101.
[102] Soules MR, Sherman S, Parrott E, et al. Executive summary: Stages of Reproductive Aging Workshop (STRAW). Fertil Steril 2001;76(5):874–8.
[103] Dennerstein L, Lehert P, Heinemann K. Global study of women's experiences of premenstrual symptoms and their effects on daily life. Menopause Int 2011;17(3):88–95.
[104] Freeman EW, Rickels K, Schweizer E, et al. Relationships between age and symptom severity among women seeking medical treatment for premenstrual symptoms. Psychol Med 1995;25(2):309–15.
[105] Freeman EW, Sammel MD, Rinaudo PJ, et al. Premenstrual syndrome as a predictor of menopausal symptoms. Obstet Gynecol 2004;103(5 Pt 1):960–6.
[106] Silva CML da, Gigante DP, Minten GC. Premenstrual symptoms and syndrome according to age at menarche in a 1982 birth cohort in southern Brazil. Cadernos de Saúde Pública 2008;24(4):835–44.
[107] Sternfeld B, Swindle R, Chawla A, et al. Severity of premenstrual symptoms in a health maintenance organization population. Obstet Gynecol 2002;99(6):1014–24.
[108] Sylvén SM, Ekselius L, Sundström-Poromaa I, et al. Premenstrual syndrome and dysphoric disorder as risk factors for postpartum depression. Acta Obstet Gynecol Scand 2013;92(2):178–84.
[109] Tschudin S, Bertea PC, Zemp E. Prevalence and predictors of premenstrual syndrome and premenstrual dysphoric disorder in a population-based sample. Arch Womens Ment Health 2010;13(6):485–94.
[110] Schweizer-Schubert S, Gordon JL, Eisenlohr-Moul TA, et al. Steroid hormone sensitivity in reproductive mood disorders: on the role of the GABAA receptor complex and stress during hormonal transitions. Front Med (Lausanne) 2021;7:479646.
[111] Meltzer-Brody S, Colquhoun H, Riesenberg R, et al. Brexanolone injection in post-partum depression: two multicentre, double-blind, randomised, placebo-controlled, phase 3 trials. Lancet 2018;392(10152): 1058–70.
[112] De Crescenzo F, Perelli F, Armando M, et al. Selective serotonin reuptake inhibitors (SSRIs) for post-partum

depression (PPD): a systematic review of randomized clinical trials. J Affect Disord 2014;152-154:39–44.

[113] Bixo M, Ekberg K, Poromaa IS, et al. Treatment of premenstrual dysphoric disorder with the GABAA receptor modulating steroid antagonist sepranolone (UC1010)-a randomized controlled trial. Psychoneuroendocrinology 2017;80:46–55.

[114] AsarinaPharma, Solna, Sweden. Asarina Pharma reports topline results from Phase IIb study in PMDD. Sepranolone. 2020. https://asarinapharma.com/sepranolone/. [Accessed 1 November 2019].

[115] Comasco E, Kopp Kallner H, Bixo M, et al. Ulipristal acetate for treatment of premenstrual dysphoric disorder: a proof-of-concept randomized controlled trial. Am J Psychiatry 2021;178(3):256–65.

[116] Kim DR, Hantsoo L, Thase ME, et al. Computer-assisted cognitive behavioral therapy for pregnant women with major depressive disorder. J Womens Health (Larchmt) 2014;23(10):842–8.

[117] Weise C, Kaiser G, Janda C, et al. Internet-based cognitive-behavioural intervention for women with premenstrual dysphoric disorder: a randomized controlled trial. Psychother Psychosom 2019;88(1):16–29.

Advances in Psychiatry and Behavioral Health 1 (2021) 107–118

ADVANCES IN PSYCHIATRY AND BEHAVIORAL HEALTH

Novel Neurosteroid Pharmaceuticals

Implications Across a Woman's Lifecycle

Leah C. Susser, MD[a,*], Clare Swanson, MD[b], Alison D. Hermann, MD[c]

[a]Department of Psychiatry, Weill Cornell Medicine, White Plains, NY, USA; [b]Department of Psychiatry, NewYork-Presbyterian Hospital/Weill Cornell, 525 East 68th Street, New York, NY 10065, USA; [c]Department of Psychiatry, Weill Cornell Medicine, 315 East 62nd Street, 5th Floor, New York, NY 10065, USA

KEYWORDS

• Allopregnanolone • Brexanolone • Ganaxolone • Zuranolone • SGE-516 • Ulipristal acetate
• Postpartum depression • Premenstrual dysphoric disorder

KEY POINTS

- Certain women are vulnerable to depression during periods of reproductive change associated with fluctuating neurosteroid levels.
- Neurosteroid pharmaceuticals are effective treatments for postpartum depression.
- Pharmaceuticals that stabilize neurosteroid levels have shown promise for treating premenstrual dysphoric disorder but warrant further study.
- The major benefit of neurosteroid pharmaceuticals is their rapid and robust effect. The major weaknesses are feasibility concerns.

INTRODUCTION

It is well established that a subgroup of women are vulnerable to affective dysregulation during times of hormonal fluctuation. This has been referred to as "reproductive depression" (RD) [1] and may occur during menarche, pregnancy, postpartum, weaning from breastfeeding, and perimenopause; or in reaction to hormonal flux such as across the menstrual cycle [1,2].

The total morbidity and mortality associated with RD across a woman's lifespan is not fully appreciated and may be best known for postpartum depression (PPD). PPD impacts 10% to 20% of new mothers [3], and suicide accounts for up to 20% of postpartum deaths [4]. While the biological factors underlying RD are not yet fully understood, there is promising research implicating neuroactive steroids—derivatives of cholesterol that act on the brain. Several neuroactive steroid compounds have been developed and studied for RD, including recently FDA-approved brexanolone. In this review, we will discuss novel neuroactive steroid pharmaceuticals, their mechanisms of action, and their advantages and disadvantages in real-world clinical settings.

BACKGROUND

Neuroactive steroids are metabolites of gonadal hormones known to modulate neuronal activity. Allopregnanolone (ALLO) is a metabolite of progesterone and a positive allosteric modulator of GABAA receptors (Gamma Aminobutyric Acid - A Rs) [5]. GABAARs are pentameric proteins that are built of heterogeneous subunits including two α-subunits, two β-subunits, and one subunit of either the γ-, δ-, ε-, π-, or θ-type

*Corresponding author. 21 Bloomingdale Road, Adult Outpatient Department, White Plains, NY 10605. *E-mail address:* Lcs7001@med.cornell.edu

https://doi.org/10.1016/j.ypsc.2021.05.017
2667-3827/21/

[6,7]. GABAAR subunit combinations mediate specific forms of inhibition in the brain. Phasic, or synaptic, inhibition involves GABAARs with γ2 subunits, while tonic inhibition is mediated by extrasynaptic receptors that usually contain a δ-subunit [8,9].

The GABAAR subunit composition changes with steroid hormone fluctuation. Withdrawal from progesterone and, therefore, ALLO, increases δ subunit expression [10], and extremely elevated levels of progesterone, such as in pregnancy, downregulate expression of δ subunits [11]. These alterations in the GABAAR subunit composition are thought to be a homeostatic mechanism maintaining appropriate levels of inhibition as neuroactive steroid levels change [12].

ALLO may have both anxiolytic and antidepressant effects [13–15]. ALLO levels have been found to be low in major depressive disorder (MDD) and to elevate with antidepressant treatment [16–18]. The hypothalamic-pituitary-adrenal (HPA) axis, which mediates the body's neuroendocrine response to stress, is tightly controlled by GABAergic signaling [19], including ALLO regulation [20,21]. Tonic GABAergic inhibition mediated by δ subunit-containing GABAARs in the paraventricular nucleus may be particularly important in regulating the expression of corticotropin-releasing hormone (CRH) and its release of corticosteroids [22,23].

GABAergic signaling may be a particularly important mechanism underlying RD because ALLO has been shown to have paradoxic effects in these populations. Smith and colleagues [24] in 2006 showed that ALLO withdrawal increased expression of the α4 subunit in the hippocampus, and reintroduction of ALLO triggered hippocampal excitability rather than inhibition in female mice. Similarly, Shen and colleagues in 2007 studied GABAAR in puberty and showed that a particular subunit configuration (α4β2δ) of GABAAR is induced by prolonged ALLO withdrawal and reverses its inhibiting effect by changing the direction of its GABA-gated current [25]. Female GABAAR δ subunit knockout mice exhibit PPD-like behaviors and deficits in maternal care that are restricted to the postpartum period [11].

There are other positive allosteric modulators of GABAARs, including benzodiazepines, which are a commonly used class of anxiolytic medications. Both neuroactive steroids and benzodiazepines modulate synaptic GABAARs containing α and γ subunits [26], so both augment phasic inhibition. Unlike benzodiazepines, neuroactive steroids also modulate extrasynaptic GABAARs, comprised of α and δ subunits, which are responsible for tonic inhibition [27,28]. Distinguishing between tonic and phasic GABAAR effects may have significant clinical consequences in terms of pharmacologic targets. It is suspected that tonic, but not phasic, inhibition is responsible for the antidepressant effect of neuroactive steroids. A recent study by Durkin and colleagues 2018, who created a knock-in mouse model that removed neuroactive steroid potentiation from α2 GABAARs subunits, revealed that the inactivated α2 subunit isoform is essential for the anxiolytic role of neuroactive steroids, but the inactivated α2 subunit isoform did not demonstrate antidepressant effects [29]. These data, in combination with the fact that other modulators of GABAARs such as benzodiazepines do not appear to exhibit antidepressant benefit, may indicate that the unique psychoactive profile of neuroactive steroids is related to their action on δ-containing receptors and, thus, augmentation of tonic inhibition [30].

Pharmaceutical agents targeting tonic GABAAR modulation for antidepressant effects have now been developed and will be discussed in detail throughout this article.

PERINATAL DEPRESSION

Selective serotonin reuptake inhibitors (SSRIs) are currently the first-line treatment for PPD but can take weeks to be effective, as their primary mechanism of action targets the presynaptic serotonin transporter [31]. PPD is associated with high maternal morbidity and mortality [32–34] and can have long-lasting adverse consequences for children [35]. Therefore, rapid treatments such as neuroactive steroid compounds are highly desirable for this population.

The perinatal period is a time of drastic changes in ALLO levels and, therefore, a strong candidate for pharmaceuticals targeting tonic GABA-A inhibition [36,37]. Several compounds (Table 1) that target this postpartum change in ALLO levels have now been studied and have been shown to have rapid, robust effects, including brexanolone, zuranolone, ganaxolone, and SGE-516.

Brexanolone

Brexanolone (SAGE-547; brand name Zulresso) is a synthetic formulation of ALLO. It has low oral bioavailability and is rapidly cleared from the body, thus is only available as an IV infusion [38]. The recommended dosing schedule is a 60-hour continuous infusion followed by a 12-hour monitoring period. Pulse oximetry is required continuously throughout the infusion and monitoring period, necessitating hospitalization in most health care systems. Clinical effect is seen as early

TABLE 1
Neurosteroids for Depression

Compound	FDA	Route	Studies	Design	Population	Results
PPD						
Brexanolone	PPD					
		IV	Kanes et al [39], 2017	Small, open label	PPD, HAMD ≥ 20	No severe adverse events
		IV	Kanes et al [40], 2017	DB-RCT	PPD, HAMD ≥ 26	60-h ΔHAMD:[a] brx90: −21.0 (SE: 2.9) Placebo: −8.8 (SE: 2.8)
		IV	Meltzer-Brody et al [41], 2018	2 DB-RCTs	PPD, 1. HAMD ≥ 26 2. HAMD: 20–25	Study 1: 60-h ΔHAMD: brx60:[a] −19.5 (SE: 1.2) brx90:[a] −17.7 (SE: 1.2) Placebo: −14.0 (SE: 1.1) Study 2: 60-h ΔHAMD: brx90:[a] −14.6 (SE: 0.8) Placebo: −12.1 (SE: 0.8) Integrated study: 60-h ΔHAMD: brx90 vs placebo:[a] −4.1 (CI: -6.0, -2.3)
Zuranolone	X					
		Oral	Hoffmann et al [43], 2019	2 dose-finding DB-RCTs	Healthy adult population	Max tolerable dose: 30 mg multidose 55 mg single dose
		Oral, 30 mg	Deligiannidis et al [44], 2019	DB-RCT	PPD, HAMD ≥ 26	Day 15 ΔHAMD:[a] Zuranolone: −17.8 Placebo: −13.6 *P* = .0028
Ganaxolone	X					
		IV 60 h, 140 μg/kg/h	Magnolia Study part 1 [50]	Placebo-controlled	PPD, HAMD≥26	60-h ΔHAMD: Ganaxolone: −16.9 Placebo: −12.7 SD: NR D 34 ΔHAMD: Ganaxolone: -15.7 Placebo: −11.6 SD: NR
		IV 6 h, 20 mg/h then 900 mg/d orally for 28 d	Magnolia Study part 2 [49]	Placebo-controlled RCT	PPD Mean HAMD: Ganaxolone 26.6 placebo 26.4	6-h ΔHAMD: Ganaxolone: −6.1 Placebo: −3.3 SD: NR 24-h ΔHAMD: Ganaxolone: −7.7 Placebo: −5.1 SD: NR D 28 HAMD: No difference reported

(*continued on next page*)

TABLE 1
(*continued*)

Compound	FDA	Route	Studies	Design	Population	Results
		Oral	Amaryllis Study [49,50]	Open label	PPD Mean HAMD: 675 mg dose 25.5 1125 mg dose 25.4	675 mg/d: D 14 ΔHAMD: Ganaxolone: −9.8 (SD: NR) D 28 ΔHAMD: Ganaxolone: -12.2 (SD: NR) 1125 mg/d: D 14 ΔHAMD: Ganaxolone: −9.3 (SD: NR) D 28 ΔHAMD: Ganaxolone: -14.5 (SD: NR)
SGE-516	X					
		Oral	Melon et al, 2018 [52]	Mouse-model	Mouse dams	• Decreased PPD-like behaviors[a] • Improved maternal care[a] • Blunted stress effects[a]
PMDD						
Dutasteride	BPH					
		Oral	Martinez et al [54], 2016	2 DB-RCT, cross-over trials	Women with and without PMDD	Follicular vs luteal ΔDRSP Irritability subscale:[a] 2.5 mg/d: 0.5 (SE: 0.3) Placebo: 1.5 (SE: 0.3) Sadness subscale:[a] 2.5 mg/d: 0.5 (SE: 0.3) Placebo: 1.5 (SE: 0.3) Anxiety subscale:[a] 2.5 mg/d: 0.6 (SE: 0.3) Placebo:1.6 (SE: 0.3)
Sepranolone	X					
		Subcutaneous, 10 mg or 16 mg	Bixo et al, 2017-part 2 [59]	DB-RCT	Women with PMDD	ΔDRSP at 1 mo[a] (10 mg and 16 mg groups combined) Sepranolone: −29 (SD: 19.94) Placebo: −22.8 (SD: 14.67)
UPA	eC [78]					
		Oral	Comasco et al [61], 2020	DB-RCT	Women with PMDD	ΔDRSP 3rd month[a] UPA: −41% (SD: 18)

(*continued on next page*)

TABLE 1
(*continued*)

Compound	FDA	Route	Studies	Design	Population	Results
						Placebo: −22% (SD: 27)
MDD						
Zuranolone	X					
		Oral, 30 mg	Mountain Study [72]	DB-RCT	Adults with MDD, MADRS≥32; HAMD≥22	D 15 ΔHAMD: Zuranolone: −12.6 Placebo: −11.2 $P = .115$
		Oral, 30 mg and 50 mg	SHORELINE study [73]	Open label	MDD, HAMD≥20	Well-tolerated D 15 ΔHAMD: 30 mg: −14.9 SD: 7.1 50 mg: no adverse events, further results pending

Abbreviations: BPH, benign prostatic hyperplasia; DB-RCT, double-blind, randomized controlled trial; eC, emergency contraceptive; NR, not reported.

[a] Statistically significant.

as 24 hours and is sustained until at least 30 days after the infusion.

Brexanolone clinical trials

The first study of brexanolone was an open-label study of four women with a Hamilton Depression Rating scale (HAMD) score greater than 20 [39]. HAMD is a clinician-administered depression rating scale. Doses were selected to mimic third trimester ALLO levels [39]. Sedation was common but transient, and there were no severe side-effects. All four women achieved rapid symptom remission.

This study was followed by a double-blind, randomized placebo-controlled trial for severe PPD (HAMD≥26, N = 21) [40]. Brexanolone infusion dose was titrated up to 90 μg/kg/h. At 60 hours, brexanolone significantly reduced HAMD by 21 points compared with 9 points for placebo, and this reduction was seen from 24 hours through 30 days without side effects.

In 2018, Meltzer-Brody and colleagues published results from two double-blind randomized placebo-controlled phase 3 trials [41]. Study 1 included 138 women with HAMD≥26, and study 2 included 108 women with HAMD of 20 to 25. In study 1, women were given brexanolone titrated to 90 μg/kg/h (brx90), brexanolone titrated to 60 μg/kg/h (brx60), or placebo. In study 2, women were given brx90 or placebo. Common side effects included headache, dizziness, and somnolence. At 60 hours, brx60 in study 1, brx90 in study 1, and brx90 in study 2 all achieved a significantly greater reduction in HAMD from baseline compared with placebo. In study 1, the reduction in HAMD for brx60 was seen from 24 hours through 30 days; for brx90, it was seen at 60 hours and at 30 days, but not at the intervening time points. In study 2, the reduction in HAMD for brx90 was observed at time points from 48 hours through 7 days, but not at 30 days. The authors then conducted an integrated analysis with all three studies, using their 2017 brx90 data, along with brx90 data from study 1 and 2 here. Using the integrated data, at 60 hours, HAMD was reduced more with brx90 than with placebo (difference of 4.1). This decrease in HAMD was statistically significant as early as 24 hours and as long as 30 days. The results from the integrated data suggest that the inconsistent results between time points in the brx90 arms in study 1 and study 2 may have been due to being underpowered. Using the integrated data, the authors also demonstrated that the brx90 group had reductions in HAMD subscales, suggesting that the benefits from brexanolone treatment are not solely related to improved sleep. Twenty-two percent of women were also on other antidepressant medications; however, change in HAMD score with brx90 was significantly higher regardless of antidepressant medication use, supporting the notion that brexanolone's clinical benefit is likely unrelated to the serotonergic medication. Finally, brexanolone treatment helped both women who developed depression in the third trimester and those with onset in the postpartum period (Meltzer-Brody and colleagues, 2018, appendix figure 4S), although most participants enrolled had depression beginning within 4 weeks postpartum [41]. In the three randomized controlled trials, few women experienced serious side effects, indicating that brexanolone is a relatively safe medication [41].

There is limited information on the safety of brexanolone during breastfeeding. In one study of 12 women receiving brexanolone infusion, ALLO breastmilk levels were undetectable 3 days after the infusion in most women, indicating that ALLO clears from breastmilk rapidly [42]. In addition, no serious adverse effects were identified [42].

These studies support that IV brexanolone is a safe and effective treatment for PPD and that the effect is rapid and sustained. As a result, in 2019, brexanolone was approved by the FDA for treatment of PPD—the first drug ever given an FDA indication specifically for PPD.

Zuranolone (SAGE-217)

Zuranolone is a GABAAR-positive allosteric modulator that was developed to address implementation challenges of IV brexanolone, such as the need for hospitalization. It is administered orally on a daily basis for 2 weeks, and then stopped. Because it has not yet achieved FDA approval, monitoring requirements have not yet been determined. Trials to date have been designed to administer the medication in the home setting. Breastfeeding while taking zuranolone is discouraged because of its increased oral bioavailability and possible associated somnolence.

Zuranolone clinical trials

Preliminary studies for zuranolone for PPD are promising. In two phase 1, double-blind, randomized placebo-controlled dose-finding studies, no serious adverse effects occurred in a healthy population [43]. Deligiannidis and colleagues in 2019 conducted a phase 3, double-blind randomized placebo-controlled trial of 151 postpartum women who had a HAMD≥26 [44]. Women were randomized to receive either zuranolone 30 mg or placebo for 14 days. At day 15, zuranolone reduced HAMD by 17.8 points compared with 13.6 points for placebo, reaching statistical significance. A difference was also seen at day 3 and day 45. Multiple secondary endpoints were achieved, including HAMD response and remission rates on day 15 and day 45 and change in MADRS score (Montgomery-Asberg Depression Rating Scale) at day 15. Side effects included somnolence, headache, dizziness, upper respiratory tract infection, diarrhea, and sedation [44].

Ganaxolone

Ganaxolone is a positive allosteric modulator of GABAAR [45,46]. It has been synthesized with the addition of a methyl group to improve oral bioavailability without affecting activity at the GABAAR [45,47,48]. It can be administered in both IV and oral formulations.

Ganaxolone clinical trials

Marinus Pharmaceuticals conducted two phase 2 studies of ganaxolone for the treatment of PPD, the Magnolia Study and the Amaryllis Study [49,50]. The Magnolia Study part 1 included patients with a baseline HAMD≥26. A 60-hour infusion of ganaxolone dosed at 140 μg/kg/h (N = 10) achieved reduced HAMD score compared with placebo at time points 48 hours through 34 days. At 48 hours, ganaxolone reduced HAMD 5.6 points more than placebo. Seventy-five percent of patients responded by day 34%, and 67% responded rapidly by 60 hours. In addition, 50% of patients were in remission at day 34, and 33% at 60 hours. Sedation and dizziness were the most common side effects, and there were no serious side effects. Subsequently, in part 2 of the Magnolia Study (N = 33), patients were treated first with a 6-hour infusion of ganaxolone 20 mg/h and then with oral ganaxolone 900 mg daily for 28 days. Women had rapid reduction of HAMD by 6 hours, although it did not differ from placebo by day 28 [49,50]. Further studies are needed to clarify whether ganaxolone's transient effect in part 2 was related to infusion length. The open-label Amaryllis Study dosed oral ganaxolone at 675 mg or titrated to 1125 mg daily for 28 days and observed a decrease in HAMD until at least day 28 with no serious side effects, although it remains unknown whether this would differ from placebo in a double-blind randomized placebo-controlled study [49,50].

SGE-516

SGE-516 is a synthetic analog of ALLO. Similar to other neuroactive steroids, it is a positive allosteric modulator of the GABAA receptor. However, the compound is synthesized with a substitution at C-21 to increase oral bioavailability while maintaining activity at GABAAR [51]. Animal studies have demonstrated that SGE-516 has potential to be both an acute and a preventive treatment for PPD, but there are no human data.

Preclinical trials

Melon and colleagues in 2018 demonstrated that SGE-516 can treat and prevent PPD in a mouse model [52].

The authors developed three mouse subtypes to mimic women sensitive to PPD: Gabrd −/− (GABAAR delta subunit knockout), Gabrd +/− (GABAAR delta subunit reduction), and KCC2/Crh, as well as wild type mice. The CRH neurons of KCC2/Crh mice lack the K+/Cl- cotransporter, which is important for GABAergic inhibition and involved in regulation of response to stress. SGE-516 was administered to the mice either chronically (end of pregnancy to 48 h postpartum) or acutely (only in the postpartum). Acute and chronic administration of SGE-516 were both associated with decreased PPD-like behaviors and improved maternal care. In addition, administration of SGE-516 blunted anticipated stress effects on the HPA-axis. Conversely, administration of clobazam, a benzodiazepine, did not prevent PPD-like behavior in Gabrd −/− or KCC2/Crh mice.

PREMENSTRUAL DYSPHORIC DISORDER

Neuroactive steroids have the potential to treat other RD, including premenstrual dysphoric disorder (PMDD). PMDD is diagnosed when affective symptoms are present during the luteal phase but absent during the follicular phase of the menstrual cycle [53]. ALLO fluctuation during the luteal phase has been implicated in PMDD in hormonally sensitive women [54]. As a result, drugs that stabilize ALLO levels or the effects of ALLO are being investigated for the treatment of PMDD. Currently FDA-approved treatments for PMDD include the SSRIs fluoxetine and sertraline, which have neuroactive steroid effects at low doses [55], and the oral contraceptive drospirenone/ethinyl estradiol, which blocks ovulation and, therefore, luteal ALLO fluctuations [56]. Clinically, many women cannot tolerate, have contraindications to, or do not respond to one or both of these first-line treatment options, and therefore, additional pharmaceuticals are necessary. Current pharmaceutical agents being investigated include dutasteride, sepranolone, and ulipristal acetate (UPA).

Dutasteride

Dutasteride is an inhibitor of 5-alpha reductase, the enzyme that catalyzes the rate-limiting step in the metabolism of progesterone to ALLO; it thus stabilizes ALLO levels (Fig. 1) [54]. It is an oral medication currently

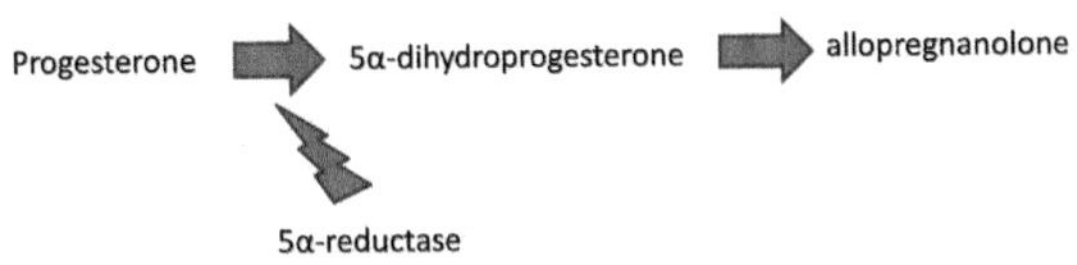

FIG. 1 Neuroactive steroid metabolism.

FDA approved for benign prostatic hyperplasia. It is a teratogen with a half-life of 5 weeks, and therefore, caution must be exercised when considering this treatment for women of reproductive age [57,58].

Dutasteride clinical trials

Martinez and colleagues in 2016 investigated whether low- or high-dose dutasteride could ameliorate PMDD symptoms [54]. The study included 16 women with PMDD with no other recent axis-1 diagnosis and 16 women without PMDD with no axis-1 diagnosis. The investigators administered dutasteride (0.5 mg or 2.5 mg/d) or placebo. Low-dose dutasteride (0.5 mg/d) failed to block luteal ALLO level changes and did not improve PMDD symptoms. Conversely, high-dose dutasteride (2.5 mg/d) prevented luteal ALLO fluctuation and decreased symptoms of PMDD compared with placebo in women with PMDD. Interestingly, it did not have an effect on women without PMDD.

Sepranolone

Sepranolone (UC1010) is a GABAAR-modulating steroid antagonist [59]. It is an analog of isoallopregnanolone, which antagonizes ALLO (rather than directly modulating the GABAAR) [59,60]. It is administered every other day subcutaneously during the luteal phase, from the day after the Luteinizing Hormone (LH) surge until the onset of menstruation [59].

Sepranolone clinical trials

Bixo and colleagues in 2017 studied subcutaneous sepranolone for the treatment of PMDD in a double-blind, randomized placebo-controlled trial, with a phase 1 study of 26 healthy women and a phase 2 trial of 106 women with PMDD [59]. In the phase 2 study, women were screened with prospective Daily Record of Severity of Problems (DRSP) ratings for 2 months for PMDD. Sepranolone (10 mg or 16 mg) or placebo was administered every other day in the luteal part of the cycle. The authors calculated the difference between luteal and follicular phase scores and, as the primary outcome, compared this difference at baseline to this difference during treatment. The primary outcome was achieved, but secondary outcomes including improvement on negative mood and impairment scales were not. However, 19 of the 106 women were found to have symptoms in the follicular phase (and, thus, did not meet criteria for PMDD), and 27 of the women did not take sepranolone as intended because of flaws in LH detection tests. In a post-hoc analysis of the 60 women who had symptoms limited to the luteal phase and who took the medication as intended, both primary and secondary outcomes reached statistical significance. Sepranolone was well tolerated, with no severe adverse effects reported [59].

Ulipristal acetate (UPA)

UPA is a selective progesterone receptor modulator that antagonizes progesterone, thereby stabilizing progesterone (and thus ALLO) levels across the menstrual cycle via anovulation [61]. It is administered daily via an oral route.

Ulipristal acetate (UPA) clinical trials

There is one double-blind, randomized placebo-controlled trial of UPA 5 mg/d for three 28-day cycles for PMDD [61]. UPA treatment lowered DRSP score in the final cycle by 41, compared with 22 for placebo. It also increased remission rate, with 50.0% of women having complete remission and 35.0% partial remission at 3 months, compared with 21.1% and 31.6% for the placebo group, respectively. Interestingly, UPA lowered psychiatric symptoms but not physical symptoms on DRSP subscales. UPA lowered progesterone levels premenstrually in the last month compared with the placebo group, supporting the hypothesis that stabilization of neuroactive steroid levels can treat PMDD. UPA was well tolerated, and the only side effect more common with UPA than placebo was nausea.

PERIMENOPAUSAL DEPRESSION

Unlike in PMDD and PPD, the link between the menopausal transition and incidence of depression is not as well established, and there has been substantially less research in this area. Several earlier cross-sectional studies found no relationship between the prevalence of MDD and menopausal status, whereas longitudinal studies have more consistently found a substantial increase in vulnerability to depressive symptoms during the menopause transition, with odds ratios ranging from 1.33 to 1.79 [62–66]. Community-based studies estimate that 20% to 40% of women will develop an episode of depression during the menopause transition [67,68].

As in other reproductive transitions, neuroactive steroids such as ALLO may have a substantive impact on perimenopausal depression risk. Owing to anovulatory cycles and erratic gonadal steroid fluctuations during the perimenopausal transition, there is significant potential for changing ALLO levels to dysregulate GABAAR functioning [69]. Consequently, neuroactive steroids may be able to ameliorate mood symptoms in the perimenopausal period in women sensitive to hormonal changes. However, while there is one small positive study of ganaxolone for postmenopausal treatment-resistant depression, to our knowledge, there are no studies of GABA-ergic compounds for the treatment of depression during the perimenopausal transition [70]. Investigation of the role of neuroactive steroids for the treatment of perimenopausal depression is needed.

OTHER PERIODS OF A WOMAN'S LIFE

Neuroactive steroids have been studied for the treatment of MDD in the general population. A preliminary double-blind, randomized placebo-controlled trial of zuranolone 30 mg for MDD found improvement in HAMD at day 15 [71].

The subsequent Mountain Study, a double-blind randomized placebo-controlled phase 3 study for MDD, found HAMD improvement with zuranolone 30 mg at day 3, 8, and 12, although not at the primary endpoint, day 15 [72]. When they excluded nonadherent patients, or when they included only severe MDD in post-hoc analyses, the primary endpoint was achieved [72]. Notably, sedation was unexpectedly uncommon, suggesting that zuranolone may have been underdosed. As a result, a subsequent study, the SHORELINE study, included a treatment arm using zuranolone 50 mg nightly [73].

The SHORELINE study, an open-label phase 3 study, found that 2-week treatment with zuranolone at doses of 30 mg and 50 mg is tolerated and a promising treatment for MDD. By day 15, zuranolone 30 mg reduced HAMD by 14.9 (SD: 7.1) [73]. Phase 3 double-blind, randomized placebo-controlled trials of zuranolone for MDD are warranted.

LIMITATIONS AND FUTURE DIRECTIONS FOR REPRODUCTIVE DEPRESSION TREATMENT WITH NEUROACTIVE STEROIDS

Neuroactive steroid pharmaceuticals hold promise for the treatment of RD across the reproductive lifespan, although current evidence is most robust for PPD. There is significant appeal for rapidly acting treatments for PPD given high rates of postpartum suicide [33], the potent and long-term impact of maternal depression on child health [35], and the normal functional demands mothers face as primary infant caregivers. Novel pharmaceuticals are additionally needed for PMDD and perimenopausal depression because many women cannot take current first-line treatments such as SSRIs and hormonal medication.

However, harnessing the full potential of neuroactive steroids may require substantive changes in health care delivery systems. Many health care systems currently lack appropriate workflows to meet FDA-required monitoring procedures for IV brexanolone in the inpatient setting, which demand medical skills and equipment that are often unavailable on behavioral health units and, alternatively, psychiatric expertise and services that are limited on medical-surgical floors. Payment models for brexanolone have faced analogous challenges.

There is considerable interest in oral neuroactive steroid formulations to avoid these challenges; however, home-based neuroactive steroid administration may present its own challenges, given its sedating effects, including concerns over impaired ability to care for infants overnight, co-sleeping risks, and other behavioral hazards such as impaired driving and concomitant use of sedating recreational or pharmaceutical substances. The rapid effects of IV formulations may still make them worthwhile and cost-effective treatments if feasibility challenges can be addressed. The postpartum is a period of increased risk for psychiatric hospitalization [74], and such a robust and rapid treatment has the potential to reduce length of stay and, consequently, maternal-infant separation. In addition, comparative efficacy of IV and oral formulations remains unknown and may be higher for IV formulations. Finally, delivery of brexanolone on mother-baby units enables inpatient psychiatric treatment for women with severe PPD, while fostering bonding and attachment, which is crucial for PPD treatment and for infant development.

For PMDD, accurate diagnosis and accurate LH detection have been challenges in clinical trials to date. It is common for women with nonreproductive mood disorders to have premenstrual worsening of mood and to inaccurately recall premenstrual symptoms [75]. Preventing fluctuations in ALLO improves premenstrual symptoms in women with PMDD, but not in women without PMDD, suggesting PMDD is distinct from premenstrual exacerbation of another mood disorder [54]. Menopausal symptom assessment has been similarly challenging, prompting the development of Stages of Reproductive Aging Workshop (STRAW) standards, although the relationship between these identified stages and RD is currently poorly characterized. It would be helpful to harness digital technologies that can accurately track symptoms in patient-friendly and clinically meaningful ways to further characterize these relationships and optimize the timing of treatment. Inquiry is also warranted into biomarkers that are accurate enough to direct treatment. Promising areas of inquiry currently are fMRI signatures and saccadic eye velocity [53,76,77].

SUMMARY

Women with mood changes during periods of hormonal fluctuation may have biologically distinct types of depression. Clinical studies of neuroactive steroid pharmaceuticals, which stabilize the neuroactive steroid changes implicated in RD, have yielded positive results. To date, brexanolone is the only neuroactive steroid FDA-indicated for the treatment of an RD. However, preliminary studies for other compounds are promising. Further investigation of neuroactive steroid compounds for RDs and their implementation is needed.

CLINICS CARE POINTS

- Certain hormonally sensitive women experience negative mood changes with fluctuations in neurosteroid levels. Stabilizing neurosteroid levels may prevent these negative mood changes.
- Brexanolone is FDA-indicated for postpartum depression (PPD).
- Preliminary studies support ganaxolone and zuranolone as potential treatments for PPD and ulipristal acetate, dutasteride, and sepranolone as potential treatments for PMDD, although large double-blind, randomized placebo-controlled trials are needed.

DISCLOSURE

A.D. Hermann is the cofounder and chief medical officer with equity stake in Iris Ob Health, Inc. and has been a paid consultant for Sage Therapeutics. L.C. Susser and C. Swanson have nothing to disclose.

REFERENCES

[1] Payne J, Palmer J, Joffe H. A reproductive subtype of depression: conceptualizing models and moving toward etiology. Harv Rev Psychiatry 2009;17:72–86.

[2] Burke C, Susser L, Hermann A. $GABA_A$ dysregulation as an explanatory model for late-onset postpartum depression associated with weaning and resumption of menstruation. Arch Womens Ment Health 2019;22:55–63.

[3] Gavin N, Gaynes B, Lohr K, et al. Perinatal Depression: a systematic review of prevalence and incidence. Obstet Gynecol 2005;106:1071–83.

[4] Lindahl V, Pearson J, Colpe L. Prevalence of suicidality during pregnancy and the postpartum. Arch Wom Ment Health 2005;8:77–87.
[5] Paul S, Purdy R. Neuroactive steroids. FASEB J 1992;6: 2311–22.
[6] Nayeem N, Green T, Martin I, et al. Quaternary structure of the native GABAA receptor determined by electron microscopic image analysis. J Neurochem 1994;62: 815–8.
[7] Klausberger T, Sarto I, Ehya N, et al. Alternate use of distinct intersubunit contacts controls GABAA receptor assembly and stoichiometry. J Neurosci 2001;21: 9124–33.
[8] Brickley SG, Mody I. Extrasynaptic GABA(A) receptors: their function in the CND and implications for disease. Neuron 2012;73:23–34.
[9] Farrant M, Nusser Z. Variations on an inhibitory theme: phasic and tonic activation of GABA(A) receptors. Nat Rev Neurosci 2005;6:215–29.
[10] Sundstrom-Poromaa I, Smith D, Gong Q, et al. Hormonally regulated $\alpha 4\beta 2\delta$ GABAA receptors are a target for alcohol. Nat Neurosci 2002;5:721–2.
[11] Maguire J, Mody I. GABA(A)R plasticity during pregnancy: relevance to postpartum depression. Neuron 2008;59:207–13.
[12] Maguire J, Mody I. Steroid hormone fluctuations and GABA(A)R plasticity. Psychoneuroendocrinology 2009; 34:S84–90.
[13] Akwa Y, Purdy R, Koob G, et al. The amygdala mediatesthe anxiolytic-like effect of the neurosteroid allopregnanolone in rat. Behav Brain Res 1999;106:119–25.
[14] Wieland S, Lan N, Mirasedeghi S, et al. Anxiolytic activity of the progesterone metabolite 5β-pregnan-3α-ol-20-one. Brain Res 1991;565:263–8.
[15] Schüle C, Nothdurfter C, Rupprecht R. The role of allopregnanolone in depression and anxiety. Prog Neurobiol 2014;113:79–87.
[16] Uzunova V, Sheline Y, Davis J, et al. Increase in the cerebrospinal fluid content of neurosteroids in patients with unipolar major depression who are receiving fluoxetine or fluvoxamine. Proc Natl Acad Sci U S A 1998;95: 3239–44.
[17] Romeo E, Strohle A, Spalletta G, et al. Effects of antidepressant treatment on neuroactive steroids in major depression. Am J Psychiatry 1998;155:901–13.
[18] Schüle C, Romeo E, Uzunov DP, et al. Influence of mirtazapine on plasma concentrations of neuroactive steroids in ma-jor depression and on 3α-hydroxysteroid dehydrogenase activity. Mol Psychiatry 2006;11:261–72.
[19] Fuzesi T, Daviu N, Wamsteeker, et al. Hypothalamic CRH neurons orchestrate complex behaviours after stress. Nat Commun 2016;7:11937.
[20] Patchev VK, Shoaib M, Holsboer F, et al. The neurosteroid tetrahydroprogesterone counteracts corticotropin-releasing hormone-induced anxiety and alters the release and gene expression of corticotropin-releasing hormone in the rat hypothalamus. Neuroscience 1994;62:265–71.
[21] Patchev V, Hassan A, Holsboer D, et al. The neurosteroid tetrahydroprogesterone attenuates the endocrine response to stress and exerts glucocorticoid-like effects on vasopressin gene transcription in the rat hypothalamus. Neuropsychopharmacology 1996;15:533–40.
[22] Sarkar J, Wakefield S, Mackenzie G, et al. Neurosteroidogenesis is required for the physiological response to stress: role of neurosteroid-sensitive GABAA receptors. J Neurosci 2011;31:18198–210.
[23] Maguire J. Neuroactive Steroids and GABAergic Involvement in the Neuroendocrine Dysfunction Associated With Major Depressive Disorder and Postpartum Depression. Front Cell Neurosci 2019;13:83.
[24] Smith S, Ruderman Y, Frye C, et al. Steroid withdrawal in the mouse results in anxiogenic effects of 3alpha, 5beta-THP: a possible model of premenstrual dysphoric disorder. Psychopharmacology 2006;186:323–33.
[25] Shen H, Gong Q, Aoki C, et al. Reversal of neurosteroid effects at $\alpha 4\beta 2\delta$ GABAA receptors triggers anxiety at puberty. Nat Neurosci 2007;10:469–77.
[26] Campo-Soria C, Chang Y, Weiss D. Mechanism of action of benzodiazepines on GABAA receptors. Br J Pharmacol 2006;148:984–90.
[27] Belelli D, Herd M, Mitchell E, et al. Neuroactive steroids and inhibitory neurotransmission: mechanisms of action and physiological relevance. Neuroscience 2006;138:821–9.
[28] Sigel E, Steinmann M. Structure, function, and modulation of GABA(A) receptors. J Biol Chem 2012;287:40224–31.
[29] Durkin E, Muessig L, Herit T, et al. Brain neurosteroids are natural anxiolytics targeting α2 subunit γ-aminobutyric acid type-A receptors. bioRxiv 2018. https://doi.org/10.1101/462457.
[30] Zorumski C, Paul S, Covey D, et al. Neurosteroids as novel antidepressants and anxiolytics: GABA-A receptors and beyond. Neurobiol Stress 2019;11:100196.
[31] Feighner J. Mechanism of action of antidepressant medications. J Clin Psychiatry 1999;60(Suppl 4):4–11.
[32] Grigoriadis S, Wilton A, Kurdyak P, et al. Perinatal suicide in Ontario, Canada: a 15-year population-based study. CMAJ 2017;189:1085–92.
[33] Shigemi D, Ishimaru M, Matsui H, et al. Suicide attempts among pregnant and postpartum women in japan: A Nationwide Retrospective Cohort Study. J Clin Psychiatry 2020;81:e1–5.
[34] Johannsen B, Larsen J, Laursen T. All-cause mortality in women with severe postpartum psychiatric disorders. Am J Psychiatry 2016;173:635–42.
[35] Weissman M, Wickramaratne P, Nomura Y, et al. Offspring of depressed parents: 20 years later. Am J Psychiatry 2006;163:1001–8.
[36] Pennell K, Woodin M, Pennell P. Quantification of neurosteroids during pregnancy using selective ion monitoring mass spectrometry. Steroids 2015;95:24–31.
[37] Luisi S, Petraglia F, Benedetto C, et al. Serum allopregnanolone levels in pregnant women: changes during pregnancy, at delivery, and in hypertensive patients. J Clin Endocrinol Metab 2000;85:2429–33.

[38] Botella G, Salituro F, Harrison B, et al. Neuroactive Steroids. 2. 3α-Hydroxy-3β-methyl-21-(4-cyano-1H-pyrazol-1′-yl)-19-nor-5β-pregnan-20-one (SAGE-217): A Clinical Next Generation Neuroactive Steroid Positive Allosteric Modulator of the (γ-Aminobutyric Acid)A Receptor. J Med Chem 2017;60:7810–9.
[39] Kanes S, Colquhoun H, Doherty J, et al. Open-label, proof-of-concept study of brexanolone in the treatment of severe postpartum depression. Hum Psychopharmacoal Clin Exp 2017;32:e2576.
[40] Kanes S, Colquhoun H, Gunduz-Bruce H, et al. Brexanolone (SAFE-547 injection) in post-partum depression: a randomized controlled trial. Lancet 2017;390:480–9.
[41] Meltzer-Brody S, Colquhoun H, Riesenberg R, et al. Brexanolone injection in post-partum depression: two multicenter, double-blind, randomized, placebo-controlled, phase 3 trials. Lancet 2018;392:1058–70.
[42] Hoffmann E, Wald J, Colquhoun H. Evaluation of breast milk concentrations following brexanolone iv administration to healthy lactating women. AJOG poster session 2019;220:S554.
[43] Hoffmann E, Nomikos G, Kaul I, et al. SAGE-217, A novel GABAA receptor allosteric modulator: clinical pharmacology and tolerability in randomized phase I dose-finding studies. Clin Pharmacokinet 2020;59: 111–20.
[44] Deligiannidis K, Lasser R, Gunduz-Bruce H, et al. A phase 3, double-blind, placebo-controlled trial of SAGE-217 in postpartum depression: assessment of depressive symptoms across multiple measures. Poster T74. Annual Meeting of ASCP 2019.
[45] Bialer M, Johannessen S, Levy R, et al. Progress report on new antiepileptic drugs: a summary of the twelfth eilat conference. Epilepsy Res 2015;111:85–141.
[46] Carter R, Wood P, Wieland S, et al. Characterization of the anticonvulsant properties of ganaxolone, a selective, high-affinity, steroid modulator of the gama-aminobutyric acidA receptor. J Pharmacol Exp Ther 1997;280:1284–95.
[47] How ganaxalone works. 2020. Available at: https://www.marinuspharma.com/our-science-pipeline/about-ganaxolone. Accessed December 4, 2020.
[48] Saporito M, Gruner J, DiCamillo A, et al. Intravenously Administered Ganaxolone Blocks Diazepam-Resistant Lithium-Pilocarpine-Induced Status Epilepticus in Rats: Comparison with Allopregnanolone. J Pharmacol Exp Ther 2019;368:326–37.
[49] Marinus Pharmaceuticals announces data from Magnolia and Amaryllis Phase 2 studies in women with postpartum depression. 2019. Available at: https://www.globenewswire.com/news-release/2019/07/23/1886335/0/en/Marinus-Pharmaceuticals-Announces-Data-from-Magnolia-and-Amaryllis-Phase-2-Studies-in-Women-with-Postpartum-Depression.html. Accessed December 7, 2020.
[50] Marinus Pharmaceuticals announces positive ganaxolone data in women with postpartum depression. 2018. Available at: https://www.globenewswire.com/news-release/2018/12/10/1664282/0/en/Marinus-Pharmaceuticals-Announces-Positive-Ganaxolone-Data-in-Women-With-Postpartum-Depression.html. Accessed December 4, 2020.
[51] Neoractive steroids. 1.Positive allosteric modulators of the GABAA receptor: structure-activity relationships of heterocyclic substitution at C-21. J Med Chem 2015;58: 3500–11.
[52] Melon L, Hammond R, Lewis M, et al. A novel, synthetic, neuroactive steroid is effective at decreasing depression-like behaviors and improving maternal care in preclinical models of postpartum depression. Front Endocrinol 2018;9:703.
[53] O'Brien P, Backstrom T, Brown C, et al. Towards a consensus on diagnostic criteria, measurement and trial design of the premenstrual disorders: the ISPMD Montreal consensus. Arch Womens Ment Health 2011;14:13–21.
[54] Martinez P, Rubinow D, Nieman L, et al. 5-alpha-reductase inhibition prevents the luteal phase increase in plasma allopregnanolone levels and mitigates symptoms in women with premenstrual dysphoric disorder. Neuropsychopharmacology 2016;41:1093–102.
[55] Pinna G, Costa E, Guidotti A. SSRIs act as selective brain steroidogenic stimulants (SBSSs) at low doses that are inactive on 5-HT reuptake. Curr Opin Pharmacol 2009; 9:24–30.
[56] De Berardis D, Serroni N, Salerno R, et al. Treatment of premenstrual dysphoric disorder (PMDD) with a novel formulation of drospirenone and ethinyl estradiol. Ther Clin Risk Manag 2007;3:585–90.
[57] Avodart. Prescribing information. 2008. Available at: https://www.accessdata.fda.gov/drugsatfda_docs/label/2008/021319s015lbl.pdf. Accessed December 4, 2020.
[58] Hirshburg J, Kelsey P, Therrien C, et al. Adverse effects and safety of 5-alpha reductase inhibitors (finasteride, dutasteride): a systematic review. J Clin Aesthet Dermatol 2016;9:56–62.
[59] Bixo M, Ekberg K, Poromaa I, et al. Treatment of premenstrual dysphoric disorder with GABAA receptor modulating steroid antagonist Sepranolone (UC1010)-A randomized controlled trial. Psychoneuroendcrinology 2017;80:46–55.
[60] Bengtsson S, Nyberg S, Hedstrom H, et al. Isoallopregnanolone antagonize allopregnanolone-induced effects on saccadic eye velocity and self-reported sedation in humans. Psychoneuroendocrinology 2015;52:22–31.
[61] Comasco E, Kallner H, Hirschberg A, et al. Ulipristal Acetate for Treatment of Premenstrual Dysphoric Disorder: A Proof-of-Concept Randomized Controlled Trial. Am J Psychiatry Adv 2020. https://doi.org/10.1176/appi.ajp.2020.20030286.
[62] McKinlay J, McKinlay S, Brambilla D. The relative contributions of endocrine changes and social circumstances to depression in mid-aged women. J Health Soc Behav 1987;28:345–63.
[63] Kaufert P, Gilbert P, Tate R. The Manitoba Project: a re-examination of the link between menopause and depression. Maturitas 1992;14:143–55.

[64] Bromberger J, Matthews K, Schott L, et al. Depressive symptoms during the menopausal transition: the Study of Women's Health Across the Nation (SWAN). J Affect Disord 2007;103(1):267–72.

[65] Freeman E, Sammel M, Liu L. Hormones and menopausal status as predictors of depression in women in transition to menopause. Arch Gen Psychiatry 2004;61:62.

[66] Woods N, Smith-DiJulio K, Percival D, et al. Depressed mood during the menopausal transition and early postmenopause: observations from the Seattle Midlife Women's Health Study. Menopause 2008;15:223–32.

[67] Cohen L, Soares C, Vitonis A, et al. Risk for new onset of depression during the menopausal transition: the Harvard study of moods and cycles. Arch Gen Psychiatry 2006;63:385.

[68] Freeman E, Sammel M, Lin H, et al. Associations of hormones and menopausal status with depressed mood in women with no history of depression. Arch Gen Psychiatry 2006;63:375.

[69] Gordon J, Girdler S, Meltzer-Brody S, et al. Ovarian hormone fluctuation, neurosteroids, and HPA axis dysregulation in perimenopausal depression: a novel heuristic model. Am J Psychiatry 2015;172:227–36.

[70] Dichtel L, Nyer M, Dording C, et al. Effects of open-label, adjunctive ganaxolone on persistent depression despite adequate antidepressant treatment in postmenopausal women: a pilot study. J Clin Psychiatry 2020;81:e1–8.

[71] Gunduz-Bruce H, Silber C, Kaul I, et al. Trial of SAGE-217 in patients with major depressive disorder. N Engl J Med 2019;381:903–11.

[72] Sage Therapeutics reports topline results from pivotal phase 3 MOUNTAIN study of SAGE-217 in major depressive disorder. 2019. Available at: https://investor.sagerx.com/news-releases/news-release-details/sage-therapeutics-reports-topline-results-pivotal-phase-3. Accessed December 5, 2020.

[73] Sage Therapeutics announces positive interim, topline zuranolone safety and tolerability data from open-label SHORELINE study in patients with MDD. 2020. Available at: https://investor.sagerx.com/news-releases/news-release-details/sage-therapeutics-announces-positive-interim-topline-zuranolone. Accessed December 5, 2020.

[74] Munk-Olsen T, Maegbaek M, Johannsen B, et al. Perinatal psychiatric episodes: a population-based study on treatment incidence and prevalence. Transl Psychiatry 2016;6:e919.

[75] Marvan M, Cortes-Iniestra C. Women's beliefs about the prevalence of premenstrual syndrome and biases in recall of premenstrual changes. Health Psychol 2001;4:276–80.

[76] O'Brien S, Sethi A, Gudbrandsen M, et al. Is postnatal depression a distinct subtype of major depressive disorder? An exploratory study. Arch Womens Ment Health 2020. https://doi.org/10.1007/s00737-020-01051-x.

[77] Sundstrom I, Backstrom T. Patients with premenstrual syndrome have decreased saccadic eye velocity compared to control subjects. Biol Psychiatry 1998;44:755–64.

[78] Ella. Prescribing information. 2018. Available at: https://www.accessdata.fda.gov/drugsatfda_docs/label/2018/022474s010lbl.pdf. Accessed December 12, 2020.

Sports Psychiatry

Advances in Psychiatry and Behavioral Health 1 (2021) 119–133

ADVANCES IN PSYCHIATRY AND BEHAVIORAL HEALTH

Mental Health in Youth Athletes

A Clinical Review

Courtney C. Walton, PhD[a,*], Simon Rice, PhD[a], R.I. (Vana) Hutter, PhD[b], Alan Currie, MD[c,d], Claudia L. Reardon, MD[e], Rosemary Purcell, PhD[a]

[a]Elite Sports and Mental Health, Orygen, 35 Poplar Road, Parkville, Victoria 3052, Australia; [b]Faculty of Behavioural and Movement Sciences, Vrije Universiteit Amsterdam, van der Boechorststraat 7-9, Amsterdam 1081 BT, the Netherlands; [c]Regional Affective Disorders Service, Cumbria; [d]Northumberland Tyne and Wear NHS Foundation Trust, Wolfson Research Centre, Campus for Ageing and Vitality, Westgate Road, Newcastle NE4 5PL, UK; [e]Department of Psychiatry, University of Wisconsin School of Medicine and Public Health, 6001 Research Park Boulevard, Madison, WI 53719, USA

KEYWORDS

• Psychiatry • Mental health • Sport • Athletes • Adolescents • Youth

KEY POINTS

- Youth sport provides an environment that can be both protective and supportive of physical and mental health. However, a range of psychosocial stressors and negative experiences can also be present.
- Potential stressors faced by elite youth athletes include pressure to perform and perfectionism, burnout, maintenance of academic and social balance, interpersonal conflict or abuse, injury and concussion, body image and weight pressures, and disrupted sleep.
- Clinicians treating a youth athlete should be conscious of the sporting context, in order to facilitate both trust and engagement with the athlete, as well as to better understand potential contributing and protective factors for distress.

INTRODUCTION

Common mental health disorders, such as depression and anxiety, are prevalent in young people. Approximately half of all mental health disorders begin by the midteens [1]. Although prevalence rates vary, an estimated 20% to 25% of adolescents and young adults in the general community experience a diagnosable disorder in any given year [2]. Puberty and the growing importance of interpersonal relationships can play a role in the potential development of a mental health disorder, along with risk factors such as abuse, neglect, bullying, and social disadvantage [2,3]. In contrast, physical exercise and sport provide benefits to the mental health of youth via multiple biological, psychological, and social effects. Biological benefits include the neurophysiologic effects of physical activity; psychological effects include the development of competence, confidence, and improved self-esteem; whereas social benefits include increased social integration, cohesion, and shared goals [4,5]. Although rates of organized sports participation vary globally, in many countries, the majority of young people are engaged in organized sport [6].

This article examines mental health within competitive youth athletes and is directed toward clinicians working with adolescent and school-aged competitive athletes, including elite junior or pathway athletes. It defines youth athletes as those aged approximately 12 to 18 years, while noting that more recent, nontraditional approaches consider the concept of youth to

*Corresponding author, *E-mail addresses:* courtney.walton@orygen.org.au; @CC_Walton; @clinpsych; @VanaHutter; @DrAlanCPsych346; @claudiareardon

https://doi.org/10.1016/j.ypsc.2021.05.011
2667-3827/21/

extend into early adulthood [7]. The article examines specific factors associated with sport that can contribute to exacerbation or causation of mental health symptoms and disorders in youth athletes, and canvasses considerations for appropriate assessment and treatment in this group.

YOUNG PEOPLE CAN THRIVE THROUGH SPORT

Sports participation contributes to physical health and psychosocial development of youth by providing a forum for building life skills, such as resilience, teamwork, leadership, and communication skills, or via intentionally developing positive mental health outcomes using positive youth development frameworks [8–11]. A recent review showed that sport can contribute to positive youth development in the form of positive self-perceptions, learning problem-solving skills, stress management, goal setting, taking personal responsibility, instilling perseverance, working hard, and independence, in addition to developing friendships, communication skills, and leadership [12]. Vella and colleagues [13] have demonstrated that the relationships between sport participation and adolescent mental health are bidirectional. Specifically, when exploring a large longitudinal sample of adolescents with assessments at 12 and 14 years of age, time involved in organized sport predicted better future mental health, and vice versa. However, these findings relate to community sport and are not necessarily a given in elite youth sport environments. Nonetheless, quality talent development environments exist in highly competitive sport (eg, European football academies), with studies reporting a positive association between the quality of the environment and the mental health outcomes of youth players [14–16].

MENTAL HEALTH AND RELATED STRESSORS IN YOUTH SPORT

Despite the proliferation of research into the mental health of elite athletes [17,18], youth sport remains under-represented [19]. Meta-analysis has shown that, for adolescents engaged in all forms of sport participation, there is a small association with lower levels of anxious and depressive symptoms [20]. In line with this, Weber and colleagues [21] showed low depression and anxiety symptoms among their sample of 12-18 year-old athletes. Seven percent and 3% were classified as possible and probable cases for anxiety, respectively, with these figures at 9.5% and 3.7% for depression. Brand and colleagues compared rates of mental health symptoms between elite student athletes (aged 12–15 years) who had recently been deselected from elite sport promotion, and nonsport students. Rates across common mental health symptoms and disorders were higher than Brand and colleagues [22] found, including generalized anxiety disorder (lifetime: men, 9.0%; women, 14.4%), social phobia (last 12 months: men, 6.7%; women, 7.4%), and depressed mood (last 12 months: men, 19.3%; women, 36.5%). In general, rates were significantly higher in deselected athletes. In addition to deselection being a risk factor, youth athletes (mean age, 14.96 years) in individual sports have reported more depressive symptoms than those in team sports (mean Center for Epidemiologic Studies Depression Scale scores of 11.55 and 9.47, respectively) [23], suggesting a range of sport-specific factors may be key to understanding rates of symptoms.

Further aspects of sport may contribute to the development or escalation of mental health symptoms or disorders in youth athletes. Salient factors that predict dropout from organized youth sport include lack of enjoyment, low perceptions of competence, social pressures, competing priorities, and physical factors such as injury [24]. These domains provide insights into contributing stressors to poor mental health, some of which may be targets of interventions to restore both sport participation and mental health. Several contextual factors and stressors related to sporting environments may also be influential to mental well-being in youth athletes, although the extant literature in this regard has focused specifically on outcomes such as sports enjoyment, dropout, performance anxiety, or burnout [5,25]. Stressors examined next in this article may not necessarily predict mental health symptoms or disorders in youth athletes but are explored in order to assist clinicians in understanding the potential negative experiences and contexts that a presenting youth athlete may be experiencing (additional references are provided in Table 1).

Pressure to Perform and Perfectionism

Youth athletes are increasingly exposed to pressures to perform at a consistent and high level, potentially encouraging or instilling high levels of perfectionism [26]. Perfectionism is a multidimensional construct, and is typically conceptualized via at least 2 key factors: (1) perfectionistic concerns, which relate to the pursuit of exacting standards imposed by significant others; and (2) perfectionistic strivings, which relate to the pursuit of self-imposed goals and standards accompanied by

TABLE 1
Stressors in Youth Sport and Corresponding Considerations for Treating Clinicians

	Clinics Care Points	Suggested Reading
Perfectionism	• Show understanding and empathy toward the exceptional standards required for success in elite sport, while conveying that harsh self-criticism can be detrimental to well-being and performance • Be aware of perfectionistic concerns and ideas relating to demanding standards or perceived negative evaluation from others • Provide psychoeducation to help the athlete identify both the positive and negative aspects of perfectionism on mental health and performance	Hill et al, [32] 2018 Hill et al, [104] 2017
Burnout and specialization	• Understand/monitor the athlete's current workload (not just the current sporting requirements but also the academic and social demands the athlete is balancing) • Assess for symptoms of burnout: physical and emotional exhaustion, reduced sense of accomplishment, and sport devaluation. These symptoms should be differentiated from depressive symptoms, although symptom overlap can occur • Work with the athletes to identify what they enjoy(ed) about their sports participation, and how this may have recently changed • Support the athlete and caregivers in reframing expectations of sports participation to emphasize that fun and development are important, even at elite youth levels. Highly specialized and demanding training regimes are not necessarily effective strategies for sporting success, and can lead to reduced well-being, burnout, and subsequent dropout • Help athletes to understand their values and potential nonsporting pursuits to expand identity and promote role balance	Pacewicz et al, [105] 2019 Brenner et al, [36] 2019[a] DiSanti et al, [37] 2019[a]
Injury	• Try to understand what is causing the distress in response to injury (eg, physical pain, frustration with rehabilitation, trauma, isolation, and fear of reinjury or not returning to prior ability) so as to inform treatment approaches • Compassion-based and acceptance-based approaches are helpful, given that injury is an almost inevitable outcome of elite sport • Help the athlete learn to transform the injury into an opportunity for growth and development	Rist et al, [106] 2020 Ross et al, [107] 2019 Baranoff et al, [108] 2019

(continued on next page)

TABLE 1
(continued)

	Clinics Care Points	Suggested Reading
Concussion	• Psychological symptoms following concussion in youth athletes are common • Athletes may be poor at recognizing, or may actively downplay, concussive symptoms. Adapted phrasing for describing concussion (using lay language or sports slang; eg, "blacked out" rather than "loss of consciousness") may assist in recognition. • Given the severe potential neurologic consequences of repetitive head trauma, treating practitioners should include specialist neuropsychologists, neurologists, sports medicine physicians, or others with relevant expertise in the assessment of symptoms and recommendations for future sport involvement	Rivara et al, [62] 2020[a] Rice et al, [59] 2018 Covassin et al, [61] 2017[a]
Interpersonal conflict	• Bullying and conflict occur in sport, and it is important to identify the athlete's key relationships that are centered in sport • Be particularly cognizant of any negative interpersonal experiences for athletes who identify as from a minority group • Collect collateral information from parents and coaches if the athlete provides consent	Wachsmuth et al, [109] 2017 Knight et al, [46] 2017[a]
Abuse and harassment	• Abuse may not be disclosed by the athlete where it exists • Aim to sensitively assess for potential experiences of trauma or maltreatment that may have gone unreported • Consider sport-specific forms of abuse such as body shaming, and encouragement to dope, cheat, or play when injured/concussed • Be conscious in considering the important consequences an athlete may perceive as a result of disclosing an abusive relationship. However, child safety must be the foremost concern	Kerr et al, [50] 2019[a] Mountjoy et al, [110] 2016 Mountjoy et al, [49] 2015 Stirling [47], 2009
Weight and body image	• Concerns around body weight and image are common in athletes, and require significant clinical attention • Screening for eating disorders following the emergence of any new body image concerns is important to reduce the potential for missed diagnoses • These concerns may relate specifically to the particular demands of the sport in question (eg, weight-dependent and aesthetic sports). Have a good awareness of, or openness to learn about, the particular requirements of the sport in order to build trust and credibility in aligning treatment goals with the athlete • Multidisciplinary care and specialist treatment are typically required for any diagnosed disorder	Wells et al, [66] 2020 Stoyel et al, [70] 2020 Karrer et al, [71] 2020[a]
Sleep	• Poor sleep is a common problem in youth athletes • Obtain accurate information about the young person's sleeping habits and any disruptions that may be present • There are many approaches to sleep extension that can be helpful, including sleep hygiene psychoeducation and cognitive behavioral approaches	Vlahoyiannis et al, [73] 2020 Kroshus et al [111], 2019[a] Gupta et al, [112] 2017[a]

Note: Clinics care points are designed to communicate evidence-based tips for treatment.
[a] Article relates predominantly to youth (including collegiate) athletes.

harsh self-criticism [27]. Perfectionistic concerns are thought to be more maladaptive to mental well-being.

Research has shown associations between perfectionistic concerns and negative outcomes in youth athletes, most commonly burnout [28–30]. Fear of failure (a construct highly related to perfectionistic concerns) is associated with psychological stress in adolescent athletes [31]. Meta-analysis has provided support that perfectionistic concerns are associated with poorer well-being and higher likelihood of anxiety, while providing no clear benefit to sporting performance [32]. There is correlational evidence that younger athletes have higher rates of perfectionistic concerns than older athletes [33], making this an area of focus for youth sport and a target for early intervention to avert negative outcomes such as burnout and dropout.

Burnout and Early Specialization

Burnout in sport can be characterized by physical and emotional exhaustion, reduced sense of accomplishment, and sport devaluation [34]. Granz and colleagues [35] identified involvement in technical, endurance, aesthetic, or weight-dependent sport, training under an autocratic or a laissez-faire coach, high subjective stress outside of sport, a low willingness to make psychological sacrifices, lack of sleep, and female sex as key contributors to youth athlete burnout. In contrast, factors that decreased the likelihood of burnout were fewer hours of training, low social pressure, low subjective stress outside of sport, a high willingness to make psychological sacrifices, and high health satisfaction [35].

Early sport specialization is becoming increasingly common as athletes, coaches, and parents quest for future success. In a review of psychosocial consequences of early sport specialization, youth athletes were considered to be at risk of social isolation, poor academic performance, increased anxiety, greater stress, inadequate sleep, decreased family time, and burnout [36]. This finding should be considered with consistent evidence that early sport specialization is not required for future elite success [37]. However, complexity as to the necessity for early specialization arises when there are clear between-sport differences, with the peak age of performance being considerably younger in some sports (eg, gymnastics) compared with others (eg, road cycling).

Peer and Parental Conflict

In adolescence, interpersonal conflict and bullying among peers is common, and a causal link exists between bullying and a range of negative mental health outcomes, such as depression, anxiety, substance use, and suicidal ideation and behaviors [38]. Although evidence suggests that bullying occurs more commonly in school settings than in sport [39], Partridge and Knapp [40] examined the role of conflict in female adolescent team sport participants, and identified jealousy, personal characteristics, and coaching influences as the key sources of interpersonal conflict. The outcomes of this conflict included performance anxiety and a range of negative emotional experiences such as sadness, embarrassment, anger, and reduced self-esteem. Among adolescent male football players, bullying was more likely to be perpetrated by those who endorsed more typically masculine traits, and it was observed that this behavior was encouraged or endorsed by influential male role models such as brothers, fathers, or coaches [41].

Parents of competitive youth athletes can be both protective of mental well-being and contribute to poor mental health. Protective aspects include providing emotional, behavioral, financial, and logistical support. However, parents of athletes can also be a key source of stress, through negative or critical feedback, anger or inappropriate behavior during training and competition, and holding unrealistic expectations for their children/athletes [42]. Qualitative investigation of clinicians' experiences in talent development pathways have highlighted the detrimental role of pushy parents in youth athlete mental health [43]. It is possible, although it has not yet been proved, that parental style (ie, authoritarian and controlling or autonomy supportive) [44] may influence athlete mental health outcomes. An assortment of factors can influence how a youth athlete perceives parental involvement in sport, including gender, goal alignment, timing of involvement, motivational climate, and relationship quality [45,46].

Abuse and Maltreatment

Abuse or maltreatment can occur in youth sport, perpetrated by coaches, parents, administrators, officials, and other athletes (Box 1) [47]. Relational maltreatment occurs within a critical relationship role in which the other has significant influence over an individual's sense of safety, trust, and fulfillment of needs [48]. Such maltreatment typically revolves around acts of neglect and/or physical, sexual, and emotional abuse. Nonrelational maltreatment does not occur within critical relationships and may include harassment, bullying, (sexual) exploitation, institutional maltreatment, and abuse or assault [47,48]. Given the importance of child safety to clinical practice, the overviews of Stirling [47]

BOX 1
Considering Culture and Minority Perspectives

Clinicians should make every effort to be aware of the potentially differing experiences of individuals who identify from groups that may experience discrimination, bullying, or abuse. In young people particularly, there is evidence that athletes identifying as from sexual, gender, or racial-ethnic minority groups can have a negative sporting experience for a range of reasons. For example, youth athletes may feel unwelcomed, be unable to express themselves, and show reduced help seeking [100–103]. Discussion of this experience should be welcomed and supported by clinicians.

and Mountjoy and colleagues [49] are recommended reading for clinicians working with youth athletes.

Central to the potential for youth athlete maltreatment is the inherent power imbalance that exists between the athletes and the adults who are responsible for decisions critical to their sporting ambitions and desires (eg, playing time, selection, medical treatment, training priority). Coaches and support staff, such as medical, nutritional, and strength and conditioning specialists, hold positions of power [50]. Parents can also become socialized into accepting a range of abusive behaviors in elite youth sport, leading to a lack of action in confronting abusive coaches [51]. In a sample of more than 4000 adult Belgian and Dutch athletes [52], the retrospective reporting of severe emotional, physical, and sexual abuse during childhood sport was predictive of mental health symptoms as an adult.

Injury and Concussion

Youth athletes are at risk of injury because of ongoing physical and physiologic changes, as well as underdeveloped coordination, skills, and perception [53]. Similar to adult elite athletes [18], injury can be a significant stressor for both acute and ongoing mental health problems in youth athletes, although accurate prevalence rates are lacking [54–56]. Distress can manifest as anger, grief, guilt, and burnout, with symptoms potentially reflective of anxiety, depression, and adjustment and posttraumatic stress disorders. These responses to injury often reflect an athlete dealing with physical pain, frustration during the rehabilitation process, traumatic flashbacks, isolation or exclusion from sport and teammates, and fear of reinjury or not returning to prior levels of ability [56–58].

The role of concussion in mental health is receiving increasing attention [59]. Concussions occur frequently in youth sport, although overall incidence varies highly between sports. Of particular concern, adolescent athletes are known to significantly underreport postconcussive symptoms, typically as a result of not wanting to leave the game, misunderstanding the severity, or not wanting to let their team down [60]. However, only limited information is available on the effects of concussion on mental health outcomes in youth athletes, including self-harm and suicide [61,62]. Anxiety has been identified in young people (aged 8–18 years) who show postconcussive symptoms for 1 month or longer, compared with those whose symptoms resolved within a week [63], and increased depressive symptoms at 2, 7, and 14 days postconcussion were reported in a sample of youth athletes [64]. In another sample of 174 young people reporting a sport-related concussion (or subsequent postconcussion syndrome), 11.5% experienced a negative postinjury mental health outcome or worsening symptoms of a preinjury mental health disorder [65].

Body Image and Weight Concerns

Disordered eating may take the form of restrictive diets, binge eating, dehydration, purging, or diet pills. It may occur with or without excessive exercise or training [66]. In a representative sample of more than 1000 adolescent athletes [67], 8% reported constantly trying to lose weight, with 12% using compensatory methods (eg, fasting, purging, and appetite suppressers), and 32.5% fulfilling criteria for an eating disorder. Little is known about comorbid mental health outcomes associated with eating disorders in youth athletes, although anxiety has been shown to be higher in those with disordered eating behaviors versus those without [68,69].

Although higher rates of eating disorder symptoms are typically found in female athletes and those competing in sports that depend on weight or aesthetics, a recent systematic review showed major inconsistencies in the literature in relation to sport-based risk factors [70], and male athletes have been neglected in the literature [71], with most interventional studies in youth athletes (>80%) focused on women [72]. Of clinical relevance, this literature suggests that successful interventions are characterized by a longer duration, higher session intensity, and targeting self-esteem and self-efficacy as well as mental disorders related to eating and nutrition.

Disrupted Sleep

The bidirectional and interdependent role of sleep and mental health is familiar to most clinicians. Athletes commonly report inadequate sleep, but additional academic and social demands in youth may accentuate this. A recent systematic review [73] showed that child and adolescent athletes had impaired sleep quality across a range of measurements, including sleep time, sleep efficiency, and waking after sleep onset, compared with young and middle-aged adults. Further, sleep onset latency was longer for elite youth athletes, compared with semi-elite. Given that 8 to 11 hours of sleep per night is recommended for young people aged 6 to 18 years [74], it is concerning that the review estimated that athletes between these ages are getting closer to 6 hours of total sleep time [73]. Although not investigated specifically in youth athletes, the use of electronic devices and screen time at night may be an important factor, particularly if athletes are away during competition. This possibility is based on moderately strong evidence for an association between screen time and depressive symptoms in young people [75].

ASSESSMENT OF YOUTH ATHLETES

Fundamental to the initial assessment of youth athletes is obtaining a clear understanding of the individual's sporting environment (Box 2). The key systems [76] that all have the potential to affect an athlete's behaviors, attitudes, and experiences are (1) the family subsystem (athlete, parents, and siblings), (2) the team subsystem (athlete, peers, and coaches), and (3) the environmental subsystem (organizations, communities, and societies) [76]. Clinicians should gather a comprehensive understanding of how each system interacts with the youth athlete and the potential protective or harmful relationships entailed within these systems.

During assessment [77], athletes should be encouraged to describe their positive and negative experiences in sport, with specific attention to key relationships with peers, coaches, and parents. Attention to the role and function of sport in the athlete's life, as well as how and why this particular sport was chosen, can help reveal proxy achievement concerns. Clinicians should be active in listening and prompting for any potential abuse or maltreatment that may be occurring, given that unguided disclosure is unlikely. Understanding the youth athlete's interpretation of perceived pressures around body image and weight, performance, and playing through injury (particularly concussion) is important, as is an understanding of the extent to which the athlete is balancing sport participation with academic and social roles. Identifying the ways in which athletes view and relate to themselves, especially with regard to athletic identity and perfectionistic concerns, is indicated given their association with mental health symptoms.

> **BOX 2**
> **Putting the Person Before the Athlete: a Brief Caution**
>
> Although sport participation is the focus of this clinical review, the authors caution against overemphasizing the role of sport when this may not be the relevant factor to the young person. Many athletes think that they are seen as the athlete throughout many interactions in social and academic life, which can lead to a reduction and rejection of their unique identities and experiences. Clinicians should be careful not to fall into this trap. Many athletes are experiencing a significant mental health problem that is related to concerns outside of sport (eg, relationship breakup, death in the family), or a long-standing condition. Any clinician working with an athlete should endeavor to work from a person-centered approach where there is capacity for the human experience to be emphasized before the athlete.

Athlete Resistance and Mental Health Stigma

Athletes commonly mask or downplay the severity of their emotional distress, given that sport is an arena where mental toughness and getting on with it is highly valued. This mentality may be particularly strong in youth athletes who are still developing confidence and self-understanding, and among those already competing in adult sport settings. Youth athletes (aged 16–23 years) in one study expressed that they should not show weaknesses, and worried about what others, including teammates, coaches, opponents, and parents, would think of their ability to perform to their best [78]. Clinicians should be conscious of the potential ramifications for help seeking or disclosure of mental health symptoms in youth athletes, including the perceived consequences, such as losing playing time or selection, or reduced trust from teammates and coaches. To enhance therapeutic engagement, some athletes respond better to treatment being framed within the context of performance optimization, rather than treatment of a disorder [17,79]. Such strategies may also be needed for parents, who could hold similarly stigmatizing views.

Assessment Tools

To our knowledge, there are no sport-specific assessment tools for mental health in youth athletes. A range of youth-appropriate general mental health screening tools are recommended by the Neurobiology in Youth

Mental Health Partnership [80], and may be used to augment sport-specific measures (developed for and normed in adult athletes). Several specific athlete-centered tools can provide valuable insights for treating clinicians as to current stressors faced by an athlete or predispositions and characteristics that may enhance case formulation and treatment approaches (eg, sports-based perfectionism). Table 2 provides a summary of measures that may be useful to consider in assessing youth athletes.

Collateral Information

Ideally, collateral information to augment the young person's self-report should be included as part of the assessment [81]. Clinicians should be sensitive to parental pressures as potential causes of distress. Because coaches identify that they have a role to play in youth athlete mental health through identifying issues and facilitating support [82], they may also provide helpful collateral information. Any information gathering should be done transparently with the young person's support and consent.

TREATMENT OF YOUTH ATHLETES

At the outset of treatment, it is important to clearly establish treatment goals in partnership with the youth athlete. Although this is good practice in youth mental health, athletes may respond particularly well to this, given goal-driven tendencies established in sport. Goals may revolve around stress control, conflict resolution, sleep and energy management, injury recovery and pain management, mental preparation, and treatment of mental health symptoms or disorders [83,84].

Psychological Approaches

Psychological approaches should be considered the first-line treatments for mental health symptoms or disorders in youth athletes, with pharmacologic treatment indicated in more severe or complex cases. Because there is a dearth of evidence regarding the efficacy of various interventions specific for youth athletes, clinicians are encouraged to extrapolate the existing evidence base and treatment guidance from the general population into the context of high-performance sport. Cognitive behavior therapies (including third-wave approaches) may be well suited to youth athletes, given a range of inherent ingredients that overlap with sport: structure, direction, practice (homework), goal setting, and self-reliance [85,86]. Given the role of parents in youth athlete support and/or stress, family therapy may be an important approach to consider in the treatment process for suitably qualified practitioners [85]. Compassion-focused therapies are increasingly relevant to athlete well-being [87,88], with enhanced self-compassion particularly suited for body image concerns [89], performance failures [90], or injury [91]. In addition, individualized education programs in schools may be helpful in the context of certain symptoms and disorders given the youth athlete's typical dual role as student.

Pharmacologic Considerations

Medication may be necessary for treatment of more severe mental health symptoms or disorders. If used in this population, medications should typically be combined with other approaches, as described earlier. In adult athletes, considerations for prescribing medications include (1) potential negative impacts on athletic performance, (2) potential performance enhancing effects, and (3) potential safety risks [18]. Those considerations also have relevance for youth athletes, although the extent to which that is the case varies by the particular sport and its demands, level of performance required, time frame within the athletic training/competition cycle, and anticipated duration of treatment [18].

Common side effects that may negatively affect athletic performance in youth include sedation, weight gain, orthostatic hypotension, tachycardia, and tremor [92]. In general, clinicians aim to minimize side effects in youth (athletes or not). The overall impact of the medication on the youth athlete's functioning and health and the salience of sport in the athlete's life all influence medication decisions. All else being equal, it is desirable to avoid performance-limiting side effects in youth athletes if possible, while not compromising on effective care.

Stimulant medications, typically prescribed for attention-deficit/hyperactivity disorder (ADHD), represent the primary group of psychiatric medications for which there are concerns about ergogenic (unfair) performance enhancement. Thus, at higher levels of competition, stimulants are typically prohibited unless an application is made for a medical exemption (called a Therapeutic Use Exemption [TUE]) [93,94]. There are typically no prohibitions at or before high school level. For youth athletes appropriately prescribed and wishing to continue stimulants and who plan to compete at certain national or international levels, clinicians may be asked to supply medical information to help youth athletes apply for a TUE [94]. A second group of medications with prohibitions in some sports are β-blockers, which are sometimes prescribed for performance anxiety. This group may improve fine motor control and

TABLE 2
Sport-specific measures for mental health and related stressors in athletes

Construct	Measure	Description
Athlete mental health: general assessment	International Olympic Committee Sport Mental Health Assessment Tool 1 [113]	• A sequential assessment guiding clinicians through identification of mental health concerns • The Athlete Psychological Strain Questionnaire [114] is used as a triage tool, and may be an appropriate option as a stand-alone measure (see below)
	Athlete Psychological Strain Questionnaire [114]	• A 10-item self-report measure assessing psychological strain related to sporting environments with the following subscales: self-regulation, performance, and coping
	Sport Interference Checklist [115]	• A 26-item self-report measure that assesses behavioral and cognitive factors that are reported to interfere with sport performance in training and competition, as well as the athletes' likelihood of seeking help for the problem
	Sport Mental Health Continuum—Short Form [116]	• A 14-item self-report measure that assesses sport-related well-being, with the following subscales: subjective, psychological, and social
Perfectionism	Sport Multidimensional Perfectionism Scale [117]	• A 34-item self-report measure with the following subscales: personal standards, concern over mistakes, perceived parental pressure, and perceived coach pressure • Although a second version of this scale exists that includes subscores for doubts about actions and organization, the value of these is negligible and the original version remains more widely used
Athletic identity	Athlete Identity Measurement Scale [118]	• A 7-item self-report measure with the following subscales: social identity, exclusivity, negative affectivity

(continued on next page)

TABLE 2
(continued)

Construct	Measure	Description
Sleep	Athlete Sleep Screening Questionnaire [119]	• A 15-item self-report measure with the following subscales: total sleep time, insomnia, sleep quality, chronotype, sleep disordered breathing, and travel disturbance
Self-compassion	Self-compassion Scale [120]	• A 26-item self-report measure with the following subscales: self-kindness, self-judgment, common humanity, isolation, mindfulness, and overidentification • Adapted wording to reflect sports environments has been used in research, and may achieve more reflective responses
Burnout	Athlete Burnout Questionnaire [121]	• A 15-item self-report measure assessing the 3 domains of athlete burnout: emotional/physical exhaustion, sport devaluation, and reduced sense of accomplishment
Body image and weight concerns	Eating Disorders Screen for Athletes [122]	• A 6-item self-report screening measure that may identify athletes at risk for an eating disorder • Unlike other sport-specific measures of disordered eating, this scale is reported to be valid with men
	Brief Eating Disorder in Athletes Questionnaire 2 [123]	• A 9-item self-report measure that can help distinguish between female athletes with or without an eating disorder

Note: these scales should supplement, rather than replace, gold-standard measures (eg, Quick Inventory of Depression Symptoms or the Generalized Anxiety Disorder Scale), for which the authors assume clinicians are already familiar. Note that the psychometric properties of many of these scales have not been rigorously assessed within adolescent samples. Therefore, clinical judgment is required when interpreting the results of these measures. The authors suggest these measures may be more useful for information collection and understanding of athletes' current experiences, rather than with the goal of assessing clinical cutoff scores.

are prohibited at higher levels of competition in certain sports, such as archery and shooting [94].

The final area of consideration regarding medications for youth athletes is safety risks. Such risks may be especially relevant for youth athletes pushing themselves to physical extremes. For example, stimulants may be a risk for heat illness [95]. They may also decrease appetite, which can be a concern if athletes are expending large amounts of energy in sport but not able to maintain appropriate dietary intake [18]. However, academic considerations are paramount in youth, and, because stimulants are often regarded as the gold-standard treatment of ADHD, they should be used when necessary if there are no other contraindications (such as cardiac disease) and adequate hydration and nutrition can be ensured [96]. Secondly, medications where blood levels need to be tightly regulated can be difficult to manage in youth athletes, because levels may fluctuate depending on hydration and perspiration [95]. In addition, β-blockers may problematically reduce blood pressure in youth athletes, who at baseline may tend to have low blood pressure [18].

Anxiety and depression can reasonably be treated with selective serotonin reuptake inhibitors (SSRIs) in youth athletes. SSRIs have not been studied in youth athletes specifically, but several are approved for use in youth in general [97]. In small studies, SSRIs have not been shown to negatively affect performance in adults [98,99], and fluoxetine may be a particularly reasonable choice in youth athletes. Little research guidance regarding specification medications is available for pharmacologic treatment of other mental health disorders in youth athletes. Accordingly, best practices for the general population of youth should be followed, with careful consideration of sport performance and sport-specific safety demands.

SUMMARY

Youth athletes represent a unique but largely neglected population in clinical mental health research. Aside from psychological performance enhancement, much remains unknown about the problems and treatment approaches specific to this group. Clinicians new to working with this population are advised to upskill as much as possible regarding contextual factors and the psychosocial stressors faced by youth athletes. A range of key psychosocial stressors and risks are identified in this article. Clinicians should consider these in the assessment and treatment of youth athlete mental health. However, given the near absence of an athlete-specific evidence base, there is a need to rely on the general nonathlete mental health research literature when making treatment decisions. By providing high-quality and timely assessment and treatment, clinicians can also play a key role in the early intervention and prevention of troubling future distress that young people may go on to experience in adulthood.

DISCLOSURE

The authors have no commercial or financial conflicts of interest to disclose. CW was supported by a McKenzie Postdoctoral Research Fellowship from the University of Melbourne (MCK2020292). SR was supported by a Career Development Fellowship from the National Health and Medical Research Council of Australia (GNT1158881), and a Dame Kate Campbell Fellowship from the Faculty of Medicine, Dentistry and Health Sciences at The University of Melbourne.

REFERENCES

[1] Kessler RC, Amminger GP, Aguilar-Gaxiola S, et al. Age of onset of mental disorders: a review of recent literature. Curr Opin Psychiatry 2007;20(4):359–64.

[2] Patel V, Flisher AJ, Hetrick S, et al. Mental health of young people: a global public-health challenge. Lancet 2007;369(9569):1302–13.

[3] Rudolph KD, Lansford JE, Rodkin PC. Interpersonal theories of developmental psychopathology. In: Cicchetti D, editor. Developmental psychopathology. New York: John Wiley & Sons Inc; 2016. p. 1–69.

[4] Eime RM, Young JA, Harvey JT, et al. A systematic review of the psychological and social benefits of participation in sport for children and adolescents: informing development of a conceptual model of health through sport. Int J Behav Nutr Phys Activity 2013;10(1):98.

[5] Vella SA. Mental Health and Organized Youth Sport. Kinesiol Rev 2019;8(3):229.

[6] Aubert S, Barnes JD, Abdeta C, et al. Global Matrix 3.0 Physical Activity Report Card Grades for Children and Youth: Results and Analysis From 49 Countries. J Phys Act Health 2018;15(S2):S251–73.

[7] Arnett JJ, Hughes M. Adolescence and emerging adulthood. Boston: Pearson; 2014.

[8] Benson PL. All kids are our kids: what communities must do to raise caring and responsible children and adolescents. New York: Jossey-Bass; 2006.

[9] Côté J, Turnnidge J, Vierimaa M. A personal assets approach to youth sport. London (UK): Routledge handbook of youth sport; 2016. p. 243–55.

[10] Scales PC, Leffert N. Developmental assets. Minneapolis (MN): Search Institute; 1999.

[11] Lerner RM, Fisher CB, Weinberg RA. Toward a science for and of the people: Promoting civil society through the application of developmental science. Child Dev 2000;71(1):11–20.

[12] Holt NL, Neely KC, Slater LG, et al. A grounded theory of positive youth development through sport based on results from a qualitative meta-study. Int Rev Sport Exerc Psychol 2017;10(1):1–49.

[13] Vella SA, Swann C, Allen MS, et al. Bidirectional Associations between Sport Involvement and Mental Health in Adolescence. Med Sci Sports Exerc 2017;49(4):687–94.

[14] Cheval B, Chalabaev A, Quested E, et al. How perceived autonomy support and controlling coach behaviors are related to well-and ill-being in elite soccer players: A within-person changes and between-person differences analysis. Psychol Sport Exerc 2017;28:68–77.

[15] Ivarsson A, Stenling A, Fallby J, et al. The predictive ability of the talent development environment on youth

elite football players' well-being: A person-centered approach. Psychol Sport Exerc 2015;16:15–23.
[16] Rongen F, McKenna J, Cobley S, et al. Psychosocial outcomes associated with soccer academy involvement: Longitudinal comparisons against aged matched school pupils. J Sports Sci 2020;38(11–12):1387–98.
[17] Poucher ZA. A Commentary on Mental Health Research in Elite Sport. Journal of Applied Sport Psychology 2021;33(1):60–82.
[18] Reardon CL, Hainline B, Aron CM, et al. Mental health in elite athletes: International Olympic Committee consensus statement (2019). Br J Sports Med 2019; 53(11):667–99.
[19] Vella SA, Swann C. Time for mental healthcare guidelines for recreational sports: a call to action. British Journal of Sports Medicine 2021;55:184–5.
[20] Panza MJ, Graupensperger S, Agans JP, et al. Adolescent Sport Participation and Symptoms of Anxiety and Depression: A Systematic Review and Meta-Analysis. J Sport Exerc Psychol 2020;42(3):1–18.
[21] Weber S, Puta C, Lesinski M, et al. Symptoms of Anxiety and Depression in Young Athletes Using the Hospital Anxiety and Depression Scale. Front Physiol 2018;9:182.
[22] Brand R, Wolff W, Hoyer J. Psychological Symptoms and Chronic Mood in Representative Samples of Elite Student-Athletes, Deselected Student-Athletes and Comparison Students. Sch Ment Health 2013;5(3):166–74.
[23] Nixdorf I, Frank R, Beckmann J. Comparison of Athletes' Proneness to Depressive Symptoms in Individual and Team Sports: Research on Psychological Mediators in Junior Elite Athletes. Front Psychol 2016;7:893.
[24] Crane J, Temple V. A systematic review of dropout from organized sport among children and youth. Eur Phys Education Rev 2015;21(1):114–31.
[25] Daniel G. The Current Youth Sport Landscape: Identifying Critical Research Issues. Kinesiol Rev 2019;8(3): 150–61.
[26] Flett GL, Hewitt PL. The perils of perfectionism in sports" revisited: Toward a broader understanding of the pressure to be perfect and its impact on athletes and dancers. Int J Sport Psychol 2014;45(4):395–407.
[27] Stoeber J. The dual nature of perfectionism in sports: relationships with emotion, motivation, and performance. Int Rev Sport Exerc Psychol 2011;4(2):128–45.
[28] Esmie PS, Andrew PH, Howard KH. Perfectionism, Burnout, and Depression in Youth Soccer Players: A Longitudinal Study. J Clin Sport Psychol 2018;12(2): 179–200.
[29] Jowett GE, Hill AP, Hall HK, et al. Perfectionism, burnout and engagement in youth sport: The mediating role of basic psychological needs. Psychol Sport Exerc 2016;24:18–26.
[30] Madigan DJ, Stoeber J, Passfield L. Perfectionism and Burnout in Junior Athletes: A Three-Month Longitudinal Study. J Sport Ecerc Psychol 2015;37(3):305.
[31] Gustafsson H, Sagar SS, Stenling A. Fear of failure, psychological stress, and burnout among adolescent athletes competing in high level sport. Scand J Med Sci Sports 2017;27(12):2091–102.
[32] Hill AP, Mallinson-Howard SH, Jowett GE. Multidimensional perfectionism in sport: A meta-analytical review. Sport Exerc Perform Psychol 2018;7(3):235–70.
[33] Jensen SN, Ivarsson A, Fallby J, et al. Depression in Danish and Swedish elite football players and its relation to perfectionism and anxiety. Psychol Sport Exerc 2018; 36:147–55.
[34] Raedeke TD. Is athlete burnout more than just stress? A sport commitment perspective. Journal of Sport and Exercise Psychology 1997;19(4):396-417.
[35] Granz HL, Schnell A, Mayer J, et al. Risk profiles for athlete burnout in adolescent elite athletes: A classification analysis. Psychol Sport Exerc 2019;41:130–41.
[36] Brenner JS, LaBotz M, Sugimoto D, et al. The Psychosocial Implications of Sport Specialization in Pediatric Athletes. J Athlet Train 2019;54(10):1021–9.
[37] DiSanti JS, Erickson K. Youth sport specialization: a multidisciplinary scoping systematic review. J Sports Sci 2019;37(18):2094–105.
[38] Moore SE, Norman RE, Suetani S, et al. Consequences of bullying victimization in childhood and adolescence: A systematic review and meta-analysis. World J Psychiatry 2017;7(1):60–76.
[39] Evans B, Adler A, MacDonald D, et al. Bullying Victimization and Perpetration Among Adolescent Sport Teammates. Pediatr Exerc Sci 2016;28(2):296.
[40] Partridge JA, Knapp BA. Mean Girls: Adolescent Female Athletes and Peer Conflict in Sport. J Appl Sport Psychol 2016;28(1):113–27.
[41] Steinfeldt JA, Vaughan EL, LaFollette JR, et al. Bullying among adolescent football players: Role of masculinity and moral atmosphere. Psychol Men Masculinity 2012; 13(4):340–53.
[42] Elliott SK, Drummond MJN. During play, the break, and the drive home: the meaning of parental verbal behaviour in youth sport. Leis Stud 2017;36(5):645–56.
[43] Hill A, MacNamara Á, Collins D, et al. Examining the Role of Mental Health and Clinical Issues within Talent Development. Front Psychol 2016;6:2042.
[44] Holt NL, Tamminen KA, Black DE, et al. Youth sport parenting styles and practices. J Sport Exerc Psychol 2009;31(1):37.
[45] Camilla JK. Revealing findings in youth sport parenting research. Kinesiol Rev 2019;8(3):252–9.
[46] Knight CJ, Berrow SR, Harwood CG. Parenting in sport. Curr Opin Psychol 2017;16:93–7.
[47] Stirling AE. Definition and constituents of maltreatment in sport: establishing a conceptual framework for research practitioners. Br J Sports Med 2009; 43(14):1091.
[48] Crooks CV, Wolfe DA. Child abuse and neglect. In: Mash EJ, Barkley RA, editors. Assessment of childhood disorders. The Guilford Press; 2007. p. 639–684.
[49] Mountjoy M, Rhind DJA, Tiivas A, et al. Safeguarding the child athlete in sport: a review, a framework and

recommendations for the IOC youth athlete development model. Br J Sports Med 2015;49(13):883–6.
[50] Kerr G, Battaglia A, Stirling A. Maltreatment in Youth Sport: A Systemic Issue. Kinesiol Rev 2019;8(3): 237–43.
[51] Kerr GA, Stirling AE. Parents' Reflections on their Child's Experiences of Emotionally Abusive Coaching Practices. J Appl Sport Psychol 2012;24(2):191–206.
[52] Vertommen T, Kampen J, Schipper-van Veldhoven N, et al. Severe interpersonal violence against children in sport: Associated mental health problems and quality of life in adulthood. Child Abuse Neglect 2018;76: 459–68.
[53] Caine D, Purcell L, Maffulli N. The child and adolescent athlete: a review of three potentially serious injuries. BMC Sports Sci Med Rehabil 2014;6:22.
[54] Truong LK, Mosewich AD, Holt CJ, et al. Psychological, social and contextual factors across recovery stages following a sport-related knee injury: a scoping review. Br J Sports Med 2020;54(19):1149.
[55] Palisch AR, Merritt LS. Depressive Symptoms in the Young Athlete after Injury: Recommendations for Research. J Pediatr Health Care 2018;32(3):245–9.
[56] Forsdyke D, Smith A, Jones M, et al. Psychosocial factors associated with outcomes of sports injury rehabilitation in competitive athletes: a mixed studies systematic review. Br J Sports Med 2016;50(9):537.
[57] te Wierike SC, van der Sluis A, van den Akker-Scheek I, et al. Psychosocial factors influencing the recovery of athletes with anterior cruciate ligament injury: a systematic review. Scand J Med Sci Sports 2013;23(5):527–40.
[58] Aron CM, Harvey S, Hainline B, et al. Post-traumatic stress disorder (PTSD) and other trauma-related mental disorders in elite athletes: a narrative review. Br J Sports Med 2019;53(12):779.
[59] Rice SM, Parker AG, Rosenbaum S, et al. Sport-Related Concussion and Mental Health Outcomes in Elite Athletes: A Systematic Review. Sports Med 2018;48(2): 447–65.
[60] Ferdinand Pennock K, McKenzie B, McClemont Steacy L, et al. Under-reporting of sport-related concussions by adolescent athletes: a systematic review. Int Rev Sport Exerc Psychol 2020;1–27.
[61] Covassin T, Elbin RJ, Beidler E, et al. A review of psychological issues that may be associated with a sport-related concussion in youth and collegiate athletes. Sport Exerc Perform Psychol 2017;6:220–9.
[62] Rivara FP, Tennyson R, Mills B, et al. Consensus Statement on Sports-Related Concussions in Youth Sports Using a Modified Delphi Approach. JAMA Pediatr 2020;174(1): 79–85.
[63] Grubenhoff JA, Currie D, Comstock RD, et al. Psychological Factors Associated with Delayed Symptom Resolution in Children with Concussion. J Pediatr 2016; 174:27–32.e21.
[64] Kontos AP, Covassin T, Elbin RJ, et al. Depression and neurocognitive performance after concussion among male and female high school and collegiate athletes. Arch Phys Med Rehabil 2012;93(10):1751–6.
[65] Michael JE, Lesley JR, Mark K, et al. Psychiatric outcomes after pediatric sports-related concussion. J Neurosurg Pediatr PED 2015;16(6):709–18.
[66] Wells KR, Jeacocke NA, Appaneal R, et al. The Australian Institute of Sport (AIS) and National Eating Disorders Collaboration (NEDC) position statement on disordered eating in high performance sport. Br J Sports Med 2020;54(21):1247–58.
[67] Giel KE, Hermann-Werner A, Mayer J, et al. Eating disorder pathology in elite adolescent athletes. Int J Eat Disord 2016;49(6):553–62.
[68] Vardar E, Vardar SA, Kurt C. Anxiety of young female athletes with disordered eating behaviors. Eat Behaviors 2007;8(2):143–7.
[69] Michou M, Costarelli V. Disordered Eating Attitudes in Relation to Anxiety Levels, Self-esteem and Body Image in Female Basketball Players. J Exerc Sci Fitness 2011; 9(2):109–15.
[70] Stoyel H, Slee A, Meyer C, et al. Systematic review of risk factors for eating psychopathology in athletes: A critique of an etiological model. Eur Eat Disord Rev 2020;28(1):3–25.
[71] Karrer Y, Halioua R, Mötteli S, et al. Disordered eating and eating disorders in male elite athletes: a scoping review. BMJ Open Sport Exerc Med 2020;6(1):e000801.
[72] Sandgren SS, Haycraft E, Plateau CR. Nature and efficacy of interventions addressing eating psychopathology in athletes: A systematic review of randomised and nonrandomised trials. Eur Eat Disord Rev 2020; 28(2):105–21.
[73] Vlahoyiannis A, Aphamis G, Bogdanis GC, et al. Deconstructing athletes' sleep: A systematic review of the influence of age, sex, athletic expertise, sport type, and season on sleep characteristics. J Sport Health Sci 2020. https://doi.org/10.1016/j.jshs.2020.03.006.
[74] Hirshkowitz M, Whiton K, Albert SM, et al. National Sleep Foundation's updated sleep duration recommendations: final report. Sleep Health 2015;1(4):233–43.
[75] Stiglic N, Viner RM. Effects of screentime on the health and well-being of children and adolescents: a systematic review of reviews. BMJ Open 2019;9(1):e023191.
[76] Dorsch TE, Smith AL, Blazo JA, et al. Toward an integrated understanding of the youth sport system. Res Q Exerc Sport 2020;1–15. https://doi.org/10.1080/02701367.2020.1810847.
[77] Currie A, Johnston A. Psychiatric disorders: The psychiatrist's contribution to sport. Int Rev Psychiatry 2016; 28(6):587–94.
[78] Gulliver A, Griffiths KM, Christensen H. Barriers and facilitators to mental health help-seeking for young elite athletes: a qualitative study. BMC Psychiatry 2012;12(1):157.
[79] Donohue B, Gavrilova Y, Galante M, et al. Controlled Evaluation of an Optimization Approach to Mental Health and Sport Performance. J Clin Sport Psychol 2018;12(2):234–67.

[80] Lavoie S, Allott K, Amminger P, et al. Harmonised collection of data in youth mental health: Towards large datasets. Aust N Z J Psychiatry 2019;54(1):46–56.
[81] Kuhn C, Aebi M, Jakobsen H, et al. Effective Mental Health Screening in Adolescents: Should We Collect Data from Youth, Parents or Both? Child Psychiatry Hum Dev 2017;48(3):385–92.
[82] Ferguson HL, Swann C, Liddle SK, et al. Investigating Youth Sports Coaches' Perceptions of Their Role in Adolescent Mental Health. J Appl Sport Psychol 2019; 31(2):235–52.
[83] Stillman MA, Glick ID, McDuff D, et al. Psychotherapy for mental health symptoms and disorders in elite athletes: a narrative review. Br J Sports Med 2019;53(12): 767–71.
[84] McDuff DR, Garvin M. Working with sports organizations and teams. Int Rev Psychiatry 2016;28(6):595–605.
[85] Stillman MA, Brown T, Ritvo EC, et al. Sport psychiatry and psychotherapeutic intervention, circa 2016. Int Rev Psychiatry 2016;28(6):614–22.
[86] Martin JT, Gillian A, Faye FD, et al. One Case, Four Approaches: The Application of Psychotherapeutic Approaches in Sport Psychology. Sport Psychol 2020; 34(1):71–83.
[87] Mosewich AD, Ferguson LJ, McHugh T-LF, et al. Enhancing capacity: Integrating self-compassion in sport. J Sport Psychol Action 2019;10(4):235–43.
[88] Walton CC, Baranoff J, Gilbert P, et al. Self-compassion, social rank, and psychological distress in athletes of varying competitive levels. Psychol Sport Exerc 2020; 50:101733.
[89] Eke A, Adam M, Kowalski K, et al. Narratives of adolescent women athletes' body self-compassion, performance and emotional well-being. Qual Res Sport Exerc Health 2020;12(2):175–91.
[90] Ceccarelli LA, Giuliano RJ, Glazebrook CM, et al. Self-Compassion and Psycho-Physiological Recovery From Recalled Sport Failure. Front Psychol 2019;10(1564): 1564.
[91] Huysmans Z, Clement D. A Preliminary Exploration of the Application of Self-Compassion Within the Context of Sport Injury. J Sport Exerc Psychol 2017;39(1):56–66.
[92] Johnston A, McAllister-Williams RH. Psychotropic drug prescribing. Sports Psychiatry 2016.
[93] Institute NCAASS. Medical exceptions procedures. 2020. Available at: https://www.ncaa.org/sport-science-institute/medical-exceptions-procedures. Accessed November 28, 2020.
[94] (WADA) WA-DA. World anti-doping agency prohibited list. 2021. Available at: https://www.wada-ama.org/sites/default/files/resources/files/2021list_en.pdf. Accessed November 9, 2020.
[95] Reardon CL. The sports psychiatrist and psychiatric medication. Int Rev Psychiatry 2016;28(6):606–13.
[96] Perrin AE, Jotwani VM. Addressing the unique issues of student athletes with ADHD. J Fam Pract 2014;63(5): E1.
[97] Creswell C, Waite P, Cooper PJ. Assessment and management of anxiety disorders in children and adolescents. Arch Dis Child 2014;99(7):674.
[98] Meeusen R, Piacentini MF, Van Den Eynde S, et al. Exercise performance is not influenced by a 5-HT reuptake inhibitor. Int J Sports Med 2001;22(05):329–36.
[99] Parise G, Bosman MJ, Boecker DR, et al. Selective serotonin reuptake inhibitors: their effect on high-intensity exercise performance. Arch Phys Med Rehabil 2001; 82(7):867–71.
[100] DeFoor MT, Stepleman LM, Mann PC. Improving Wellness for LGB Collegiate Student-Athletes Through Sports Medicine: A Narrative Review. Sports Med Open 2018;4(1):48.
[101] Ballesteros J, Tran AGTT. Under the face mask: Racial-ethnic minority student-athletes and mental health use. J Am Coll Health 2020;68(2):169–75.
[102] Gorczynski P, Currie A, Gibson K, et al. Developing mental health literacy and cultural competence in elite sport. J Appl Sport Psychol 2020;1–30.
[103] Castaldelli-Maia JM, Gallinaro JGdMe, Falcão RS, et al. Mental health symptoms and disorders in elite athletes: a systematic review on cultural influencers and barriers to athletes seeking treatment. Br J Sports Med 2019; 53(11):707–21.
[104] Hill AP, Madigan DJ. A short review of perfectionism in sport, dance and exercise: out with the old, in with the 2×2. Curr Opin Psychol 2017;16:72–7.
[105] Pacewicz CE, Mellano KT, Smith AL. A meta-analytic review of the relationship between social constructs and athlete burnout. Psychol Sport Exerc 2019;43:155–64.
[106] Rist B, Glynn T, Clarke A, et al. The Evolution of Psychological Response to Athlete Injury Models for Professional Sport. J Sci Med 2020;2(4):1–14.
[107] Ross W, Kylie R-D, Lynne E, et al. Sport Psychology Consultants' Perspectives on Facilitating Sport-Injury-Related Growth. The Sport Psychol 2019;33(3):244–55.
[108] Baranoff J, Appaneal RN. In: Henriksen K, Hansen J, Larsen CH, editors. Helping the Injured Athlete to Accept and Refocus. Mindfulness and Acceptance in Sport: How to Help Athletes Perform and Thrive under Pressure. Routledge; 2019.
[109] Wachsmuth S, Jowett S, Harwood CG. Conflict among athletes and their coaches: what is the theory and research so far? Int Rev Sport Exerc Psychol 2017; 10(1):84–107.
[110] Mountjoy M, Brackenridge C, Arrington M, et al. International Olympic Committee consensus statement: harassment and abuse (non-accidental violence) in sport. Br J Sports Med 2016;50(17):1019.
[111] Kroshus E, Wagner J, Wyrick D, et al. Wake up call for collegiate athlete sleep: narrative review and consensus recommendations from the NCAA Interassociation Task Force on Sleep and Wellness. Br J Sports Med 2019;53(12):731.
[112] Gupta L, Morgan K, Gilchrist S. Does Elite Sport Degrade Sleep Quality? A Systematic Review. Sports Med (Auckland, NZ) 2017;47(7):1317–33.

[113] Assessment Tool 1 (SMHAT-1) and Sport Mental Health Recognition Tool 1 (SMHRT-1): towards better support of athletes' mental health. British journal of sports medicine, 55(1), 30–7.

[114] Rice S, Olive L, Gouttebarge V, et al. Mental health screening: severity and cut-off point sensitivity of the Athlete Psychological Strain Questionnaire in male and female elite athletes. BMJ Open Sport Exerc Med 2020;6(1):e000712.

[115] Donohue B, Galante M, Maietta J, et al. Empirical development of a screening method to assist mental health referrals in collegiate athletes. J Clin Sport Psychol 2019;13(4):561–79.

[116] Brian JF, Graig MC. Development of the Sport Mental Health Continuum—Short Form (Sport MHC-SF). J Clin Sport Psychol 2019;13(4):593–608.

[117] Dunn JG, Dunn JC, Syrotuik DG. Relationship between multidimensional perfectionism and goal orientations in sport. Journal of Sport and Exercise Psychology 2002:24(4):376-95.

[118] Brewer BW, Cornelius A. Norms and factorial invariance of the Athletic Identity Measurement Scale. Acad athletic J 2001;15(2):103–13.

[119] Samuels C, James L, Lawson D, et al. The Athlete Sleep Screening Questionnaire: a new tool for assessing and managing sleep in elite athletes. Br J Sports Med 2016;50(7):418.

[120] Neff KD. The development and validation of a scale to measure self-compassion. Self Identity 2003;2(3): 223–50.

[121] Raedeke TD, Smith AL. Development and preliminary validation of an athlete burnout measure. J Sport Exerc Psychol 2001;23(4):281–306.

[122] Hazzard VM, Schaefer LM, Mankowski A, et al. Development and validation of the Eating Disorders Screen for Athletes (EDSA): A brief screening tool for male and female athletes. Psychol Sport Exerc 2020;50:101745.

[123] Martinsen M, Holme I, Pensgaard AM, et al. The development of the brief eating disorder in athletes questionnaire. Med Sci Sports Exerc 2014;46(8): 1666–75.

Advances in Psychiatry and Behavioral Health 1 (2021) 135–143

ADVANCES IN PSYCHIATRY AND BEHAVIORAL HEALTH

Diagnosis and Management of Substance Use Disorders in Athletes

Pamela Walters, MB BCh, MRCPysch[a,b,*], Bradley Hillier, BM BCh, MA, MFFLM, FRCPsych[c], Filippo Passetti, MD, PhD, MRCPsych[d], Anju Soni, MB, BS, MRCPsych[e], Ian Treasaden, MB, BS, LRCP, MRCS, FRCPsych, LLM[f]

[a]Substance Misuse and Mental Health Services, The Forward Trust Edinburgh House, 170 Kennington Lane, Vauxhall, London SE11 5DP, UK; [b]SLaM NHS Trust, HMP Wandsworth, Wandsworth SW18 OHU, UK; [c]West London NHS Trust, 1 Armstrong Way, Southall UB2 4SD, UK; [d]Cognacity, 54 Harley Street, Marylebone, London W1G 9PZ, UK; [e]Broadmoor Hospital, West London NHS Trust and Imperial College London, 1 Armstrong Way, Southall UB2 4SD, UK; [f]West London NHS Trust and Bucks New University, 1 Armstrong Way, Southall UB2 4SD, UK

KEYWORDS

• Substance misuse • SUD • Athlete • Treatment • Recovery • Addiction • Sport

KEY POINTS

- Substance misuse and substance use disorder (SUD) in athletes varies by country, sex, age, ethnicity, sport, and competitive level.
- There are inconsistencies in the application of World Anti-Doping Agency (WADA) rules.
- No clinical trials for the treatment of SUDs have been done in athletes.
- Stigma is evident for athletes with SUD.
- Often those athletes who go on to develop SUD have problematic usage as students.

INTRODUCTION

The objective of this review is to evaluate current treatment approaches for substance misuse and substance use disorders (SUDs) among athletes as defined in *Diagnostic and Statistical Manual of Mental Disorders* (Fifth Edition) (DSM-5) [1], including use involving alcohol, cannabis, nicotine, cocaine, opioids, and stimulants. This article will not address performance-enhancing drugs (PEDs) and their role in SUDs as much has been written about their misuse in athletes to date [2–4].

The literature was reviewed for the following:

- Better understanding risks, neurobiological correlates, drivers, and current management of substance misuse within athletes.
- Evaluating the assessment and screening process for athletes.
- Collating evidence where available and making recommendations for optimal management of athletes with vulnerabilities to or diagnosed with SUD. This step will include highlighting evidence-based pharmacologic and psychosocial interventions for SUD for athletes (where possible), and where absent, describing interventions used in the general population that would seemingly be applicable to athletes.

BACKGROUND

Substance misuse was responsible for 11 million deaths in 2017, or 1 in 5 deaths globally [5]. Although in general athletes are inherently health-conscious individuals, as optimal physical health is directly related to enhanced performance by as much as 5% [2], substance

*Corresponding author, *E-mail addresses:* pamela.walters@forwardtrust.org.uk; @pamelaw70013748

https://doi.org/10.1016/j.ypsc.2021.06.001
2667-3827/21/

misuse can hinder performance by as much as 11% [6]. With the most minuscule of margins differentiating between achieving a medal or not, optimizing performance is important for the individual, teams, and the countries the athletes represent.

Stigma for athletes is evident. There are inconsistencies in the application of World Anti-Doping Agency (WADA) rules. For example, for those in recovery from opiate use disorder, WADA prohibits use of methadone and does not give provisions for therapeutic use exemptions in training and competition. In contrast, WADA can approve attention-deficit/hyoeractivity disorder medication in the form of stimulants—which are otherwise prohibited—on therapeutic grounds.

Athletes use substances for a variety of reasons, including [2,6–9]:

- Injury (self-treatment)
- Mental health problems (self-treatment)
- Adverse childhood experiences
- Peer pressure
- Culture of particular forms of sport
- Stress management
- Genetic vulnerabilities
- Performance enhancement
- Coping with transition phases or training stressors
- Lack of good alternative means of managing boredom/structuring nontraining time
- Celebrating wins or consoling losses postcompetition

Athletes can normatively use substances for relaxation and recreational purposes, but if use escalates to heavy and hazardous usage, there are increased risks of dependence and other manifestations of SUDs [2].

Neurobiological Correlates: Athletes and Addictive Behaviors

There are parallels between the period of vulnerability to developing a SUD and the timing of becoming an elite athlete during adolescence and high school [3]. Early substance use (before age 14 years) is associated with the highest risk of developing SUD [3]. As individuals continue to mature between 13 and 21 years, the likelihood of lifetime substance misuse/use disorder drops 4% to 5% for each year that initiation of substance use is delayed [3]. It is therefore key to provide both psychoeducation and adequate screening for young athletes in schools and colleges about the risks of SUD and how to access rapid treatment.

Diagnostic Criteria for Substance Use Disorder

A list of 11 symptoms of SUDs is provided in the DSM-5 (Box 1) [2]. Where only 2 or 3 symptoms are seen, the misuse is defined as mild in severity. If there are 4 or 5 symptoms, this is defined as moderately severe, and when there are 6 or more symptoms, this is categorized as severe.

Common substances of misuse have varying effects on performance in athletes and varying relationships to different types of sport (Table 1).

Assessment

There are currently no specific instruments for screening, assessment, and management of SUD in athletes. It is encouraging to see the recent developments of the International Olympic Committee Sports Mental Health Assessment Tool 1 and Sports Mental Health Recognition Tool 1 [20]. These tools incorporate assessment for and consideration of substance use concerns and a variety of comorbidities in athletes.

The following can be useful in providing an assessment of athletes with SUD given the comorbidity with other mental illnesses:

- PHQ-9 to assess for symptoms of depression [24].
- GAD-7 to assess for symptoms of anxiety [25].

Table 2 illustrates the likely comorbidities for different substances of misuse. For example, the presence of cocaine use disorder predicts a very high likelihood of the comorbid presence of alcohol use disorder.

PHARMACOLOGIC INTERVENTIONS

Background

There is a paucity of evidence-based research as to what interventions work best for athletes with SUD. The following evidence-based research findings relate to the general population and consequently have not been validated for use in athletes.

Alcohol

Management

The AUDIT (Alcohol Use Disorders Identification Test) [20] is considered by some to be the gold standard test for screening, validated across cultures and also indicating severity with 10 questions and a maximum score of 40. Scores of 8 to 15 indicate hazardous drinking, scores of 16 to 19 indicate harmful drinking, and athletes with scores of greater than 20 can be offered a medically assisted detox with long-acting benzodiazepines [26], for example, chlordiazepoxide or diazepam.

Detoxification medication is tailored according to the Clinical Institute Withdrawal Assessment for Alcohol Scale, Revised (CIWA-Ar) [27,28] scoring and is usually administered for several days. Thiamine

BOX 1
Diagnostic Criteria: Substance Use Disorder

1. Taken in larger amounts or over a longer period than was intended.
2. Persistent desire or unsuccessful efforts to cut down or control use.
3. A great deal of time is spent in activities necessary to obtain the substance, use it, or recover from its effects.
4. Craving, or a strong desire or urge to use.
5. Failure to fulfill major role obligations at work, school, or home.
6. Continued use despite persistent or recurrent social or interpersonal problems.
7. Important social, occupational, or recreational activities are given up or reduced.
8. Recurrent use in situations in which it is physically hazardous.
9. Continued use despite knowledge of a persistent or recurrent physical or psychological problem that is likely to have been
10. Tolerance, as defined by either of the following:
    - A need for markedly increased amounts to achieve intoxication or desired effect
    - A markedly diminished effect with the same amount of the substance.
11. Withdrawal, as manifest by either of the following:
    - The characteristic withdrawal syndrome for that substance
    - Substance (or closely related substance) is taken to relieve or avoid withdrawal symptoms.

(oral or parenteral) should be offered with alcohol detoxification to prevent Wernicke encephalopathy and Korsakoff syndrome [29,30].

Postdetoxification, relapse prevention anticraving agents can assist in the recovery of athletes with moderate to severe levels of dependence [29]. Naltrexone [31], an opiate antagonist, works by blocking the release of endogenous opioids and dopamine in the mesolimbic system and can be started when athletes are still drinking or during medically assisted withdrawal. Liver function monitoring should continue for 6 months with tailored community follow-up treatment [29]. Acamprosate inhibits glutamine transmission at the *N*-methyl-D-aspartate receptors and can be initiated during detoxification because it is thought to have neuroprotective effects. The treatment effect is most pronounced at 6 months, and the effect is significant for up to 12 months [29,32]. Acamprosate should be initiated as soon as possible after abstinence is achieved. Disulfiram has been available since the 1940s and works by irreversibly inhibiting the aldehyde dehydrogenase enzyme, converting ethanol to acetaldehyde. Excess acetaldehyde leads to unpleasant effects of headache, tachycardia, perspiration, flushed skin, and nausea. On average, the disulfiram reaction lasts 30 to 60 minutes. Nalmefene [29] (a competitive antagonist at the opioid receptor) is sometimes suggested for problematic binge-type drinking, although the evidence base is minimal.

Gabapentin, an antiepileptic drug, has shown some promise in the management of alcohol use disorder. Gabapentin can be helpful for those with intractable insomnia and mood instability [33]. Caution should be exercised due to some emerging evidence that it may have dependence-producing potential [44].

Alcohol use disorder and comorbid mental health symptoms and disorders

Depression and anxiety may predate SUD or result from alcohol usage [34]. A month after detoxification, anxiety and depressive symptoms often diminish considerably. For athletes with alcohol misuse and anxiety, it is advisable, although not imperative, that the clinician waits 8 weeks before reassessing anxiety symptoms toward the end of determining if long-term treatment of a potential underlying anxiety disorder may be needed [35].

Acamprosate and baclofen [29] are beneficial in reducing anxiety and cravings postalcohol detox. One meta-analysis suggests that buspirone is effective in reducing anxiety, but not alcohol consumption [29,35].

For athletes with depression, relapse prevention medication should be considered in combination with antidepressants. A study [36] showed that the combination of sertraline (200 mg/d) with naltrexone (100 mg/d) had superior outcomes—improved drinking outcomes and better mood—compared with

TABLE 1
Management of Substance Use Disorders in Athletes

	Performance Effects	In Competition Considerations	Training Considerations	Sports With Disproportionate Use of the Substance and/or with Unique Impacts Due to Use of It
Alcohol	CNS depressant [10] Sleep disruption Reduced endurance, strength and power [6]	WADA prohibition in certain sports, eg, archery, motorcycling, skydiving [7]. Violations at alcohol concentrations of 0.10 g/L or more if used in air sports, archery, automobile racing, and powerboating [7]	Aerobic capacity reduced by as much as 11%; hangover can affect training [6] Increased injury risk, prolonged healing [6] Can be problems with hormonal imbalance of testosterone and cortisol [6]	Team sports disproportionately consume, especially hockey and rugby [5]
Cannabinoids	CNS depressant, which may be ergolytic [11,12] May have analgesic effects centrally and peripherally [11] Reduced motivation [11]	Subjective effects of well-being, calmness [11] WADA prohibition in competition except cannabidiol [7] Anxiolysis before competition [11]	Exercise increases endocannabinoid receptors [11] Commonly used for analgesic effects [11] Perception of relaxation and improved sleep posttraining [13] Increased injury risk [13]	Cycling, skeleton, ice hockey, and bobsleigh disproportionately consume [11,13] Common in collegiate athletes, across a large array of sport [14] In cycling, there were noted reductions in cycling time, until exhaustion [13]
Nicotine	CNS stimulant. Perception of ergogenicity via improved endurance and strength [6], cognitive functions, and fine motor and reaction times [10]	Withdrawing: cravings, irritability, poor effects on performance [6] Insomnia reports in some athletes Spit tobacco commonly used for postgame relaxation [15]	Smoking reduces aerobic performance [2] Dental checks being used preseason as opportunity to offer brief intervention work to assist with quitting [15]	Widespread usage across American football, ice hockey, skiing, baseball, gymnastics, and wrestling [16]
Stimulants	Ergogenic [10]. Increased aerobic performance [10]. Improved reaction times and alertness [6] Paradoxic problems with attention and concentration and impairment in motor tasks [17–20] Impulse control problems & thermoregulation issues [14]	Increased self- confidence, aggression, hostility and competitiveness [14] The most common stimulants detected in antidoping tests: amphetamines, cocaine, ecstasy, methylphenidate TUE through WADA for athletes with ADHD [7].	Interference with timing in technical events [14] Increased injury risk, excess confidence, aggression, and loss of judgment [14]	Lacrosse athletes highest likelihood of using cocaine (last year 22% men and 6% women)[44] The numbers of student-athletes testing positive for stimulant medications use, has increased[45] Requests for therapeutic exemption up for major baseball league representing 8% of their cohort [21,22]

Opioids	This group of drugs cause CNS-depressant effects [6] For sports injuries, analgesic effects [2] Overdose potential in those without tolerance to opioids, due to respiratory depression [6]	WADA prohibition on all opioids, aside from minor groups, eg, tramadol, codeine [7] Systematic review, involving 11 studies and 226,256 athletes noted opioid usage at any time for professional athletes to range from 4.4%–4.7%. Opioid use over an NFL career was 52% [23]. For high school athletes, lifetime opioid use was 28%–46%	Pain and depression during training, associated with higher opioid use [23] Playing at least one high school sport with opioid use for injury puts individual at risk of lifetime opioid prescription use [23]	Ice hockey greater odds of heroin use. Higher injury risks [16] Risks for opioid use: Caucasian, male, contact sports, postretirement unemployment, undiagnosed concussion [23] By having a better understanding of sports commonly associated with different substances of misuse, this will allow targeted, clinical, psychoeducation, screening, and support both during an active career and into retirement

Abbreviation: CNS, central nervous system.

TABLE 2
Comorbid Substance use Disorders

	Percentage of Individuals Who Also Have:					
Among Individuals With:	**Alcohol Use Disorder**	**Nicotine Dependence**	**Marijuana Use Disorder**	**Cocaine Use Disorder**	**Prescription Opioid Use Disorder**	**Heroin Use Disorder**
Alcohol use disorder	-	23.8	9.5	3.3	3.9	0.9
Nicotine dependence	12.9	-	4.3	1.4	2.7	1.3
Marijuana use disorder	38.7	32.6	-	4.8	7.9	1.8
Cocaine use disorder	59.8	47.7	21.3	-	16.4	13.4
Prescription opioid use disorder	35.2	45.4	17.6	8.2	-	11.2
Heroin use disorder	24.5	66.3	12.3	20.9	34.9	-

From National Institute on Drug Abuse (NIDA); National Institutes of Health; U.S. Department of Health and Human Services. What are some approaches to diagnosis?. National Institute on Drug Abuse website. https://www.drugabuse.gov/publications/research-reports/common-comorbidities-substance-use-disorders/what-are-some-approaches-to-diagnosis. May 27, 2020 Accessed November 30, 2020.

placebo and compared with each drug alone. Citalopram showed no benefit when added to naltrexone [36–39].

Cannabis

Management

Cannabis withdrawal does not usually require pharmacologic intervention [29]. If anxiety, agitation, or even psychosis is evident, benzodiazepines and antipsychotics may be useful. The mainstay of management is psychosocial interventions.

Nicotine

Management

In the absence of athlete-specific research, management of nicotine misuse and use disorder includes psychoeducation measures, self-help, behavioral support, and replacement therapy. Supporting athletes to reduce or stop use mirrors treatments available to nonathletes. The odds ratio (OR) of abstinence for any form of NRT (nicotine replacement therapy) compared with placebo is 1.84.

Reduction in spit-tobacco use among baseball players has been associated with preseason dental and physical examination screening for heavy use; where positive, a brief intervention by a dental technician or substance counselor experienced in nicotine cessation has been associated with up to 15% reduction of use [25]. Drugs used to treat nicotine use disorder include varenicline, a selective nicotinic acetyl cholinergic receptor partial agonist. In a 2017 study, varenicline was more effective than a nicotine patch in depressed smokers.

Bupropion is an antagonist at the nicotinic acetylcholinergic receptor. Bupropion seems to be of similar efficacy as single-product NRT (risk ratio 0.99) and less effective for quitting compared with varenicline and combination NRT. Combination NRT (ie, combining 2 formulations such as a patch and an oral/nasal product) is more effective than using a single NRT product.

Quit rate for varenicline compared with placebo is 2.24. Varenicline is more effective when compared with bupropion (OR 1.39) and single-product NRT (OR 1.25) and is similarly effective compared with combination NRT [11]. In smokers with mental illness, bupropion improved the odds of quitting by four times compared with placebo [40].

Stimulants

Management

Management of stimulant use disorder is primarily through psychological measures [41]. Given cocaine's short half-life and the binge nature of cocaine use, athletes essentially detoxify themselves regularly unaided. For those with comorbid mental health problems, antidepressants have a role in treating major depressive disorder associated with stimulant use [29] as do antipsychotics for amphetamine-associated psychosis [29].

For cocaine use disorder, there is some evidence that substitute psychostimulants improve sustained cocaine abstinence, and one trial supports the use of 300 mg/d of modafinil [31].

Opioids

Management

The Opioid Risk Tool [ORT] [42] is a brief self-reported screening tool, for use and validated in persons prescribed opioids in the context of chronic pain. Although not yet validated in athletes, this can be considered as a screen for athletes with opioid use disorder problems in the context of chronic pain. Otherwise, more generally, NIDA and DAST screening tools [31] can be used to screen for opioid use not related to chronic pain.

Clinicians should establish the length of opioid usage, quantity, route of administration and frequency of opioid use, form, and use of street drugs such as heroin versus prescription opioids. The COWS [43] is used to guide administration of opioid substitution treatment [17,29]. A urine drug screen is normally taken, but oral and hair samples can additionally be used.

Methadone and buprenorphine are the mainstay of pharmacotherapy for opioid use disorder alongside psychosocial interventions [29].

Methadone is a long-acting full agonist at opioid μ receptors, whereas buprenorphine is a partial agonist at the μ-receptor. Higher doses of methadone (60–100 mg/d) are often recommended, as they are more effective than lower dosages in treatment retention [17]. About half of those entering treatment will also meet the criteria for depression. These athletes may require 20% to 50% higher doses of methadone to stabilize [29].

Opioids are prohibited "in-competition" by WADA, which uniquely places this athlete group in what some would potentially view as a stigmatized situation where they would need to take time off from training or competition. This is unlike athletes [10] with ADHD who require stimulant pharmacotherapy for their illness and are able to apply for therapeutic use exemptions to be able to take otherwise prohibited stimulants.

Use of naltrexone, an opioid antagonist, for this group has been suggested where a break or training and competition is not possible [10,29]. There needs to be a washout period between stopping the opioid and commencing naltrexone; the exact amount of time depends on the opioid used, duration of use, and amount taken as a last dose [17,29]. However, the evidence base is clear that opioid substitution, as opposed to naltrexone, is the treatment of choice for most individuals with longstanding opioid use disorder [29,32]. Thus, this creates a conflict for those clinicians treating significant opioid use disorder in high-level athletes.

Buprenorphine, available in oral and depot formulations, is a long-acting synthetic partial opioid agonist with low intrinsic activity and high affinity at opioid μ receptors. Buprenorphine produces less euphoria than full opioid agonists even at saturating doses and simultaneously blocks the action of other opioids. It is an effective treatment for use in maintenance treatment at doses between 12 and 24 mg daily [17,29].

Psychosocial Interventions

A meta-analysis of psychosocial treatments for SUDs looked at the effect size for various types of psychosocial treatments, as well as abstinence and treatment retention rates for cannabis, cocaine, opiate, and polysubstance use disorder treatment trials. A total of 34 well-controlled treatment conditions—5 for cannabis, 9 for cocaine, 7 for opioid, and 13 for polysubstance users—representing the treatment of 2340 people was examined [41]. Psychosocial treatments evaluated included contingency management, relapse prevention, general cognitive behavior therapy, and treatments combining cognitive behavior therapy and contingency management. Approximately one-third of participants across all psychosocial treatments dropped out before completion compared with 44.6% for the control condition [41].

Overall, the data indicated that psychosocial treatments provide a moderate effect in line with comparable treatments in other areas of psychiatry. Interventions were most efficacious for cannabis use and least for polysubstance use. The strongest effects were in contingency management interventions [41]. Contingency management is the application of 3-term contingency, which uses stimulus control and consequences to change behavior.

SUMMARY

Considerable progress has been made to reduce stigma around non–substance-related mental health issues affecting athletes; frustratingly, the same cannot be said for SUD in athletes. Stigma in athletes with substance use concerns continues, requiring a global discussion and a cohesive approach to understand the treatment needs of these athletes better. The evidence base reflects this because there is scant research regarding optimal interventions for athletes with SUD. Thus, by necessity, we have drawn upon the evidence base for the general population with regard to optimal management for SUD.

Opioids can be considered ergolytic [2] and stimulants ergogenic [2]. Given the prevailing situation regarding WADA's therapeutic exemptions, we suggest this warrants further careful consideration to improve fairness and reduce the entrenched stigma for athletes with SUD.

There is some evidence to suggest that those vulnerable to SUD manifest difficulties early on as students. Prevention and psychoeducation have to be at the forefront of management, including using ambassadors from the sporting world to relay their powerful, unique stories of recovery. For some, the human cost of an intense, brief career in athletics might be a chronic SUD, as seen in some athletes postretirement.

Given the high rates of substance misuse among athletes, we advocate for a greater emphasis on preventative measures by clubs, trainers, and sporting organizations, including psychoeducation, access to mental health services, and relevant improved means of managing stressors both on and off the playing field. We note that although there is awareness of substance misuse in the world of sport, the true scale of the problem and the best ways for identifying, managing, and preventing substance misuse have been minimally researched and inadequately understood. Sportspeople are motivated individuals and are therefore well placed to engage with and benefit from treatment.

CLINICS CARE POINTS

- Athletes should be screened for substance use concerns on a regular basis.
- Athletes who have confirmed substance use problems should also be screened for the presence of mental illness given the high levels of comorbidity.
- Athletes with substance use concerns should undergo psychosocial/psychotherapeutic interventions.
- In some cases, pharmacological interventions for substance use concerns in athletes should be offered, taking care to consider athlete-specific issues that arise with certain medications. e.g. WADA prohibited list.
- Telemedicine should be utilised more in this group to allow greater accessibility to assessment, treatment and reducing stigma.
- It is essential that an evidence base is established for these athletes with SUD to optimise recovery.

ACKNOWLEDGMENTS

Kind acknowledgments to Mr Carl Wright Forward Trust for his support with this article and Mr Dennis Walters, my constant source of inspiration.

DISCLOSURE

Contributors: All authors contributed to the review article. All other authors were responsible for the critical review of the article. All authors read and approved the final version of the article.

Funding: No funding has been received for the production of this article.

Competing interests: None declared.

REFERENCES

[1] Diagnostic and statistical manual of mental disorders (5th Edition). 5th edition. American Psychiatric Association; 2013.
[2] Dunn M, Thomas JO, Swift W, et al. Recreational substance use among elite Australian athletes. Drug Alcohol Rev 2011;30(1):63–8.
[3] De Grace LA, Knight CJ, Rodgers WM, et al. Exploring the role of sport in the development of substance addiction. Psychol Sport Exerc 2017;28:46.
[4] United Nations, Department of Economic and Social Affairs, Population Division. World population Prospects: the 2017 Revision, DVD Edition 2017. Available at: https://esa.un.org/unpd/wpp/Download/Standard/Population/.
[5] Walters P, Hearn A, Currie A. Substance misuse, sports Psychiatry, Chapter 5. Oxford Psychiatry Library; 2016 ISBN- 97801987328.
[6] Kingsland M, Wiggers JH, Vashum KP, et al. Interventions in sports settings to reduce risky alcohol consumption and alcohol- related harm: A systematic review. Syst Rev 2015;5:12.
[7] World Anti-Doping Agency Prohibited List. Available at: https://www.wada-ama.org/sites/default/files/wada_2020_english_prohibited_list_0.pdf. Accessed November 21, 2020.
[8] Shirreffs S, Maughan R. Restoration of fluid balance after exercise-induced dehydration: Effects of alcohol consumption. J Appl Physiol 1997;83(4):1152–8.
[9] Shirreffs SM, Maughan RJ. The effect of alcohol on athletic performance. Nutrition 2006;5:192–6.
[10] McDuff D, Stull T, Castaldelli-Maia JM, et al. Recreational and ergogenic substance use and substance use disorders in elite athletes: a narrative review - *British*. J Sports Med 2019;53:754–60.
[11] Docter S, Khan M, Gohal C, et al. Cannabis Use and Sport: A Systematic Review. Sports Health 2020;12(2): 189–99.
[12] CORE alcohol and drug Survey. Available at: https://core.siu.edu/_common/documents/2013.pdf.
[13] Brisola-Santos MB, Gallinaro JG, Gil F, et al. Prevalence and correlates of cannabis use among athletes-A systematic review. Am J Addict 2016;25(7):518–28.
[14] Avois L, Robinson N, Saudan C, et al. Central nervous system stimulants and sport practice. Br J Sports Med 2006;40(Suppl 1):i16–20.
[15] Reardon CL, et al. Br J Sports Med 2019;53:667–99.

[16] Pesta DH, Angadi SS, Burtscher M, et al. The effects of caffeine, nicotine, ethanol, and tetrahydrocannabinol on exercise performance. Nutr Metab (Lond) 2013;10:71.

[17] NIDA. Comorbidity: Substance Use Disorders and Other Mental Illnesses DrugFacts. National Institute on Drug Abuse website; 2018. Available at: https://www.drugabuse.gov/publications/drugfacts/comorbidity-substance-use-disorders-other-mental-illnesses. Accessed December 14, 2020.

[18] Department of Health. Drug misuse and dependence: UK guidelines on clinical management 2017. Available at: https://www.gov.uk/government/publications/drug-misuse-and-dependence-uk-guidelines-on-clinical-management.

[19] Rice SM, Purcell R, De Silva S, et al. The Mental Health of Elite Athletes: A Narrative Systematic Review. Sports Med 2016;46(9):1333–53.

[20] Babor TF, Higgins-Biddle JC, Saunders JB, et al. AUDIT: the alcohol Use disorders Identification test: guidelines for Use in primary health Care. 2nd ed. Geneva: World Health Organization; 2001.

[21] Shaikin B. Los Angeles Times. Baseball's 2008 drug test results released in report. 2009. Available at: http://articles.latimes.com/2009/jan/10/sports/sp-newswire10. Accessed September 17, 2010.

[22] Gouttebarge V, Bindra A, Blauwet C, et al. International Olympic Committee (IOC) Sport Mental Health Assessment Tool 1 (SMHAT-1) and Sport Mental Health Recognition Tool 1 (SMHRT-1): towards better support of athletes' mental health. Br J Sports Med 2020. https://doi.org/10.1136/bjsports-2020-102411.

[23] Ekhtiari S, Yusuf I, AlMakadma Y, et al. Opioid Use in Athletes: A Systematic Review. Sports Health 2020; 12(6):534–9.

[24] Kroenke K, Spitzer RL, Williams JB. The PHQ-9: validity of a brief depression severity measure. J Gen Intern Med 2001;16(9):606–13.

[25] Spitzer RL, Kroenke K, Williams JB, et al. A brief measure for assessing generalized anxiety disorder: the GAD-7. Arch Intern Med 2006;166(10):1092–7.

[26] Amato L, Minozzi S, Vecchi S, et al. Benzodiazepines for alcohol withdrawal. Cochrane Database Syst Rev 2010;3: CD005063.

[27] Sullivan JT, Sykora K, Schneiderman J, et al. Assessment of alcohol withdrawal: the revised clinical institute withdrawal assessment for alcohol scale (CIWA-Ar). Br J Addict 1989;84(11):1353–7.

[28] Donoghue K, Elzerbi C, Saunders R, et al. The efficacy of acamprosate and naltrexone in the treatment of alcohol dependence, Europe versus the rest of the world: a meta-analysis. Addiction 2015;110(6):920–30.

[29] Lingford-Hughes AR, Welch S, Peters L, et al, British Association for Psychopharmacology, Expert Reviewers Group. BAP updated guidelines: evidence-based guidelines for the pharmacological management of substance abuse, harmful use, addiction and comorbidity: recommendations from BAP. J Psychopharmacol 2012;26(7): 899–952.

[30] National Institute for Health and Care Excellence. Alcohol use disorders: diagnosis, assessment and management of harmful drinking and alcohol dependence. Clin Guidance 2011;115.

[31] Skinner HA. The drug abuse screening test. Addict Behav 1982;7(4):363–71.

[32] Taylor DM, Barnes TRE, Young AH. The Maudsley prescribing guidelines in Psychiatry. United Kingdom: Wiley; 2018.

[33] Anton RF, Latham P, Voronin K, et al. Efficacy of Gabapentin for the Treatment of Alcohol Use Disorder in Patients with Alcohol Withdrawal Symptoms: A Randomized Clinical Trial. JAMA Intern Med 2020;180(5):728–36.

[34] Ipser JC, Wilson D, Akindipe TO Sager C, et al. Pharmacotherapy for anxiety and comorbid alcohol use disorders. Cochrane Database Syst Rev 2015;(1):CD007505.

[35] Foulds JA, Adamson SJ, Boden JM, et al. Depression in patients with alcohol use disorders: Systematic review and meta-analysis of outcomes for independent and substance-induced disorders. J Affective Disord 2015;185:47–59.

[36] Pettinati HM, Oslin DW, Kampman KM, et al. A double-blind, placebo-controlled trial combining sertraline and naltrexone for treating co-occurring depression and alcohol dependence. Am J Psychiatry 2010;167(6):668–75.

[37] McCartney D, Benson MJ, Desbrow B, et al. Cannabidiol and Sports Performance: a Narrative Review of Relevant Evidence and Recommendations for Future Research. Sports Med - Open 2020;6:27.

[38] Jayaram-Lindström N, Hammarberg A, Beck O, et al. Naltrexone for the treatment of amphetamine dependence: a randomized, placebo-controlled trial. Am J Psychiatry 2008;165(11):1442–8.

[39] Kaufman KR, Bajaj A, Schiltz JF. Attention deficit/hyperactivity disorder (ADHD) in gymnastics: preliminary findings. Apunts Medicina de l'Esport 2011;46:89-85.

[40] Cahill K, Stevens S, Perera R, et al. Pharmacological interventions for smoking cessation: an overview and network meta-analysis. Cochrane Database Syst Rev 2013;(5):CD009329.

[41] Dutra L, Stathopoulou G, Basden SL, et al. A meta-analytic review of psychosocial interventions for substance use disorders. Am J Psychiatry 2008;165(2):179–87.

[42] Opioid risk tool, NIDA. Webster LR, Webster R. Predicting aberrant behaviours in Opioid-treated patients: preliminary validation of the Opioid risk too. Pain Med 2005;6(6):432.

[43] Wesson DR, Ling W. The Clinical Opiate Withdrawal Scale (COWS). J Psychoactive Drugs 2003;35(2):253–9.

[44] Leung JG, Hall-Flavin D, Nelson S, et al. The Role of Gabapentin in the Management of Alcohol Withdrawal and dependence. Annals of Pharmacotherapy 2015;49(8): 897–906. https://doi.org/10.1177/1060028015585849.

[45] National college athletic association NCAA guidelines to document ADHD treatment with banned medications. Addendum to the Jan 2009 guideline 2010. Available at: http://lagrange.edu/resources/pdf/athletics/athletictraining/FAQ.pdf. Accessed June 23, 2021.

Advances in Psychiatry and Behavioral Health 1 (2021) 145–148

ADVANCES IN PSYCHIATRY AND BEHAVIORAL HEALTH

Sex Differences in Psychiatric Diagnosis and Management of Athletes

Danielle Kamis, MD*
Stanford University, Palo Alto, CA, USA

KEYWORDS
• Female athlete • Psychopathology • Sex differences in athletes • Sports psychiatry

KEY POINTS

- Female athletes are more likely than men to be diagnosed with several psychiatric conditions.
- Risk may be moderated by the type of sport.
- An interdisciplinary team comprising a sports psychiatrist, sports medicine physician, counselors, coach, and trainers is necessary to support the mental health care needs of athletes.

SEX DIFFERENCES IN PSYCHOPATHOLOGY

Mood Disorders

Previous research has found that the incidence of mild depression in the overall athletic population is 23.7%, and moderate to severe depression is 6.3%. When separating by sex, female athletes were found to have a higher incidence of mild depression at 28.1% and moderate to severe depression at 7.5% [1]. Thus, the most recent data indicate that female athletes are at greater risk of depression than their male counterparts. Not only is the rate of depression higher among female athletes, but it has also been found to be greater than in the general population of nonathletic females [2]. Additionally, the incidence of depression varies sport by sport. Some examples are highlighted in Table 1, and interestingly when categorizing by sport, track and field rates one of the highest incidences of depression [1].

The incidence of depression within each specific sport is higher for females than for their male counterparts. In addition, when analyzing the incidence of depression by sport, the data suggest that sports that put a premium on individual performance and low body weight tend to have a higher incidence of depression [2], and these factors may affect females differently than males.

Anxiety Disorders

Generalized anxiety disorder (GAD), characterized by persistent worry in many areas of life, is the most prevalent disorder found in male and female athletes and is especially prominent in aesthetic sports (eg, figure skating, diving, and gymnastics). Specifically, 38.9% of women in aesthetic sports had a lifetime prevalence of GAD compared with only 10.3% of women in other sports. In comparison, 16.8% of men in aesthetic sports were found to have a lifetime prevalence of GAD compared with 6.8% of men in other sports. This female-to-male GAD prevalence ratio resembles that typically reported in large population studies.

The Female Athletic Triad

The female athlete triad is a medical condition observed in physically active females involving 3 key

*164 Main Street, Suite 201, Los Alto, CA 94022. *E-mail address:* dkamis@stanford.edu

https://doi.org/10.1016/j.ypsc.2021.05.012
2667-3827/21/

TABLE 1
Incidence of Depression by Sport

	Incidence of Depression, Female	Incidence of Depression, Male
Track and Field	25%	38%
Soccer	13%	31%
Lacrosse	125	17%

components: low energy availability with or without an eating disorder, menstrual disturbance such as amenorrhea, and bone loss or full osteoporosis. In the healthy athlete, an optimal balance between energy availability, bone health, and menstrual function exists, and as a consequence, energy deficiency is the main *cause* of the female athlete triad. An energy deficiency is an imbalance between the amount of energy consumed and the amount of energy expended during exercise. Often, this deficiency can involve a conscious restriction of food intake, problems with body image, and a high drive for thinness. Sometimes, these conditions can lead to disordered eating or more serious eating problems, such as anorexia nervosa or bulimia nervosa. Low energy availability is associated with hypothalamic dysfunction and subsequently will negatively affect menstrual function and bone health. The most serious menstrual problem associated with the triad is amenorrhea, defined as no menstrual period for 3 months or more. However, athletes who have irregular (but still present) menstrual cycles are also susceptible to the effects of the triad. Additionally, women with the triad are at higher risk for low bone mass leading to osteoporosis in its severe form. When there is insufficient energy to fuel the athlete's normal bodily processes, the reproductive system is shut down to conserve energy, and as a consequence, the body stops producing estrogen. Without estrogen, the body cannot build bone mass, resulting in a loss of bone mineral density. This type of bone loss can cause an increased risk of fractures, including stress fractures.

While the simultaneous prevalence of all 3 components tends to be rather low and shows a high level of variation (0%–16%), the presence of 1 or 2 concurrent components approaches 50% to 60% in female sports [3]. Athletes who engage in sports where low body weight and lean physique are desired (eg, dancers, gymnasts, and runners) are at the greatest risk of the female athletic triad, but no sport is immune. The consequences of the female athlete triad may not be reversible, so prevention and early intervention are critical. Additionally, some health care providers in the field are using a more recently developed term, relative energy deficiency in sport, to conceptualize a similar set of symptoms that are not limited to female athletes [4].

Eating Disorders

The inadequate intake component of the female athlete triad may or may not represent an eating disorder, and thus eating disorders bear separate consideration. Eating disorders among athletes have been relatively well studied and include anorexia nervosa and bulimia nervosa. Anorexia nervosa is characterized by a refusal to maintain a minimum healthy weight, whereas bulimia nervosa involves repeated episodes of binge eating followed by compensatory behaviors such as self-induced emesis or the use of laxatives, diuretics, extra exercise, or fasting. The incidence of eating disorders is strongly sex-dependent, and females are much more likely than males to have had anorexia nervosa or bulimia nervosa during their lifetimes. In fact, some studies show an incidence of eating disorders as high as 60% in highly competitive female athletes [5].

The most common sports in which female athletes develop eating disorders are considered "leanness sports" such as those mentioned in the female athlete triad section above. In leanness sports, male athletes have about a 33% lower likelihood than females of developing eating disorders.

Substance Use

Trends in substance use by male and female college-level athletes show many similarities [6]. Data reported for the years 2005, 2009, and 2013 show a consistently high rate of alcohol use over the past 12 months by collegiate athletes. Although similar percentages of male and female student-athletes report using alcohol, males use other social and ergogenic (or performance-enhancing) substances at higher rates than females. Altogether, female college sports show substantially less substance use than male sports. However, the patterns and trends in the use of specific substances can be very similar. Among women, ice hockey shows the most overall substance use, exhibiting the highest levels of past-year alcohol use in women's programs. Women's basketball, track, and gymnastics rank lowest for total substance use among collegiate athletes.

Surprisingly, women's collegiate soccer, tennis, and basketball players all show a greater prevalence of past-year alcohol use than participants in men's programs. At the same time, marijuana was used less frequently by women than men across all sports, with women's ice hockey players exhibiting the highest level of use (25.3%). Cigarette smoking by female collegiate athletes was most common among lacrosse players (16.7%), followed by softball players, and for smokeless tobacco use, ice hockey was once again the top sport (11.8%).

Clinical Case

Kelly Catlin was highly gifted [7–15]. At 7, she was an accomplished violin player. Within 2 years of taking up bike racing, she was invited to the national team workout facility. There, though she was not an especially large person, she put out more power on an erg than any woman before her. She and her team were in the hunt for gold in the Olympics; some had them favored. She had a perfect score on the SATs. She was enrolled in a graduate program at Stanford—computational mathematics—fulfilling a lifelong obsession with numbers. She was positioning herself to have a high-level job in Silicon Valley after her racing days were over. Unfortunately, Kelly lost her life to suicide.

Her father, a pathologist, blamed her suicide on a combination of factors, including a success-at-all cost personality, overtraining stress, and athletic injuries. The breaking point was reportedly a concussion she sustained during a training ride. She had previously had a failed suicide attempt by enclosing herself in a car filled with helium.

As highlighted in this case, in order to help facilitate care, it is crucial that a multidisciplinary support team is present for highly trained athletes. An interdisciplinary team comprising a sports psychiatrist, sports medicine physician, therapist (if different from the psychiatrist), coach, and trainers involved in the athlete's care is necessary in order to identify and treat any psychiatric symptoms that may be present and help prevent future athlete suicides. Female athletes are more likely than men to be diagnosed with several psychiatric diagnoses and may be more susceptible than their male counterparts to difficulties encountered in their environment. Important variations in these occurrences by type of sport convey the demands and pressures associated with the practice of particular sports, and when these demands and pressures are combined with particular personalities and genetic predispositions, they may act as significant socioenvironmental risk factors facilitating the development of specific disorders.

SUMMARY AND FUTURE DIRECTION

While a large body of literature exists on sex differences in psychopathology for the general population, such large-scale psychological data on female versus male athletes are scarce. Some studies report exercise as a protective factor, which may lead to surmising that psychopathology would be less frequent in the athletic population, including female athletes. Others attest that the stress of sports leads to higher levels of psychopathology, with female athletes disproportionately affected across several mental illnesses. Further studies must be completed in order to discern this incongruency. In the meantime, biological and psychosocial differences in the sexes should be considered when diagnosing and managing mental illness in athlete populations.

DISCLOSURE

The authors have nothing to disclose.

REFERENCES

[1] Wolanin A, Hong E, Marks D, et al. Prevalence of clinically elevated depressive symptoms in college athletes and differences by gender and sport. Br J Sports Med 2016;50:167–71.

[2] Castaldelli-Maia JM, Gallinaro JGDME, Falcão RS, et al. Mental health symptoms and disorders in elite athletes: a systematic review on cultural influencers and barriers to athletes seeking treatment. Br J Sports Med 2019;53: 707–21.

[3] Committee on Adolescent Health Care. The Female Athlete Triad. Am Coll Obstetricians Gynecologists 2017 Number 702.

[4] Mountjoy M, Sundgot-Borgen J, Burke L, et al. The IOC consensus statement: beyond the Female Athlete Triad—Relative Energy Deficiency in Sport (RED-S) British. J Sports Med 2014;48:491–7.

[5] Schaal K, Tafflet M, Nassif H, et al. Psychological balance in high level athletes: gender-based differences and sport-specific patterns. PLoS One 2011;6(5):e19007.
[6] Mental Health. NCAA.org - The Official Site of the NCAA. Available at: www.ncaa.org/sport-science-institute/mental-health.
[7] Olympic Cyclist Kelly Catlin Seemed Destined for Glory. Then She Killed Herself. New York Times 2019.
[8] Jones TV. Predictors of perceptions of mental illness and averseness to help: a survey of elite football players. J Ment Health 2016;25(5):422–7.
[9] Lopez R, Levy J. Barriers to help seeking checklist, counseling, and psychotherapy preferences questionnaire. J Coll Couns 2013;16.
[10] Harmison R. Athletes Attitudes toward seeking sports psychology consultation questionnaire 2000 Thesis at University of North Texas.
[11] Hausenblas H, Symons Downs D. Comparison of body image between athletes and non athletes review. J Appl Sport Psychol 2001.
[12] Assisting athletes in Distress, Guide for Coaches and athletic trainer. Le Moyne College.
[13] Sarac N, Sarac B, Pedroza A, et al. Epidemiology of mental health conditions in incoming division I collegiate athletes. Phys Sportsmed 2018;46(2):242–8.
[14] Turner JC, Victor Leno E, Keller A. Causes of Mortality Among American College Students: A Pilot Study. J Coll Student Psychotherapy 2013;27(1):31–42.
[15] Storch EA. Self-Reported psychopathology in athletes: A comparison of intercollegiate student athletes and non-student athletes. J Sports Behav 2005.

Advances in Psychiatry and Behavioral Health 1 (2021) 149–160
ADVANCES IN PSYCHIATRY AND BEHAVIORAL HEALTH

Anxiety Disorders in Athletes

A Clinical Review

Claudia L. Reardon, MD[a,*], Paul Gorczynski, PhD[b], Brian Hainline, MD[c], Mary Hitchcock, MA, MS[d], Rosemary Purcell, PhD[e,f], Simon Rice, PhD[f,g], Courtney C. Walton, PhD[f,g]

[a]Department of Psychiatry, University of Wisconsin School of Medicine and Public Health, 6001 Research Park Boulevard, Madison, WI 53719, USA; [b]School of Sport, Health and Exercise Science, University of Portsmouth, Spinnaker Building, Cambridge Road, Portsmouth, Hampshire PO1 2ER, UK; [c]National Collegiate Athletic Association, 700 West Washington Street, PO Box 6222, Indianapolis, IN 46206, USA; [d]University of Wisconsin-Madison, Ebling Library for the Health Sciences, 2339 Health Sciences Learning Center, 750 Highland Avenue, Madison, WI 53705, USA; [e]Research and Translation, Orygen, 35 Poplar Road, Parkville, Melbourne, Australia; [f]Centre for Youth Mental Health, The University of Melbourne, Locked Bag 10, Parkville, Melbourne, Australia; [g]Orygen, 35 Poplar Road, Parkville, Melbourne, Australia

KEYWORDS

• Anxiety • Athletes • Sport • Performance anxiety • Psychiatry • Generalized anxiety • Panic disorder • Obsessive-compulsive disorder

KEY POINTS

- Athletes experience anxiety symptoms and disorders at rates similar to those in the general population.
- Sport and nonsport factors may incite or perpetuate anxiety symptoms and disorders in athletes.
- Nuanced considerations that take into account athletes' psychosocial context and physiology are necessary when implementing treatment of anxiety symptoms and disorders in this population.

INTRODUCTION/BACKGROUND

Contrary to the perceptions of some people, athletes are not protected from mental health symptoms and disorders [1]. Among these are anxiety and related disorders, including generalized anxiety disorder (GAD), panic disorder, social anxiety disorder, and obsessive-compulsive disorder (OCD), and, although not specifically a diagnosis in the Diagnostic and Statistical Manual of Mental Disorders, competitive performance anxiety [1]. Many factors contribute to anxiety in this population [2]. Furthermore, there may be athlete-specific manifestations of anxiety symptoms and disorders and particular considerations when it comes to diagnosing and managing such conditions in this demographic [1].

Despite these athlete-specific considerations, a comprehensive review on clinical aspects of anxiety disorders in athletes has not been written. Anxiety disorders are some of the most common and enduring mental health disorders across countries and cultures [3], with earlier onsets than most other mental health disorders [4]. Increasing attention is being paid to the importance of safeguarding athlete mental health, given that this population experiences significant mental health stigma, is vulnerable in many ways, and experiences barriers to accessing mental health care [5]. This article provides a clinical review on GAD, panic disorder, social anxiety disorder, OCD, and competitive performance anxiety in athletes. Posttraumatic stress disorder in athletes is an anxiety-related condition that has been covered elsewhere in a recent review [6].

An experienced academic librarian (M.H.) developed a search strategy using PubMed, SportDiscus, PsycINFO,

*Corresponding author, *E-mail address:* clreardon@wisc.edu

https://doi.org/10.1016/j.ypsc.2021.05.010
2667-3827/21/

Scopus, and Cochrane databases from inception until October 2020. Additional articles were reviewed for possible inclusion based on reference lists of the original articles found. Studies were selected if they included information on athletes and anxiety-related symptoms or disorders and excluded if they were not published in English. General mental health articles were included where athlete-specific research was not available.

GENERAL INFORMATION

Anxiety disorders in combination reportedly affect athletes in a past 12-month prevalence of approximately 9% [7], fairly similar to the rates reported to affect the general population (11%–12%) [8,9]. Preliminary research has examined comparative rates of anxiety in different sports. Individual sport athletes may be at greater risk for anxiety than are team sport athletes [10,11]. Starting at younger ages, motivations for athletes to join team sports disproportionately include a desire to have fun, whereas motivations to join individual sports disproportionately include goal-oriented reasons such as obtaining a scholarship or controlling weight [10]. The latter reasons may be anxiogenic or associated with an underlying anxious predisposition. Individual sport athletes may also be more likely to internalize failure after loss, set intense personal goals, exhibit perfectionism, receive less social support, train year-round in a single sport, and experience injuries, all of which may contribute to anxiety [12,13]. Among specific individual sports, those for which judges determine success (eg, gymnastics, figure skating, and dance) are correlated with the highest rates of anxiety in athletes [7]. These athletes describe feeling significant pressure to differentiate themselves from the competition in the pursuit of perfection and judges' approval [7].

Several other factors have been described as precipitating or exacerbating anxiety in athletes (Table 1).

As in the general population, anxiety disorders in athletes commonly occur with comorbid mental health symptoms and disorders. Among athletes, depression and eating disorders may be particularly common comorbidities [7,22–26]. This finding is unsurprising, given that depression is as prevalent in athletes as in nonathletes [27], eating disorders are disproportionately common in athletes [22–24], and comorbidities among these conditions are common in the general population [28,29].

Anxiety symptoms and disorders can affect sport performance. For example, higher ratings of self-reported anxiety are associated with negative performance outcomes and skill errors in elite athletes [30–32]. Anxiety is known to affect attention, executive function, stimulus processing, information selection, and muscle tension, all of which are important in sport competition [2]. Furthermore, feelings of stress and worry before competition are normal to some degree in athletes, but the athlete's interpretation of those emotions may mediate the functional impact on performance [33]. For example, if the athlete interprets the feelings as facilitative in getting psyched up to face an opponent or execute a skill, that may be functionally helpful. Alternatively, if the athlete perceives the feelings as detrimental, then behavioral responses are less adaptive, and performance may be negatively affected [34,35]. In addition, anxiety in athletes is one of the most researched and consistent variables associated with sport injury occurrence [36].

GENERALIZED ANXIETY DISORDER

GAD in athletes seems to be as common as in the general population, ranging in prevalence from 6.0% for a clinician-confirmed diagnosis [7] to 14.6% using self-report measures [37]. Paralleling the general population, female athletes report experiencing GAD more frequently [38–44]. Aesthetic sports (eg, gymnastics, figure skating, synchronized swimming) across genders reportedly confer a higher risk for GAD among elite athletes [7]. Athletes in such sports have described a feeling of lacking control, including over the outcome of their sport performances, which are judged by others, as well as over other aspects of their sport [45]. In contrast, high-risk sports, which include sliding sports (eg, luge), aerial sports, and motor sports, are associated with the lowest risk for GAD among elite athletes [7]. These sports have a high risk of lethal accidents, and participants in them have been described as thrill seekers [46,47]. In addition, these athletes may cope better with stressful or frightening situations [48].

PANIC DISORDER

By self-report, panic disorder symptoms are estimated to affect 4.5% of athletes [49], which is similar to rates in the general population [50]. Exercise has been shown to have an overall anxiolytic effect, but some research shows that exercise can trigger acutely heightened anxiety and panic attacks, with up to one-third of patients with panic disorder and/or agoraphobia reporting increased anxiety during acute exercise [51]. Thus, people with panic disorder may avoid exercise [52]. The association between exercise and panic attacks may relate to the physical sensations of exercise (eg, heart beating

TABLE 1
Factors that Precipitate and/or Perpetuate Anxiety in Athletes

Domain of Factors that Precipitate/Perpetuate Anxiety in Athletes	Specific Factors
Sport specific	• Sense of pressure to perform [14] • Public scrutiny [14] • Sporting career uncertainty or dissatisfaction [15,16] • Injury [17–19] • Harassment and abuse in sport [20]
Non–sport-specific	• Female [2,11] • Younger age [2] • Recent experience of adverse life events [2] • Behavioral inhibition [21] • Social withdrawal or avoidance [21] • Rumination [21]

faster and shortness of breath). These sensations mimic those of panic, and thus exercisers who experience panic attacks worry that they are going to have a panic attack, which exacerbates further symptoms of panic [53]. The association of panic attacks with exercise in athletes specifically has not been studied. However, if an athlete presents with panic attacks, and concomitant with development of that condition is considering dropping out of sport, the clinician should evaluate whether the athlete's panic seems worse when exercising [24].

SOCIAL ANXIETY DISORDER

By self-report, symptoms of social anxiety disorder are estimated to affect 14.7% of athletes [49], which is similar to rates in the general population [50]. A pattern of fear of social evaluation, especially if extending to social venues outside of sport, warrants evaluation for social anxiety disorder [24]. There may be a correlation between social anxiety and avoidance of individual sports (where athletes may perceive they singularly are being watched by many people), but not team sports (where public viewing is dispersed across multiple athletes) [54]. It is important to distinguish social anxiety disorder from competitive performance anxiety. In social anxiety disorder, the focus of fears is interaction with and fear of negative evaluation by others, whereas, in competitive performance anxiety, the symptoms are limited to sport participation, with fear of scrutiny by others not typically a primary factor [55]. Athletes with social anxiety disorder may avoid team meetings and meals and services such as rehabilitation exercises in the athletic training room. Together with a cognitive focus on self rather than sport task, these factors may result in a negative impact of social anxiety on sport performance [56].

OBSESSIVE-COMPULSIVE DISORDER

By self-report, OCD is estimated to affect 5.2%% of athletes [57], which appears to be higher than rates in the general population [50,58]. Moreover, in that same study of athletes (collegiate), nearly 35% reported OCD symptoms without meeting full OCD criteria [57]. Dysfunction from OCD can ensue in sport if intrusive thoughts interfere with present moment attention or if the athlete cannot stop the obsessive-compulsive routine to engage in sport performance [56]. It is important not to overdiagnose OCD in athletes who may manifest superstitious rituals. Such rituals are common in sport [59,60], and idiosyncratic mannerisms or routines alone do not merit a diagnosis of OCD if they do not cause distress or dysfunction [1]. These behaviors may serve to offer a sense of predictability and reassurance to athletes, for whom other aspects of their competitive environment (eg, the

TABLE 2
Differentiation Between Normal Competition-Induced Hyperarousal, Competitive Performance Anxiety, and Anxiety Disorders [1,24,56]

	Normal Competition-Induced Hyperarousal	Competitive Performance Anxiety	Anxiety Disorder (eg, GAD)
Pattern of symptom onset	Mild hyperarousal symptoms (eg, feeling mildly nervous) typically starting during the day before/of or during sport performance	Hyperarousal symptoms starting any time before or during sport performance	Anxiety symptoms present most days irrespective of performance times (although symptoms might become even worse before/during performance). In GAD, symptoms have been present at least 6 mo [61]
Source of worry	Performance in sport	Performance in sport	Worries that are often multiple (in the case of GAD) and that are not solely sport related
Duration	Typically <24 h	Variable; can be a week or more before performances	Ongoing
Severity	No negative impact on functioning or significant distress, and arousal to a certain degree may optimize performance according to the inverted-U hypothesis [62]	Detrimental impact on sport performance and/ or significant distress	Detrimental impact on life functioning outside of (and sometimes within) sport and/or significant distress

weather, what their opponent or spectators will do) are unpredictable [24]. However, if pericompetition rituals start to take up more time (eg, extending increasing amounts of time before competition) or extend outside of the sport realm, clinicians should be on the alert for OCD [24]. To be diagnosed as OCD, there is typically at least an hour per day of obsessions and/ or compulsions in a manner that causes significant distress and/or dysfunction [61].

COMPETITIVE PERFORMANCE ANXIETY

Competitive performance anxiety in sport is defined as fear an athlete has occurring around the time of sport participation, especially competition, that they will not be able to perform in the desired manner, that the situation will be too challenging, and/or that it will be dangerous or harmful, thus resulting in anxious cognitive appraisals, behavioral responses, and/or physiologic arousals. It can be difficult to distinguish among competitive performance anxiety, normal degrees of competition-induced hyperarousal, and overt anxiety disorders. Patterns of symptom onset, duration, and severity should be used to differentiate these 3 possibilities (Table 2). Complicating things further, competitive performance anxiety (often considered a state, or circumstantial and temporary, form of anxiety) and specific anxiety disorders such as GAD (considered trait, or more enduring, forms of anxiety) can overlap [30,63]. Thus, diagnosis of competitive performance anxiety should prompt careful evaluation for specific anxiety disorders.

Competitive performance anxiety often has many physical symptoms, which can also occur in other types of anxiety. These symptoms include the typical fight-or-flight response symptoms, such as rapid heart rate and breathing, dry mouth, trembling, and sweaty hands. In addition, gastrointestinal disturbances, such as urges to defecate, diarrhea, and even vomiting, are fairly common during training and competition, especially among endurance athletes, and may relate to competitive performance anxiety [64].

Even though, by definition, competitive performance anxiety is limited to sport in its impact, it can be highly distressing and problematic for athletes. It can lead to slumps (an extended period of performance at a level less than demonstrated capabilities) or chokes (acute performance much lower than predicted by skill level, especially referring to high-stakes moments) [55]. Athletes and clinicians in the field sometimes reference what they call the yips, a term used to describe a possible variant of a choke in which there is an involuntary movement during a sport-specific task, especially in sports such as golf, cricket, shooting, bowling, or darts that require finely controlled motor skills [65]. Nonsport analogies include writer's cramp and musician's hand [65]. For example, a golfer may develop a problematic posture, tremor, or jerk during attempted putting, chipping, or full swing [66]. Studies on the yips phenomenon in athletes have been limited, but the condition may be common and underdiagnosed in sports such as golf [66]. There may be a spectrum of causes for the yips, ranging from competitive performance anxiety to a focal dystonia, with a continuum between the two [65,66]. Some investigators hypothesize that the 2 causes may be distinguishable depending on whether the involuntary movement occurs in nonstressful settings (eg, informal sports practices), with focal dystonia a more prominent factor if it occurs even in nonstressful settings [65]. Ultimately, any manifestations of competitive performance anxiety can result in burnout and losses that are important to athletes [55,67], including loss of continued participation in sport, financial support (in the form of scholarships, sponsorships, appearance fees, or salary), ability to ascend to the next competitive level, or medals or other recognitions in sport.

Risk factors for competitive performance anxiety in athletes have been reported to include female gender, younger age, lower athletic experience [68], and athlete perception of coaching behaviors as controlling versus autonomy supporting [69]. In addition, social media use preceding or during competition, especially if push notifications are enabled on the athlete's phone, is associated with higher rates of competitive performance anxiety [70]. It is hypothesized that such media use could serve to increase comparisons with others in an anxiogenic way; that use interferes with mental preparation and thus leaves athletes feeling less confident in competition; or that use is a marker for anxious, unconfident trait anxiety at baseline [70].

OTHER ANXIETY-RELATED DISORDERS

The authors found no studies examining other anxiety-related disorders, including specific phobia, agoraphobia, obsessive-compulsive personality disorder, or adjustment disorder with anxiety, in athletes. Given many transient, sport-specific stressors in the athlete population, adjustment disorder with anxiety may be common in this population [71].

GENERAL PRINCIPLES OF DIAGNOSIS AND MANAGEMENT

There are no known comprehensive, validated, athlete-specific anxiety screening tools. However, recently the International Olympic Committee published its Sports Mental Health Assessment Tool 1 (SMHAT-1), which includes several screening tools packaged together for use in athletes [72]. The GAD-7 is the anxiety screening tool included in the SMHAT-1 and thus seems an acceptable choice for athletes [72]. It would be reasonable to incorporate the entire SMHAT-1, or the GAD-7 if primarily concerned about anxiety, into preparticipation physical examinations, and to repeat such screening at high-risk times such as after injury. In addition, there are tools such as the Sport Anxiety Scale-2 available for screening specifically for competitive performance anxiety [73].

Before initiating treatment of anxiety symptoms or disorders in athletes, clinicians should consider possible nonpsychiatric medical contributors to the symptoms (Table 3) [24].

Psychotherapy is often first-line treatment of mild to moderate mental health symptoms and disorders, including anxiety, in athletes [1,82]. Although this is often the case in the general population too, it is important in this population for whom medication side effects can be impairing in the patient's major role or occupation as an athlete [1]. Athletes often express preferences for psychotherapists with familiarity with the culture of sport [83]. Athletes with anxiety disorders may be particularly good candidates for cognitive-behavior therapy, given their familiarity with receiving instruction (from coaches), following rules, and completing homework (eg, via memorizing plays, studying film of the opponent, and so forth) [82]. Specific psychological factors that are considered necessary for success in high level sport (affect regulation, maintenance of motivation, self-confidence, adaptive coping strategies, and maintenance of supportive interpersonal relationships [84]) simultaneously help in management of anxiety symptoms [2]. Thus, focus on these aspects serves multiple means to the end of optimized sport performance in athletes with anxiety. In the case of panic attacks exacerbated by physiologic sensations during exercise, treating the panic disorder and not

TABLE 3
Common Nonpsychiatric Medical Conditions that May Contribute to Anxiety Symptoms in Athletes [74]

Nonpsychiatric Medical Condition	Signs/Symptoms that May Mimic Anxiety in Athletes	Relevance to Athletes	Typical Evaluation	Management
Anemia	• Shortness of breath • Tachycardia • Fatigue	• Endurance athletes and athletes with eating disorders may be at risk for anemia	• Hemoglobin and ferritin laboratory tests	• Increased dietary iron intake • Iron supplements
Asthma	• Shortness of breath that may contribute to a sense of anxiety, panic, or impending doom • Tachycardia	• Asthma may be exercise induced • Athletes in certain sports (eg, swimming) may have high rates of asthma [75]	• Lung auscultation • Pulmonary function testing	• Beta-agonists (some are prohibited at higher levels of competition without therapeutic use exemptions) [76] • Other daily controller medications
Caffeine overuse	• Nervousness • Restlessness • Jitteriness • Insomnia • Tachycardia	• Athletes may overuse caffeine to increase energy or enhance performance [77]	• Clinical interview	• Taper caffeine (athletes consuming large doses may experience short-term withdrawal effects that may temporarily exacerbate anxiety)
Concussion [78]	• Nervousness • Irritability • Trouble concentrating • Insomnia • Fatigue	• Athletes experience SRC • Anxiety symptoms may be multifactorial after SRC	• Immediate clinical neurologic assessment • Serial symptom assessment • Possible neuropsychological testing • Possible neuroimaging	• Gradual return-to-sport and return-to-learn protocols • Symptom-targeted pharmacology as needed • Psychotherapy if mental health symptoms are persistent or severe
Hypoglycemia [79]	• Acute episodes of nervousness, jitteriness, irritability, and/or sweating	• High training demands with insufficient or poorly timed caloric intake may occur in athletes • Eating disorders may be associated with hypoglycemia	• Glucose laboratory test while symptomatic	• Improved timing and composition of meals and snacks

(*continued on next page*)

TABLE 3
(*continued*)

Nonpsychiatric Medical Condition	Signs/Symptoms that May Mimic Anxiety in Athletes	Relevance to Athletes	Typical Evaluation	Management
Thyroid dysfunction [80]	• Palpitations • Tremors • Restlessness • Insomnia • Fatigue	• Overtraining in female athletes is associated with thyroid dysfunction • Iron deficiency (common in some athlete populations) is commonly comorbid with hypothyroidism • Athletes may use exogenous thyroid hormone to attempt to improve performance	• Thyroid function laboratory tests	• Typically medication • Sometimes radioactive thyroid ablation or thyroidectomy
EILO [81]	• Episodic shortness of breath that can lead to acute anxiety/panic	• Symptoms occur during exercise, resolve within minutes of stopping exercise, and are especially common in adolescent female athletes	• Referral to otolaryngology • Spirometry before/after bronchodilator and bronchoprovocation challenge, with confirmation via continuous laryngoscopy during exercise	• Behavioral management with speech-language pathologist • Manage psychosocial stressors related to EILO episodes

Abbreviations: EILO, exercise-induced laryngeal obstruction; SRC, sport-related concussion.

encouraging phobic avoidance of sport and exercise is recommended [24]. Mindfulness-based stress reduction and mindfulness-based cognitive therapy have shown efficacy for anxiety symptoms in the general population [85] and are increasingly popular for, and may be effective for, stress and other symptoms that may be associated with anxiety in athletes [86]. In addition, nutritional support may be helpful for athletes experiencing gastrointestinal manifestations of anxiety during sport [64].

Anxiolytic medications should be considered as a potential treatment modality, especially in cases of moderate to severe symptoms of GAD, panic disorder, social anxiety disorder, and OCD [1]. However, side effects that may lead to performance impairment or compromised safety in sport must be considered [87]. Antidepressants are the most common pharmacologic treatments for anxiety, and selective serotonin reuptake inhibitors tend to be top choices for this population [88]. Specifically, escitalopram, sertraline, and fluoxetine are the top choices of sports psychiatrists for anxiety in athletes [88]. Among these, fluoxetine has received some study of performance impact and not been shown to cause a detrimental effect [89,90], although sample sizes, participant diversity, performance measures, and duration of study were limited. Escitalopram and sertraline have not been studied in athletes, but clinicians working with athletes use them without significant concern [88]. Tricyclic antidepressants (TCAs) are another class of antidepressants sometimes used for anxiety in general populations, but they too have received little study in athletes. Monitoring of blood levels in anyone taking tricyclic antidepressants is important, because blood levels that are too high may result in toxicity, including dangerous cardiac consequences [1]. In theory, this may have particular relevance for athletes exercising to high cardiac intensity. Moreover, eating disorders, which are common in athletes and a common comorbidity with anxiety, are typically regarded as a reason to avoid TCAs if possible [91].

Thus, TCAs should be used with caution, if at all, in athletes with anxiety [1].

Buspirone is another anxiolytic sometimes used in athletes. One small study suggested impaired performance in recreational athletes, but only a single 45-mg dose was tested, not a dosing strategy reflective of real-world use [92].

Medications are not indicated for competitive performance anxiety in athletes [1]. Quick-acting options such as benzodiazepines may impair performance. They have muscle relaxant properties and may slow reaction time and cause sedation [55,93–95]. β-Blockers such as propranolol may reduce blood pressure and cause dizziness in athletes who may already have low blood pressure [1] and may decrease cardiopulmonary capacity in endurance athletes [96]. Moreover, the World Anti-Doping Agency prohibits β-blockers at all times (out of competition and in competition) for athletes in archery and shooting, and in competition for athletes in automobile, billiards, darts, golf, some skiing/snowboarding, and some underwater sports [76]. In these types of sports, β-blockers may reduce tremor and thus improve fine motor control and therefore could create an unfair performance advantage [1]. Consequently, psychotherapeutic approaches are often the only reasonable option for management of competitive performance anxiety [55]. Athletes need practice in management and interpretation of the feelings of being pumped up before and during performance just as they need practice in the other physical and technical aspects of sport. In addition, although sometimes used, pharmacologic interventions such as benzodiazepines and botulinum toxin have received little study in the treatment of the yips. [66] In the yips, various behavioral strategies have been used, including, depending on sport, change in grip technique, change in length/type of golf club or other implement used, development of a new biomechanical routine while engaging in the problematic aspect of sport, and hypnosis, but none have undergone rigorous study [66].

Especially for athletes at higher levels of competition (eg, collegiate, professional, and other elite levels), care must be taken if any nonregulated supplements are taken to attempt to treat anxiety. Although athletes might be drawn to the idea of taking a natural product, these levels of competition have strict prohibitions against certain substances [76], and supplements may be unknowingly tainted with prohibited substances [1]. Ignorance of ingredients or improper labeling are not typically regarded as valid excuses for adverse analytical findings on drug tests [1]. If supplements (eg, melatonin, which is commonly used by athletes for insomnia associated with anxiety) are taken, they should be obtained from a reputable company [1]. Moreover, several other supplements marketed for anxiety (eg, kava, valerian) may cause sedation [74], which could be problematic for performing athletes. Recently, cannabidiol has been marketed to athletes as helpful for anxiety, among other conditions, but there is inadequate research on this substance for anxiety [97]. In addition, athletes consuming it risk ingesting tetrahydrocannabinol, which may contaminate the product and is prohibited at several levels of competition [76].

DISCUSSION

Athletes may experience a broad swath of anxiety symptoms and disorders. Knowledge of and attention to the reported risk factors for anxiety in athletes can help clinicians to have heightened awareness of the possibility of anxiety symptoms or disorders in this population. For example, if an athlete is experiencing an acute injury, reports dissatisfaction with the role as an athlete, or is primarily motivated in sport by prospects of obtaining a scholarship, the clinician should be particularly certain to screen for anxiety and arrange for treatment if needed. Early intervention can then be used, which may help prevent progression from symptoms to outright disorders, such as from competitive performance anxiety to an all-encompassing disorder. This approach depends on health care systems and sports organizations ensuring services are designed and delivered in a manner that is truly accessible and embraces diversity.

Treatment recommendations should take into account athletes' unique resources, strengths, and physiology. Anecdotally, athletes sometimes express concern that treatment of their anxiety symptoms might have a negative impact on performance via a detrimental impact on fear-driven work ethic and conscientiousness; however, the authors found no evidence to substantiate this concern. However, clinicians must be aware of potential impacts on sport performance of pharmacologic choices. Daily controller medication such as selective serotonin reuptake inhibitors have not been shown to have detrimental impacts on sport performance, but research methodology to date has been limited, and reports from individual athletes about how they perceive medications to be affecting them should be sought and taken seriously.

An understanding of the culture of sport by clinicians providing care for athletes with anxiety is important. Athletes may not respond well to clinicians who are naive to the world of sport, and who, for example, advise quitting of sport because of mental health symptoms such as competitive performance anxiety. These athletes may think they have to do too much teaching in session about the sport environment. Their response may be that the clinician does not understand, with resultant premature cessation of mental health treatment. Clinicians thus must find an adequate balance between not unhelpfully jumping to a stance of recommending retirement from sport in the face of symptoms, most of which improve with evidence-based interventions, while also validating current suffering and being alert for problematic circumstances in sport (eg, abuse, playing through serious injuries) that do warrant intervention. In addition, clinicians should be aware of the apparent mental health benefits of sport when it is pursued for the fun and enjoyment it affords (more often the case in team sports), versus the more negative effects when it is associated with anxiogenic, lonely pursuits of individual perfection and internal attribution after failure (more often the case in individual sports). Clinicians should appreciate the sense of powerlessness (a triggering factor for anxiety in athletes and nonathletes alike) that athletes in certain sports, such as aesthetic ones that are judged by others, may disproportionately feel. Although clinicians should not disparage the athlete's choice of sport, there may be utility to helping the athlete develop insight into the anxious tendencies, how the particular sport may perpetuate those tendencies, and how such tendencies can be counteracted.

SUMMARY

Athletes are not protected from anxiety symptoms and disorders through their sporting roles. Numerous sport and nonsport risk factors promote anxiety in this population. Effective treatment has nuances in this population, and should be used in haste just as in nonathlete populations.

CLINICS CARE POINTS

- Screen for more pervasive anxiety disorders if an athlete presents with competitive performance anxiety.
- Assess for potential nonpsychiatric medical causes of anxiety symptoms in athletes before assuming an anxiety disorder is present.
- Recommend psychotherapy (with a provider familiar with the sporting context) for treatment of anxiety symptoms and disorders in athletes.
- Consider medications for treatment of moderate to severe anxiety symptoms and disorders in athletes, taking into consideration potential side effects, safety issues, and sport governing body regulations of relevance to athletes.

DISCLOSURE

The authors have no commercial or financial conflicts of interest or funding sources to disclose.

REFERENCES

[1] Reardon CL, Hainline B, Aron CM, et al. Mental health in elite athletes: International Olympic Committee consensus statement (2019). Br J Sports Med 2019; 53(11):667–99.
[2] Rice SM, Gwyther K, Santesteban-Echarri O, et al. Determinants of anxiety in elite athletes: a systematic review and meta-analysis. Br J Sports Med 2019;53:722–30.
[3] Whiteford HA, Ferrari AJ, Degenhardt L, et al. The global burden of mental, neurological and substance use disorders: an analysis from the of disease study 2010. PLos One 2015;10:e0116820.
[4] Kessler RC, Berglund P, Demler O. Lifetime prevalence and age-of-onset distributions of DSM-IV disorders in the national comorbidity survey replication. Arch Gen Psychiatry 2005;62(6):593–602.
[5] Gulliver A, Griffiths KM, Christensen H. Barriers and facilitators to mental health help-seeking for young elite athletes: a qualitative study. BMC Psychiatry 2012;12:157.
[6] Aron CM, Harvey S, Hainline B, et al. Post-traumatic stress disorder (PTSD) and other trauma-related mental disorders in elite athletes: a narrative review. Br J Sports Med 2019;53(12):779–84.
[7] Schaal K, Tafflet M, Nassif H, et al. Psychological balance in high level athletes: gender-based differences and sport-specific patterns. PLoS One 2011;6:e19007.
[8] Somers JM, Goldner EM, Waraich P, et al. Prevalence and incidence studies of anxiety disorders: a systematic review of the literature. Can J Psychiatry 2006;51:100–13.
[9] Wittchen H-U, Jacobi F. Size and burden of mental disorders in Europe—a critical review and appraisal of 27 studies. Eur Neuropsychopharmacol 2005;15:357–76.
[10] Pluhar E, McCracken C, Griffith KL, et al. Team sport athletes may be less likely to suffer anxiety or depression than individual sport athletes. J Sports Med Sci 2019; 18(3):490–6.
[11] Correia M, Rosado A. Anxiety in athletes: gender and type of sport differences. Int J Psychol Res 2019;12(1): 9–17.
[12] Nixdorf I, Frank R, Hautzinger M, et al. Prevalence of depressive symptoms and correlating variables among German elite athletes. J Clin Sport Psychol 2013;7(4): 313–26.

[13] Nixdorf I, Frank R, Beckmann J. Comparison of athletes' proneness to depressive symptoms in individual and team sports: research on psychological mediators in junior elite athletes. Front Psychol 2016;7:893.
[14] Hodge K, Smith W. Public expectation, pressure, and avoiding the choke: a case study from elite sport. Sport Psychol 2014;28:375–89.
[15] Brown CJ, Webb TL, Robinson MA, et al. Athletes' retirement from elite sport: a qualitative study of parents and partners' experiences. Psychol Sport Exerc 2019;40: 51–60.
[16] Gustafsson H, Hassmén P, Kenttä G, et al. A qualitative analysis of burnout in elite Swedish athletes. Psychol Sport Exerc 2008;9:800–16.
[17] Lavallée L, Flint F. The relationship of stress, competitive anxiety, mood state, and social support to athletic injury. J Athl Train 1996;31(4):296–9.
[18] Ivarsson A, Johnson U. Psychological factors as predictors of injuries among senior soccer players. A prospective study. J Sports Sci Med 2010;9(2):347–52.
[19] Kiliç Ö, Aoki H, Goedhart E, et al. Severe musculoskeletal time-loss injuries and symptoms of common mental disorders in professional soccer: a longitudinal analysis of 12-month follow-up data. Knee Surg Sports Traumatol Arthrosc 2018;26:946–54.
[20] Mountjoy M, Brackenridge C, Arrington M, et al. International Olympic Committee consensus statement: harassment and abuse (non-accidental violence) in sport. Br J Sports Med 2016;50:1019–29.
[21] Leach LS, Christensen H, Mackinnon AJ, et al. Gender differences in depression and anxiety across the adult lifespan: the role of psychosocial mediators. Soc Psychiatry Psychiatr Epidemiol 2008;43:983–98.
[22] Gouttebarge V, Aoki H, Verhagen EALM, et al. A 12-month prospective cohort study of symptoms of common mental disorders among European professional footballers. Clin J Sport Med 2017;27:487–92.
[23] Hulley AJ, Hill AJ. Eating disorders and health in elite women distance runners. Int J Eat Disord 2001;30:312–7.
[24] Reardon CL. Psychiatric comorbidities in sports. Neurol Clin 2017;35:537–46.
[25] Kerr ZY, DeFreese JD, Marshall SW. Current physical and mental health of former collegiate athletes. Orthop J Sports Med 2014;2:232596711454410–232596711454419.
[26] Junge A, Prinz B. Depression and anxiety symptoms in 17 teams of female football players including 10 German first league teams. Br J Sports Med 2019;53:471–7.
[27] Gorczynski PF, Coyle M, Gibson K. Depressive symptoms in high-performance athletes and non-athletes: a comparative meta-analysis. Br J Sports Med 2017; 51(18):1348–54.
[28] Blinder BJ, Cumella EJ, Sanathara VA. Psychiatric comorbidities of female inpatients with eating disorders. Psychosom Med 2006;68(3):454–62.
[29] Kaye WH, Bulik CM, Thornton L, et al. Comorbidity of anxiety disorders with anorexia and bulimia nervosa. Am J Psychiatry 2004;161(12):2215–21.
[30] Halvari H, Gjesme T. Trait and state anxiety before and after competitive performance. Percept Mot Skills 1995; 81(3_suppl):1059–74.
[31] Morgan WP, O'Connor PJ, Ellickson KA, et al. Personality structure, mood states, and performance in elite male distance runners. Int J Sport Psychol 1988;19:247–63.
[32] Turner PE, Raglin JS. Variability in precompetition anxiety and performance in college track and field athletes. Med Sci Sports Exerc 1996;28:378–85.
[33] Rice SM, Purcell R, De Silva S, et al. The mental health of elite athletes: a narrative systematic review. Sports Med 2016;46:1333–53.
[34] Hatzigeorgiadis A, Chroni S. Pre-competition anxiety and in-competition coping in experienced male swimmers. Int J Sports Sci Coach 2007;2:181–9.
[35] Jones G, Hanton S, Swain A. Intensity and interpretation of anxiety symptoms in elite and non-elite sports performers. Pers Individ Dif 1994;17:657–63.
[36] Ford JL, Ildefonso K, Jones ML, et al. Sport-related anxiety: current insights. Open Access J Sports Med 2017;8: 205–12.
[37] Du Preez EJ, Graham KS, Gan TY, et al. Depression, anxiety, and alcohol use in elite rugby league players over a competitive season. Clin J Sport Med 2017;27:530–5.
[38] Junge A, Feddermann-Demont N. Prevalence of depression and anxiety in top-level male and female football players. BMJ Open Sport Exerc Med 2016;2: e000087.
[39] Brand R, Wolff W, Hoyer J. Psychological symptoms and chronic mood in representative samples of elite student-athletes, deselected student-athletes and comparison students. Sch Ment Health 2013;5:166–74.
[40] Yang J, Peek-Asa C, Corlette JD, et al. Prevalence of and risk factors associated with symptoms of depression in competitive collegiate student athletes. Clin J Sport Med 2007;17:481–7.
[41] Lancaster MA, McCrea MA, Nelson LD. Psychometric properties and normative data for the brief symptom Inventory-18 (BSI-18) in high school and collegiate athletes. Clin Neuropsychol 2016;30:321–33.
[42] Weber S, Puta C, Lesinski M, et al. Symptoms of anxiety and depression in young athletes using the hospital anxiety and depression scale. Front Physiol 2018;9:1–12.
[43] Gerber M, Holsboer-Trachsler E, Pühse U, et al. Elite sport is not an additional source of distress for adolescents with high stress levels. Percept Mot Skills 2011; 112:581–99.
[44] Ivarsson A, Johnson U, Podlog L. Psychological predictors of injury occurrence: a prospective investigation of professional Swedish soccer players. J Sport Rehabil 2013;22:19–26.
[45] Kerr G, Goss J. Personal control in elite gymnasts: the relationships between locus of control, self-esteem and trait anxiety. J Sport Behav 1997;20:69–82.
[46] Carton S, Morand P, Bungenera C, et al. Sensation-seeking and emotional disturbances in depression: relationships and evolution. J Affect Disord 1995;34:219–25.

[47] Michel G, Carton S, Jouvent R. Sensation seeking and anhedonia in risk taking. Study of a population of bungy jumpers. Encephale 1997;23:403–11.

[48] Larkin M, Griffiths M. Dangerous sports and recreational drug-use: rationalizing and contextualizing risk. J Commun Appl Soc Psychol 2004;14:215–32.

[49] Gulliver A, Griffiths KM, Mackinnon A, et al. The mental health of Australian elite athletes. J Sci Med Sport 2015; 18:255–61.

[50] Bandelow B, Michaelis S. Epidemiology of anxiety disorders in the 21st century. Dialogues Clin Neurosci 2015; 17:327–35.

[51] Cameron OG, Hudson CJ. Influence of exercise on anxiety level in patients with anxiety disorders. Psychosomatics 1986;27:720–3.

[52] Broocks A, Meyer TF, Bandelow B, et al. Exercise avoidance and impaired endurance capacity in patients with panic disorder. Neuropsychobiology 1997;36:182–7.

[53] Strohle A, Graetz B, Scheel M, et al. The acute antipanic and anxiolytic activity of aerobic exercise in patients with panic disorder and healthy control subjects. J Psychiatr Res 2009;43:1013–7.

[54] Northon PJ, Burns JA, Hope DA. Generalization of social anxiety to sporting and athletic situations: gender, sports involvement, and parental pressure. Depress Anxiety 2000;12:193–202.

[55] Patel DR, Omar H, Terry M. Sport-related performance anxiety in young female athletes. J Pediatr Adolesc Gynecol 2010;23:325–35.

[56] Chang CJ, Putukian M, Aerni G, et al. Mental health issues and psychological factors in athletes: detection, management, effect on performance, and prevention: American Medical Society for Sports Medicine Position Statement. Clin J Sport Med 2020;30(2):e61–87.

[57] Cromer L, Kaier E, Davis J, et al. OCD in college athletes. Am J Psychiatry 2017;174:595–7.

[58] Goodman WK, Grice DE, Lapidus KAB, et al. Obsessive-compulsive disorder. Psychiatr Clin North Am 2014;37: 257–67.

[59] Bleak JL, Frederick CM. Superstitious behavior in sport: levels of effectiveness and determinants of use in three collegiate sports. J Sport Behav 1998;21:1–15.

[60] Dömötör Z, Ruíz-Barquín R, Szabo A. Superstitious behavior in sport: a literature review. Scand J Psychol 2016;57:368–82.

[61] American Psychiatric Association. Diagnostic and statistical manual of mental disorders (DSM-5). Washington, DC: American Psychiatric Publishing; 2013.

[62] Yerkes RMD, Dodson JD. The relation of strength of stimulus to rapidity of habit formation. J Comp Neurol Psychol 1908;18(5):459–82.

[63] Guillén F, Sánchez R. Competitive anxiety in expert female athletes: sources and intensity of anxiety in national team and first division Spanish basketball players. Percept Mot Skills 2009;109:407–19.

[64] Wilson PB. The psychobiological etiology of gastrointestinal distress in sport: a review. J Clin Gastroenterol 2020;54(4):297–304.

[65] Adler CH, Temkit M, Crews D, et al. The yips: methods to identify golfers with a dystonic etiology/golfer's cramp. Med Sci Sports Exerc 2018;50(11):2226–30.

[66] Dhungana S, Jankovic J. Yips and other movement disorders in golfers. Mov Disord 2013;28(5):576–81.

[67] Martorell MS, Ponseti FJ, Prats AN, et al. Competitive anxiety and performance in competing sailors. Retos 2021;39:187–91.

[68] Rocha VVS, Osório FdeL, FdL O. Associations between competitive anxiety, athlete characteristics and sport context: evidence from a systematic review and metaanalysis. Arch Clin Psychiatry 2018;45:67–74.

[69] Cho S, Choi H, Youngsook K. The relationship between perceived coaching behaviors, competitive trait anxiety, and athlete burnout: a cross-sectional study. Int J Environ Res Public Health 2019;16(8):1424.

[70] Encel K, Mesagno C, Brown H. Facebook use and its relationship with sport anxiety. J Sports Sci 2017;35(8): 756–61.

[71] McDuff DR. Adjustment and anxiety disorders. In: Currie A, Owen B, editors. Sports psychiatry. Oxford, United Kingdom: Oxford University Press; 2016. p. 1–16.

[72] Gouttebarge V, Bindra A, Blauwet C, et al. International Olympic Committee (IOC) Sport Mental Health Assessment Tool 1 (SMHAT-1) and Sport Mental Health Recognition Tool 1 (SMHRT-1): towards better support of athletes' mental health. Br J Sports Med 2020;55(1):30–7.

[73] Smith RE, Smoll FL, Cumming SP, et al. Measurement of multidimensional sport performance anxiety in children and adults: the Sport Anxiety Scale-2. J Sport Exerc Psychol 2006;28(4):479–501.

[74] Locke AB, Kirst N, Shultz C. Diagnosis and management of generalized anxiety disorder and panic disorder in adults. Am Fam Phys 2015;91(9):617–24.

[75] Fisk MZ, Steigerwald MD, Smoliga JM, et al. Asthma in swimmers: a review of the current literature. Phys Sportsmed 2010;38(4):28–34.

[76] World anti-doping agency prohibited list, 2021. In: World Anti-Doping Agency (WADA). Available at: https://www.wada-ama.org/sites/default/files/resources/files/2021list_en.pdf. Accessed November 9, 2020.

[77] Pickering C, Kiely J. What should we do about habitual caffeine use in athletes? Sports Med 2019;49(6):833–42.

[78] Reardon CL. Psychiatric manifestations of sport-related concussion. Curr Psychiatr 2020;19(7):22–8.

[79] Brun JF, Dumortier M, Fedou C, et al. Exercise hypoglycemia in nondiabetic subjects. Diabetes Metab 2001; 27(2 Pt 1):92–106.

[80] Luksch J, Collins PB. Thyroid disorders in athletes. Curr Sports Med Rep 2018;17(2):59–64.

[81] Wilson JJ, Wilson EM. Practical management: vocal cord dysfunction in athletes. Clin J Sport Med 2006;16(4): 357–60.

[82] Stillman MA, Glick ID, McDuff D, et al. Psychotherapy for mental health symptoms and disorders in elite athletes: a narrative review. Br J Sports Med 2019;53(12):767–71.

[83] Castaldelli-Maia JM, de Mello e Gallinaro JG, Falcao RS, et al. Mental health symptoms and disorders in elite athletes: a systematic review on cultural influences and barriers to athletes seeking treatment. Br J Sports Med 2019; 53:707–21.

[84] Burns L, Weissensteiner JR, Cohen M. Lifestyles and mindsets of Olympic, Paralympic and world champions: is an integrated approach the key to elite performance? Br J Sports Med 2018;53(13):818–24.

[85] Hofmann SG, Gomez AF. Mindfulness-based interventions for anxiety and depression. Psychiatr Clin North Am 2017;40(4):739–49.

[86] Moreton A, Wahesh E, Schmidt CD. Indirect effect of mindfulness on psychological distress via sleep hygiene in division I college student athletes. J Am Coll Health 2020;1–5.

[87] Reardon CL, Factor RM. Sport psychiatry: a systematic review of diagnosis and medical treatment of mental illness in athletes. Sports Med 2010;40:961–80.

[88] Reardon CL, Creado S. Psychiatric medication preferences of sports psychiatrists. Physicians Sportsmed 2016;44(4):397–402.

[89] Parise G, Bosman MJ, Boecker DR, et al. Selective serotonin reuptake inhibitors: their effect on high-intensity exercise performance. Arch Phys Med Rehabil 2001;82: 867–71.

[90] Meeusen R, Piacentini M, Van Den Eynde S, et al. Exercise performance is not influenced by a 5-HT reuptake inhibitor. Int J Sports Med 2001;22:329–36.

[91] Marvanova M, Gramith K. Role of antidepressants in the treatment of adults with anorexia nervosa. Ment Health Clin 2018;8(3):127–37.

[92] Marvin G, Sharma A, Aston W, et al. The effects of buspirone on perceived exertion and time to fatigue in man. Exp Physiol 1997;82:1057–60.

[93] Johnston A, McAllister-Williams RH. Psychotropic drug prescribing. In: Currie A, Owen B, editors. Sports psychiatry. Oxford: Oxford University Press; 2016. p. 133–43.

[94] Paul MA, Gray G, Kenny G, et al. Impact of melatonin, zaleplon, zopiclone, and temazepam on psychomotor performance. Aviat Space Environ Med 2003;74: 1263–70.

[95] Charles RB, Kirkham AJ, Guyatt AR, et al. Psychomotor, pulmonary and exercise responses to sleep medication. Br J Clin Pharmacol 1987;24:191–7.

[96] Cowan DA, abuse D, Harries M, et al. Oxford textbook of sports medicine. New York: Oxford University Press; 1994. p. 314–29.

[97] Lachenmeier DW, Diel P. A warning against the negligent use of cannabidiol in professional and amateur athletes. Sports (Basel) 2019;7(12):251.

Neurosciences

Advances in Psychiatry and Behavioral Health 1 (2021) 161–172

ADVANCES IN PSYCHIATRY AND BEHAVIORAL HEALTH

Neuropsychiatric Manifestations of COVID-19

A Review

Moein Foroughi, MD[a,1], Rishab Gupta, MD[b], Amvrine Ganguly, MD[a], Junaid Mirza, MD[a], Aryandokht Fotros, MD[c,*,1]

[a]Department of Psychiatry and Behavioral Sciences, SUNY Downstate Health Sciences University, 450 Clarkson Avenue, Brooklyn, NY 11203, USA; [b]Department of Psychiatry, Brigham and Women's Hospital, Harvard Medical School, 75 Francis Street, Boston, MA 02115, USA; [c]Department of Psychiatry and Human Behavior, Brown University, Providence, RI, USA

KEYWORDS

• COVID-19 • SARS-CoV-2 • Neuropsychiatry • Psychiatry • Review

KEY POINTS

- COVID-19 is associated with increased manifestation of neuropsychiatric symptoms.
- The presence of neuropsychiatric symptoms may worsen prognosis in COVID-19 infection.
- Screening for neuropsychiatric symptoms in patients with COVID-19 will help with early identification and management of these symptoms and may improve patient outcome.

INTRODUCTION

A pandemic, as defined by the World Health Organization [1], is an epidemic occurring worldwide, or over a very wide area, crossing international boundaries and usually affecting a large number of people. Presently, the COVID-19 pandemic is raging through the USA, and as time is progressing, the larger undercurrent of neuropsychiatric ailments and disorders is making its presence felt. At the time of writing this paper, in the last week of November 2020, 1 year after the detection of the first case of COVID-19 in Wuhan, China, there have been over 57.8 million cases and 1.3 million deaths worldwide [2]. Most patients with COVID-19 present initially with fever (83%–99%), cough (59%–82%), fatigue (44%–70%), anorexia (40%–84%), and shortness of breath (31%–40%) [3]. However, the signs and symptoms present at the illness onset may vary widely and involve various organ systems. Recent literature is beginning to shed light on the impact of COVID-19 on the nervous system and its neuropsychiatric sequelae.

Studies describing the association between COVID-19 and neuropsychiatric symptoms are limited. Large-scale cohort studies are currently not available in the extant literature. A recent study assessing the potential relationship between COVID-19 and psychiatric disorders found a reciprocal relationship between the two [4]. This study included 62,354 patients diagnosed with COVID-19 with the primary outcomes being the incidence and hazard ratios for psychiatric disorders, dementia, and insomnia during the first 14 to 90 days after a diagnosis of COVID-19 was established. The authors observed that the patients recovering from COVID-19 had a significantly higher rate of psychiatric disorders.

[1] These authors contributed equally to this work.

*Corresponding author. 593 Eddy Street, Potter Building 2, Providence, RI 02903. *E-mail address:* Fotros@brown.edu

https://doi.org/10.1016/j.ypsc.2021.05.003
2667-3827/21/

There was a 5.8% probability of being newly diagnosed with a psychiatric illness within 90 days post COVID-19 diagnosis. The most frequently acquired psychiatric diagnosis was anxiety disorder, with a probability of outcome within 90 days of 4.7%. Among anxiety disorders, adjustment disorder, generalized anxiety disorder (GAD), posttraumatic stress disorder (PTSD), and panic disorder were the most frequent. The probability of a new diagnosis of mood disorder within 14 to 90 days after COVID-19 diagnosis was 2%. Interestingly, previous psychiatric illness was found to be independently associated with an increased risk of being diagnosed with COVID-19. A diagnosis of a psychiatric disorder 1 year prior to the onset of the COVID-19 pandemic was associated with a 65% increased risk of COVID-19 compared with a cohort matched for established physical risk factors for COVID-19, but without a psychiatric diagnosis. This finding held ground in sensitivity analyses.

In this article, we will review and discuss the existing evidence regarding various neuropsychiatric manifestations of COVID-19, including delirium, cognitive impairment, psychosis, depression, suicide, mania, and anxiety in patients with COVID-19 and COVID-19 survivors. We will also discuss the neurobiological mechanisms that are hypothesized to be involved in developing neuropsychiatric symptoms. Furthermore, we will discuss the potential role of medications used for treatment of COVID-19 in causing/worsening neuropsychiatric symptoms. Lastly, we will review the psychosocial factors contributing to the psychiatric presentations of infected individuals considering how important psychosocial factors are in the occurrence of primary psychiatric disorders.

METHODS

We performed a comprehensive search on PubMed and Google Scholar to find all relevant publications on COVID-19 and various neuropsychiatric disorders for this review which were available until November 30, 2020. We used the following keywords for our search: COVID-19 or SARS-CoV-2 and survivors, neuropsychiatry, psychiatry, psychosis, delusion, hallucination, anxiety, mood, depression, suicide, mania, delirium, and cognition. We focused primarily on the studies that described neuropsychiatric symptoms among COVID-19 survivors, as well as patients with active COVID-19 infection.

COVID-19 AND DELIRIUM

Compared to patients with delirium secondary to other comorbid conditions, delirium in COVID-19 patients has been reported with higher frequency, higher mortality, worse agitation, and a greater likelihood of presenting with specific features, such as catatonia [5]. The incidence of delirium in COVID-19 patients has been reported to be 30% to 50% in various studies [6–9]. One in five patients who died of COVID-19 suffered from encephalopathy [10]. The mortality rate in COVID-19 patients who experienced delirium has been reported to be as high as 55% in comparison to 30% in nondelirious patients [8]. In a study by Garcez and colleagues [8], delirium was determined using the Chart-based Delirium Identification Instrument (CHART-DEL) and it was found to be an independent predictor of in-hospital death. In a case series from Massachusetts General Hospital, the authors reported that in addition to the typical features of delirium, patients displayed significant agitation, increased tone or rigidity, abulia, alogia, and evidence of significant systemic inflammatory response [5]. In a case series from France, out of 58 COVID-19 patients admitted to ICU, 26 scored positive on the Confusion Assessment Method for the Intensive Care Unit (CAM-ICU) scale. Agitation, corticospinal tract signs, and dysexecutive syndrome were seen in 40, 39, and 14 patients, respectively [7]. Diagnostic accuracy in most of these studies appears to be limited as most used retrospective chart reviews for delirium diagnosis or relied on self-report questionnaires from the patients [9].

Delirium and mental status changes in patients with COVID-19 could be due to involvement of various pathways: primary central nervous system (CNS) invasion, secondary to hypoxemia and oxidative stress, or a combination of both. Regarding primary CNS invasion, there are reported cases of encephalitis in patients with COVID-19 with positive cerebrospinal fluid (CSF) PCR, and one reported specific MRI findings [11–13]. The underlying mechanism in these cases could be similar to the pathophysiology of herpes simplex virus (HSV) encephalitis, where the virus spreads via a synapse-connected route to the medullary cardiorespiratory center from the mechanoreceptors and chemoreceptors in the lungs and lower respiratory airways [14]. It is noteworthy that the presence of the SARS-CoV-2 virus in CSF is not required for the occurrence of delirium or encephalitis [7,15]. The other possible mechanism for direct invasion of CNS is via invasion of the olfactory bulb. This hypothesis is based on the observation that patients with COVID-19 have high rates of anosmia and ageusia. It is reported that more than 85% of patients may report anosmia [16]. Delirium could also occur secondary to a systemic response to acute infection, similar to other acute infectious and metabolic diseases. Hypoxemia, oxidative stress, hypoperfusion, uremia, and acute respiratory distress syndrome (ARDS) that occur in hospitalized patients with COVID-19 are known causes of delirium. Acute full-blown inflammatory response and cytokine storm could be another possible mechanism to explain the high rate of delirium in this population. A combination of both primary and secondary CNS involvement could also occur, similar to encephalopathy due to HIV [5].

Delirium is highly comorbid in patients with COVID-19 and is a significant prognostic factor for poorer outcomes and increased mortality. The risk factors associated with increased rates of delirium in COVID-19 patients and increased risk of death in these patients are not fully understood yet. Some suggest that guidelines for assessment of COVID-19 should include delirium as a presenting feature and its screening should be the standard of care [17].

COVID-19 AND COGNITIVE DEFICITS

In addition to increased risk of altered mental status and delirium, there is some evidence supporting COVID-19's impact on cognitive functioning. This effect has been shown in patients with no prior cognitive impairment, as well as in those with a history of dementia. In their prospective study of 58 patients with COVID-19, Raman and colleagues reported impaired cognitive performance, specifically in the executive and visuospatial domains, relative to controls [18].

Results from previous studies investigating long-term neuropsychological outcomes in patients with medical conditions requiring ventilation indicated declines in several domains of cognitive function. Impairment was shown in memory, verbal fluency, processing speed, and executive functioning. These impairments were noted in 78% of patients, 1 year after discharge, and in around half of the patients, up to 2 years [19–21]. Another study reported memory problems persisting up to 5 years after ARDS, and significantly impacting daily functioning [22]. Moreover, previous studies of sepsis and pneumonia found that mild cognitive impairment and dementia were common in survivors, regardless of infection severity. Given the similarity of acute manifestations of severe COVID-19 and sepsis in general, survivors of severe COVID-19 are anticipated to experience similar cognitive sequelae to sepsis survivors [23].

A small case-control study investigating cognitive impairments in COVID-19 survivors posthospitalization noted cognitive impairment in the domain of sustained attention in the individuals who had recovered from COVID-19 [24]. However, it was not clear to us whether the study patients had severe illness or not. Additionally, the authors did not use a comprehensive neuropsychological test battery and cognitive deficits in other domains might have been missed.

The mechanisms underlying cognitive impairment in COVID-19 are yet to be investigated. Some speculations include direct damage of COVID-19 to the hippocampus [25], postintensive care syndrome [26], and increased risk of cognitive impairment due to delirium and systemic disease [27]. Raman and colleagues noted tissue changes in thalamus, posterior thalamic radiations, and sagittal stratum on the brain MRIs of patients with COVID-19 who showed impairment in their cognitive functioning [18].

Patients with dementia are more vulnerable to SARS-CoV2 infection and are more likely to have severe disease compared to other individuals [28]. This is mostly due to the shared risk factors of the two diseases, including age, obesity, cardiovascular disease, hypertension, smoking, and diabetes mellitus [29]. COVID-19 can also potentially lead to more severe cognitive impairment in elderly patients, individuals with a history of cognitive impairment, or other comorbid conditions [28].

Overall, the identification of at-risk populations, monitoring of cognitive function for both at-risk and general populations, and study of persistent cognitive impairment and long-term cognitive functioning in patients with COVID-19 appear to be important aspects of addressing neuropsychiatric manifestations of COVID-19.

COVID-19 AND PSYCHOSIS

There are currently few reports of new-onset psychosis in patients with COVID-19 infection. This could likely be explained by two main hypotheses of direct pathophysiological mechanisms and the effect of psychological stressors [30]. A UK study investigating neuropsychiatric symptoms in a COVID-19 database reported new-onset psychosis. In this study, 23 out of 125 patients fulfilled the clinical case definition for psychiatric diagnoses. It was noted that 10 (43%) out of 23 patients with neuropsychiatric disorders had new-onset psychosis [31]. However, such a high prevalence of psychosis was not replicated in other studies, though there have been case reports and case series published on this. One case series reported three COVID-19 patients who presented with new-onset psychotic symptoms but were otherwise asymptomatic [32]. There are also several case reports of COVID-19 patients who presented initially with psychotic symptoms. These include case reports of patients with SARS-CoV-2-positive test results and no prior psychiatric history who presented with psychosis [33], a COVID-19 patient who presented with command auditory hallucinations [34], and a case report of exacerbated paranoia in a COVID-19 patient with a history of schizophrenia [35].

Neuroinflammatory processes are one of the possible mechanisms of action proposed for inducing psychosis with coronavirus. In a recent rapid review, the authors concluded that exposure to SARS, H1N1, MERS, and coronavirus immune reactivity were associated with recent psychosis [36]. Prior to the current pandemic, some studies suggested infection with certain coronaviruses is associated with recent-onset psychotic symptoms [37,38]. The interaction between psychosis and COVID-19 may be further complicated by the treatment of COVID-19 with high doses of steroids to modulate the inflammatory response since steroids are known to trigger psychotic symptoms [39,40].

In summary, the relationship between COVID-19 and psychosis is not yet established. Most of the available evidence has been gathered through individual case reports and case series. Large-scale systematic studies are needed to elaborate on the relationship between the two.

COVID-19 AND DEPRESSION

COVID-19 has been found to be associated with increased rates of depression in the general population [41], and especially in COVID-19 survivors [42]. Studies of COVID-19 survivors found the prevalence of depression to be 31% to 43% [42–44]. However, in all those studies, depression was assessed using self-rated questionnaires, and not by clinical interview, the gold-standard for diagnosing major depression.

A few studies have attempted to understand the biological mechanisms underlying depressive symptoms in patients with COVID-19. Among these is a study of 402 adult patients who were tested for several inflammatory markers during an ED visit for COVID-19-related systemic or respiratory symptoms, and evaluated various psychiatric disorders after 1-month follow-up in those who were diagnosed with COVID-19 [42]. The inflammatory markers assessed were C-reactive protein (CRP), neutrophil/lymphocyte ratio, monocyte/lymphocyte ratio, and Systemic Immune-inflammation Index (SII). The majority of these patients were hospitalized due to clinical deterioration. No correlation was seen between inflammatory markers and depression, except for a positive association between baseline SII and depression. The SII highlights the balance between systemic inflammation and immune response. It is a ratio reflecting product from platelets, neutrophils, and lymphocytes, which are all involved in various immune/inflammatory response pathways [45]. In one study, higher SII levels were associated with major depressive disorder (MDD) [46]. Another study [47] compared total and differential WBC counts, neutrophil ratio, lymphocyte ratio, monocyte ratio, eosinophil ratio, basophilic granulocyte ratio, neutrophil-to-lymphocyte ratio (NLR), CRP, and IL-6 between cured COVID-19 patients with and without self-reported depression. They found that WBC count, neutrophil count, NLR, and CRP levels were higher in the self-reported depression group than in the normal group. In a study by Guo and colleagues, no association was seen between depressive symptoms and inflammatory indicators among the entire COVID-19 patient group [48]. However, in this study the patients had mild illness, the inflammatory markers measured were different from the study by Mazza and colleagues [42], and a control group was also used for comparison. This study measured CRP and other inflammatory markers (mainly different white blood cell counts). One interesting finding was that the depressive symptoms were more severe than anxiety symptoms in patients with COVID-19. Among those patients with baseline depressive symptoms (self-reported Patient Health Questionnaire-9 (PHQ-9) score greater than 4), CRP levels positively correlated with PHQ-9 scores. The change of CRP level from baseline negatively correlated with the PHQ-9 score, suggesting that the improved CRP level may have resulted in less depressive symptoms.

It can be safely concluded that more studies are required to elucidate the biological mechanism of the occurrence of depression in COVID-19 patients. There is a possibility that systemic inflammation may be mediating depressive symptoms. This has been noted in previous studies linking inflammation and depression. However, there is no consensus till date regarding which biomarker predicts the occurrence of depression and its severity.

COVID-19 AND SUICIDE

Both clinicians and researchers have anticipated that COVID-19 may lead to an increase in suicidal ideation and suicide attempts. This concern stems from the studies conducted during previous pandemics and infectious disease-related public health emergencies. A systematic review indicated increased suicide rates among older adults during the SARS outbreak, in the year following the epidemic, and associations between SARS/Ebola exposure and increased suicide attempts [49].

Various psychosocial complications pertaining to COVID-19 may serve to increase the risk of suicide among the general population and patients. For example, lockdowns and social distancing leading to isolation and feelings of loneliness, rising rates of depression, anxiety, substance use, domestic violence, limited access to health services, worsening of physical illnesses, and the trauma of losing family and friends are likely significant factors. Misconceptions, fear, stigma related to COVID-19, as well as financial hardship due to loss of employment may also play a role in increasing the risk of suicide [50]. A recent survey from the Centers for Disease Control and Prevention indicated more than a twofold increase in suicidal ideation of responders in June 2020 compared to a similar survey in 2018. In this survey, 10.7% of 5412 adults reported serious consideration of suicide in the previous 30 days, whereas the 2018 survey reports 4.3% of 10.7 million adults with serious suicidal ideation in the previous 12 months [51]. However, it remains to be seen whether COVID-19 has actually led to an increased number of suicides. Studies that have been conducted to date in Australia [52] and the USA [53] have not yet reported an increase in the number of suicides or suicidal behavior during the COVID-19 pandemic. Similarly, a recent systematic review by John and colleagues [54] did not show an increase in suicide rate or suicidal behavior during the COVID-19 pandemic. Two case reports from India and Bangladesh described two patients who died by suicide and mentioned COVID-19-related stigma as the key driver of the suicides [55,56]. Currently there are no studies which have systematically assessed the risk of suicide in COVID-19 survivors. A meta-analysis of the studies investigating various psychiatric disorders in COVID-19 survivors did not find suicide as its complication/manifestation [57].

So far, no study has evaluated any direct biological mechanism behind suicide risk in those with COVID-19 infection. Considering the tremendous impact of COVID-19 on the global population, it may be too early to conclude that COVID-19 does not increase the risk of suicide. More studies are needed to understand the immediate- and long-term risk of self-harm behavior in patients with COVID-19 and those suffering from its psychosocial impact.

COVID-19 AND MANIA

Numerous studies have linked COVID-19 to depression, whereas the data on mania occurring in COVID-19 patients are scarce. Only a few reports [33,58,59] are available in the literature describing mania after COVID-19 infection. Interestingly, in all those cases, mania occurred for the first time in their lives, and they had very few to none of the risk factors associated with mania. Furthermore, the participants in the study were in the age range of 30s–50s, which is not typical for first-episode mania. One common thread that tied all the cases was the appearance of manic symptoms concurrent with ongoing COVID-19 symptoms.

The neurobiological processes underlying manic symptoms in patients with COVID-19 are unknown. Future studies should carefully survey the occurrence of manic symptoms during COVID-19 infection and in the follow-up period to see if there is a true association between the two disorders.

COVID-19 AND ANXIETY

COVID-19 may increase anxiety symptoms and anxiety disorders in both COVID-19 patients and the general population [41,60,61]. It has also been demonstrated that non-COVID-19 subjects with a preexisting anxiety disorder were more negatively impacted by COVID-19, compared to those with no history of mental illness [62]. A cross-sectional study assessing 402 adults who survived COVID-19 found the prevalence of PTSD, anxiety, and obsessive-compulsive symptoms in 28%, 42%, and 20% of the subjects, respectively [42]. In another study from China, Bo and colleagues reported a significantly high rate of posttraumatic stress symptoms among hospitalized patients. They reported that 96.2% of 714 hospitalized patients with COVID-19 scored higher than the threshold value on the posttraumatic stress disorder checklist-civilian version (PCL-CV) [63].

An increase in anxiety and related disorders may occur through the devastating psychosocial effects of the pandemic and affect various subgroups. These effects are discussed later in this review. However, it is important to note a higher likelihood of the occurrence of PTSD, GAD, panic disorder, and obsessive-compulsive disorder, both as new-onset disorders in vulnerable populations and exacerbation of these disorders among those who already carry these diagnoses. A recent systematic review by Pappa and colleagues showed a higher prevalence of anxiety disorders in healthcare workers [64].

The neurobiological mechanisms underlying an increase in anxiety symptoms in patients with COVID-19 remain to be explored. It has been hypothesized that anxiety in patients with COVID-19 could be due to primary CNS invasion impacting neural circuits related to anxiety, hypoxemia, and oxidative stress, or a combination [42]. In a study by Mazza and colleagues [42], the authors noted that PTSD, anxiety, and obsessive-compulsive symptoms were not associated with oxygen saturation level or inflammatory markers, but were correlated with baseline SII. The SII was also positively associated with anxiety scores at follow-up. However, further studies are needed to investigate infection-triggered changes in the immune system that may also induce anxiety disorders.

PROPOSED NEUROBIOLOGICAL MECHANISMS

The COVID-19 pandemic is novel in its protean manifestation, including the neuropsychiatric ones. Several mechanisms have been proposed for neurotropism of this virus and resultant clinical presentations [65]. Various mechanisms have been proposed for the CNS affliction of SARS-CoV-2, including direct viral invasion, cytokine storm, molecular mimicry, and through systemic illness.

Direct viral injury to the neurons may occur akin to the herpes simplex virus encephalitis. SARS-CoV-2 binds to angiotensin-converting enzyme 2 (ACE2) receptors. These receptors, although highly expressed in epithelial cells of the respiratory and digestive systems, are also expressed in neurons and glial cells in the CNS. These receptors are also highly expressed in endothelial cells, which may serve as a route of entry into the CNS [66].

Cytokine storm may lead to acute or subacute CNS involvement, including encephalopathy. Cytokine storm is a hyperactive immune response characterized by a rapid release of inflammatory mediators [67]. Several studies suggest an association between chronic neuroinflammation and high levels of cytokines and chemokines is involved in the pathogenesis of neurodegenerative diseases such as multiple sclerosis, Parkinson's disease, and Alzheimer's disease [68]. Neuroinflammation has also been found to play a role in the pathogenesis of psychiatric diseases, including mood disorders, schizophrenia spectrum disorders, and substance use disorders, especially alcohol use disorder [69]. Proinflammatory cytokine dysregulation can induce changes in neurotransmitter metabolism, cause hypothalamic–pituitary–adrenal axis dysregulation, or alter neuroplasticity [70].

Molecular mimicry may lead to bystander effect, such as in the case of Guillain–Barré syndrome [71]. In susceptible individuals, an aberrant immune response may cross-react with both viral antigens and self-antigens [72].

Systemic illness leading to CNS manifestations may also be contributory. For example, peripheral myeloid cells infected by SARS-CoV-2 may subsequently transmigrate to CNS under conditions of increased blood–brain barrier permeability due to inflammation and psychological stress [73].

NEUROPSYCHIATRIC ADVERSE EFFECTS OF MEDICATIONS USED TO TREAT COVID-19

Neuropsychiatric complications can potentially occur as adverse effects of COVID-19 treatment agents. The mechanistic details underlying these complications are largely unknown, and it is often difficult to determine causality. In this section, we will review the evidence regarding the neuropsychiatric side effects of currently used treatment agents for COVID-19.

As of November 2020, the FDA had approved only one drug, remdesivir, for the treatment or prevention of COVID-19, and had authorized the use of a few unapproved drugs under Emergency Use Authorization (EUA). Chloroquine phosphate, hydroxychloroquine sulfate, and COVID-19 convalescent plasma are among the treatment agents that have been granted EUA for treatment of hospitalized patients with COVID-19 [74,75]. Other widely used investigational agents include steroids, IL-6 pathway inhibitors, such as tocilizumab, sarilumab and siltuximab, interferons, favipiravir, ivermectin, and azithromycin [76–78]. A recent study described the role of fluvoxamine, an antidepressant, in preventing serious illness among COVID-19 outpatients [79].

There are no reported major neuropsychiatric events associated with remdesivir to this date [80]. Remdesivir is a nucleotide analogue that blocks the virus replication. In the fact sheet issued by its makers, there is no report of known neuropsychiatric adverse effects in clinical trials [81]. In an open-label cohort of 61 patients diagnosed with COVID-19 and treated with remdesivir, delirium was reported in two patients [82]. However, the causality could not be determined since delirium could be induced by the viral infection itself, or other confounding factors. Other major studies did not report any neuropsychiatric complications induced by remdesivir. A large clinical trial of 532 subjects using remdesivir versus 516 control subjects reported 12 cases of delirium and altered mental status in the remdesivir group, compared to 12 cases in the control group [83]. The limited available data from other smaller studies do not indicate any major neuropsychiatric side effects associated with remdesivir [84]. However, this drug is still at the investigational stage and the possibility of any neuropsychiatric complications cannot be convincingly excluded.

Neuropsychiatric adverse effects of corticosteroids are common, with a relatively high incidence rate of 13% to 62% [85]. These are complex, unpredictable, and often severe, ranging across most categories of psychopathology, including psychotic, manic, or depressive episodes, or their admixture, cognitive deficits, and minor psychiatric disturbances (irritability, insomnia, anxiety, labile mood). These adverse effects are usually dose dependent. The timing of their appearance is unpredictable, and they could happen immediately after initiation or even after discontinuing treatment. Short-course, high-dose corticosteroid treatment, commonly used in the treatment of COVID-19 infection, may cause delirium and mood changes, with manic symptoms more frequently reported than depressive symptoms [86]. That being said, steroids have also been used to successfully treat COVID-19-associated encephalopathy [87].

There is some evidence concerning the neuropsychiatric side effects of hydroxychloroquine. Both hydroxychloroquine and chloroquine are antimalarial agents with antiinflammatory and immunomodulatory activity. They are known to have neuropsychiatric side effects, most notably, psychosis. Hospitalized patients with COVID-19 are more prone to their side effects, compared to patients with malaria. This increased vulnerability is likely associated with advanced age and possible medical comorbidities of hospitalized patients, such as hepatic and renal insufficiency, which alter the metabolism and clearance of these drugs. Hydroxychloroquine is more widely used, and at present more research is published on the treatment of COVID-19 with hydroxychloroquine, compared to chloroquine, mostly due to its favorable side effect profile [88]. Garcia and colleagues reviewed all psychiatric adverse effects with hydroxychloroquine in 1754 COVID-19 patients registered in VigiBase, the WHO's global database of individual case safety reports, among which they found 56 counts of psychiatric adverse effects. Half of these adverse effects were serious, including four completed suicides, three cases of intentional self-injury, and 12 cases of psychotic disorder with hallucinations. They also found that the use of hydroxychloroquine was associated with an increased risk of psychiatric disorders compared with remdesivir, tocilizumab, or lopinavir/ritonavir [89]. Moreover, chloroquine and hydroxychloroquine are mild inhibitors of CYP2D6, and have potential interactions with numerous psychotropic medications.

Tocilizumab's neuropsychiatric effects have not been widely studied in the context of COVID-19 treatment. It is a recombinant humanized monoclonal antibody that is used for treating rheumatoid arthritis. It blocks the IL-6 pathway, which could contribute to reducing the inflammatory cascade secondary to cytokine storm seen in many patients with COVID-19 infection. Currently, there is no evidence of induced or increased psychiatric symptoms in patients treated with tocilizumab [90,91]. On the contrary, it has been shown that tocilizumab might have a positive effect on cognition, when used as an adjunctive agent for the treatment of schizophrenia [92].

PSYCHOSOCIAL FACTORS ASSOCIATED WITH COVID-19 AS RISK FACTORS FOR NEUROPSYCHIATRIC DISORDERS

The psychosocial complications associated with COVID-19 are wide ranging, from emotional factors such as loss of loved ones to increased financial burden, while the usual coping and support systems are severely compromised [93]. It is still early for any large-scale study to show how various countries tackling the pandemic are coming up with different and often shifting guidelines [94]. Box 1 lists various psychosocial factors associated with COVID-19 which may increase the risk of psychiatric disorders.

DISCUSSION

The evidence for the increased occurrence of various neuropsychiatric disorders due to COVID-19 infection is still limited but is accumulating with time. Keeping that in mind and based on our knowledge gathered from the studies carried out in the context of previous pandemics and infectious outbreaks, we must anticipate and screen for various neuropsychiatric symptoms among those who carry a diagnosis of COVID-19. Moreover, it is worthwhile remembering that individuals with preexisting neuropsychiatric disorders are more vulnerable to this infection and are likely to experience a more severe course of the disease.

In 1918, during the Spanish flu pandemic, Karl Menninger presented 80 patients with "mental disturbances"

BOX 1
Psychosocial Factors Associated with COVID-19

PTSD/trauma from morbid hospitalization/ICU stay/medical procedures
Experiencing a near-death situation due to COVID-19
Experiencing/witnessing death/morbidity in other family members/friends/colleagues who also suffered from COVID-19
Societal/perceived stigma/isolation (due to quarantine or some other reasons) experienced by patients with COVID-19
Loss of employment due to contracting COVID-19
Grave injuries while self-treating COVID-19, leading to morbidity
Discontinuing (intentional or due to nonavailability of doctors) previous psychiatric/medical treatments leading to recurrence/relapse of preexistent psychiatric disorders
Stress of COVID-19 leading to exacerbation/relapse of preexisting psychiatric disorder

that he associated with influenza. Of those, 16 had delirium, 25 had dementia praecox, 23 had other types of psychosis, and the remaining 16 were unclassified. In his follow-up study, carried out over a period of 5 years, most patients with dementia praecox improved [95]. Similarly, the HIV pandemic is well known to have a significant effect on the brain [96] and is associated with a host of neurologic and psychiatric disorders. From time to time, several virological illnesses with a relatively small area of spread have been shown to cause neuropsychiatric symptoms. Most of these viruses, if not all, are encephalopathic and neurotropic. Examples include West Nile virus, enterovirus 71, Chikungunya, and Nipah [97–99]. Though lethal in their presentation, their effect is offset by limited geographic presence and variable modes of transmission.

Before the COVID-19 pandemic, coronaviruses caused two noteworthy outbreaks: severe acute respiratory syndrome (SARS) in 2002, and Middle East respiratory syndrome (MERS) in 2012. A systematic review and meta-analysis reported the neuropsychiatric presentations of individuals with suspected or laboratory-confirmed coronavirus infection (SARS coronavirus, MERS coronavirus, or SARS coronavirus) [57]. One study reported psychosis in 13 (0.7%) of the 1744 patients with SARS in the acute stage of the disease [100]. Therefore, it is not surprising that our review also indicates possible increased risk of delirium, cognitive impairment, psychosis, anxiety, and mood symptoms in patients with COVID-19.

Some of the strengths of our paper are its timeliness and our focus on elucidation of biological mechanisms underlying neuropsychiatric symptoms due to COVID-19, compared to most other review papers which conflated psychiatric disorders among those at risk of COVID-19 and those who actually got infected with COVID-19. However, this paper should by no means be considered comprehensive in this area. There are several noteworthy limitations to our study. We omitted all non-English language papers, and our search strategy was limited to the two most widely used search engines.

During this acute phase of the pandemic, mental health professionals are facing unique challenges including caring for patients with serious mental illness and COVID-19 infection [101–103], preventing infection spread in acute psychiatric units, and providing emergency mental health services. In the outpatient world, the practice of psychiatry has transformed over weeks, if not months [104]. Telepsychiatry, which used to account for a small portion of psychiatric services [105], has now become a new norm. A similar transition to telemedicine is also underway for consultation-liaison services [106], and even for emergency psychiatry and inpatient psychiatry units.

The wave of deaths precipitated by COVID-19, its traumatic aftermath, coupled with numerous psychological complications has the potential to change the praxis of psychiatry. In order to serve the needs of our patients and of society, psychiatrists and researchers will need to remain nimble, forward-thinking, and ready to adapt to new situations. Like other medical disciplines, psychiatry will continue to contribute to the constant endeavor of betterment of mankind.

To conclude, there remains a huge knowledge gap in the field of neuropsychiatric disorder and COVID-19, and further studies are required to clearly understand the epidemiology of various psychiatric disorders associated with COVID-19. Additionally, the studies on the etiopathogenesis of those disorders may shed light on their treatments and also help take psychiatric research forward in the process. We remain hopeful of the ability of our profession to help protect humanity from the dangerous impact of COVID-19.

DISCLOSURE

The authors report no commercial or financial conflicts of interest. No funding source was used for writing this article.

REFERENCES

[1] Kelly H. The classical definition of a pandemic is not elusive. Bull World Health Organ 2011;89:540–1.

[2] Home. Johns Hopkins Coronavirus Resource Center. Available at: https://coronavirus.jhu.edu/. Accessed December 4, 2020.

[3] Cennimo DJ, Bergman JS, Olsen KM. Coronavirus Disease 2019 (COVID-19): Practice Essentials, Background, Route of Transmission. In: Bronze MS. ed. Medscape. Available at: https://emedicine.medscape.com/article/2500114-overview. Accessed December 4, 2020.

[4] Taquet M, Luciano S, Geddes JR, et al. Bidirectional associations between COVID-19 and psychiatric disorder: retrospective cohort studies of 62 354 COVID-19 cases in the USA. Lancet Psychiatry 2020. https://doi.org/10.1016/S2215-0366(20)30462-4.

[5] Beach SR, Praschan NC, Hogan C, et al. Delirium in COVID-19: A case series and exploration of potential mechanisms for central nervous system involvement. Gen Hosp Psychiatry 2020;65:47–53.

[6] Mao L, Jin H, Wang M, et al. Neurologic Manifestations of Hospitalized Patients With Coronavirus Disease 2019 in Wuhan, China. JAMA Neurol 2020;77(6):683–90.

[7] Helms J, Kremer S, Merdji H, et al. Neurologic Features in Severe SARS-CoV-2 Infection. N Engl J Med 2020; 382(23):2268–70.

[8] Garcez FB, Aliberti MJ, Poco PC, et al. Delirium and adverse outcomes in hospitalized patients with COVID-19. J Am Geriatr Soc 2020;68(11):2440–6.

[9] Zazzara MB, Penfold RS, Roberts AL, et al. Probable delirium is a presenting symptom of COVID-19 in frail, older adults: a cohort study of 322 hospitalized and 535 community-based older adults. Age Ageing 2020. https://doi.org/10.1093/ageing/afaa223.

[10] Chen T, Wu D, Chen H, et al. Clinical characteristics of 113 deceased patients with coronavirus disease 2019: retrospective study. BMJ 2020;368:m1091.

[11] Moriguchi T, Harii N, Goto J, et al. A first case of meningitis/encephalitis associated with SARS-Coronavirus-2. Int J Infect Dis 2020;94:55–8.

[12] Bernard-Valnet R, Pizzarotti B, Anichini A, et al. Two patients with acute meningoencephalitis concomitant with SARS-CoV-2 infection. Eur J Neurol 2020. https://doi.org/10.1111/ene.14298.

[13] Huang YH, Jiang D, Huang JT. SARS-CoV-2 Detected in Cerebrospinal Fluid by PCR in a Case of COVID-19 Encephalitis. Brain Behav Immun 2020;87:149.

[14] Li Y-C, Bai W-Z, Hashikawa T. The neuroinvasive potential of SARS-CoV2 may play a role in the respiratory failure of COVID-19 patients. J Med Virol 2020;92(6): 552–5.

[15] Al Saiegh F, Ghosh R, Leibold A, et al. Status of SARS-CoV-2 in cerebrospinal fluid of patients with COVID-19 and stroke. J Neurol Neurosurg Psychiatry 2020; 91(8):846–8.

[16] Lechien JR, Chiesa-Estomba CM, De Siati DR, et al. Olfactory and gustatory dysfunctions as a clinical presentation of mild-to-moderate forms of the coronavirus disease (COVID-19): a multicenter European study. Eur Arch Oto-rhino-laryngol 2020;277(8):2251–61.

[17] O'Hanlon S, Inouye SK. Delirium: a missing piece in the COVID-19 pandemic puzzle. Age Ageing 2020; 49(4):497–8.

[18] Raman B, Cassar MP, Tunnicliffe EM, et al. Medium-term effects of SARS-CoV-2 infection on multiple vital organs, exercise capacity, cognition, quality of life and mental health, post-hospital discharge. medRxiv 2020. https://doi.org/10.1101/2020.10.15.20205054.

[19] Hopkins RO, Weaver LK, Pope D, et al. Neuropsychological sequelae and impaired health status in survivors of severe acute respiratory distress syndrome. Am J Respir Crit Care Med 1999;160(1):50–6.

[20] Hopkins RO, Weaver LK, Collingridge D, et al. Two-year cognitive, emotional, and quality-of-life outcomes in acute respiratory distress syndrome. Am J Respir Crit Care Med 2005;171(4):340–7.

[21] Mikkelsen ME, Christie JD, Lanken PN, et al. The adult respiratory distress syndrome cognitive outcomes study: long-term neuropsychological function in survivors of acute lung injury. Am J Respir Crit Care Med 2012; 185(12):1307–15.

[22] Adhikari NKJ, Tansey CM, McAndrews MP, et al. Self-reported depressive symptoms and memory complaints in survivors five years after ARDS. Chest 2011;140(6): 1484–93.

[23] Prescott HC, Girard TD. Recovery From Severe COVID-19: Leveraging the Lessons of Survival From Sepsis. JAMA 2020;324(8):739–40.

[24] Zhou H, Lu S, Chen J, et al. The landscape of cognitive function in recovered COVID-19 patients. J Psychiatr Res 2020;129:98–102.

[25] Ritchie K, Chan D, Watermeyer T. The cognitive consequences of the COVID-19 epidemic: collateral damage? Brain Commun 2020. https://doi.org/10.1093/braincomms/fcaa069.

[26] Desai SV, Law TJ, Needham DM. Long-term complications of critical care. Crit Care Med 2011;39(2):371–9.

[27] Korupolu R, Francisco GE, Levin H, et al. Rehabilitation of critically Ill COVID-19 survivors. J Int Soc Phys Rehabil Med 2020;3(2):45–52.

[28] Ibanez A, Kosik KS. Latin America and the Caribbean Consortium on Dementia (LAC-CD). COVID-19 in older people with cognitive impairment in Latin America. Lancet Neurol 2020;19(9):719–21.

[29] Korczyn AD. Dementia in the COVID-19 Period. J Alzheimers Dis 2020;75(4):1071–2.

[30] Fusar-Poli P, McGorry PD, Kane JM. Improving outcomes of first-episode psychosis: an overview. World Psychiatry 2017;16(3):251–65.
[31] Varatharaj A, Thomas N, Ellul MA, et al. Neurological and neuropsychiatric complications of COVID-19 in 153 patients: a UK-wide surveillance study. Lancet Psychiatry 2020;7(10):875–82.
[32] Ferrando SJ, Klepacz L, Lynch S, et al. COVID-19 Psychosis: A Potential New Neuropsychiatric Condition Triggered by Novel Coronavirus Infection and the Inflammatory Response? Psychosomatics 2020;61(5):551–5.
[33] Noone R, Cabassa JA, Gardner L, et al. Letter to the Editor: New onset psychosis and mania following COVID-19 infection. J Psychiatr Res 2020;130:177–9.
[34] Mirza J, Ganguly A, Ostrovskaya A, et al. Command Suicidal Hallucination as Initial Presentation of Coronavirus Disease 2019 (COVID-19): A Case Report. Psychosomatics 2020;61(5):561–4.
[35] Fischer M, Coogan AN, Faltraco F, et al. COVID-19 paranoia in a patient suffering from schizophrenic psychosis – a case report. Psychiatry Res 2020;288:113001.
[36] Brown E, Gray R, Lo Monaco S, et al. The potential impact of COVID-19 on psychosis: A rapid review of contemporary epidemic and pandemic research. Schizophr Res 2020;222:79–87.
[37] Severance EG, Dickerson FB, Viscidi RP, et al. Coronavirus immunoreactivity in individuals with a recent onset of psychotic symptoms. Schizophr Bull 2011;37(1):101–7.
[38] Troyer EA, Kohn JN, Hong S. Are we facing a crashing wave of neuropsychiatric sequelae of COVID-19? Neuropsychiatric symptoms and potential immunologic mechanisms. Brain Behav Immun 2020;87:34–9.
[39] Wada K, Yamada N, Sato T, et al. Corticosteroid-induced psychotic and mood disorders: diagnosis defined by DSM-IV and clinical pictures. Psychosomatics 2001;42(6):461–6.
[40] Russell CD, Millar JE, Baillie JK. Clinical evidence does not support corticosteroid treatment for 2019-nCoV lung injury. The Lancet 2020;395(10223):473–5.
[41] Salari N, Hosseinian-Far A, Jalali R, et al. Prevalence of stress, anxiety, depression among the general population during the COVID-19 pandemic: a systematic review and meta-analysis. Glob Health 2020;16. https://doi.org/10.1186/s12992-020-00589-w.
[42] Mazza MG, De Lorenzo R, Conte C, et al. Anxiety and depression in COVID-19 survivors: Role of inflammatory and clinical predictors. Brain Behav Immun 2020;89:594–600.
[43] Cai X, Hu X, Ekumi IO, et al. Psychological distress and its correlates among COVID-19 survivors during early convalescence across age groups. Am J Geriatr Psychiatry 2020;28(10):1030–9.
[44] Ma Y-F, Li W, Deng H-B, et al. Prevalence of depression and its association with quality of life in clinically stable patients with COVID-19. J Affect Disord 2020;275:145–8.
[45] Huang H, Liu Q, Zhu L, et al. Prognostic Value of Preoperative Systemic Immune-Inflammation Index in Patients with Cervical Cancer. Sci Rep 2019;9. https://doi.org/10.1038/s41598-019-39150-0.
[46] Zhou L, Ma X, Wang W. Inflammation and Coronary Heart Disease Risk in Patients with Depression in China Mainland: A Cross-Sectional Study. Neuropsychiatr Dis Treat 2020;16:81–6.
[47] Yuan B, Li W, Liu H, et al. Correlation between immune response and self-reported depression during convalescence from COVID-19. Brain Behav Immun 2020;88:39–43.
[48] Guo Q, Zheng Y, Shi J, et al. Immediate psychological distress in quarantined patients with COVID-19 and its association with peripheral inflammation: A mixed-method study. Brain Behav Immun 2020;88:17–27.
[49] Zortea TC, Brenna CTA, Joyce M, et al. The Impact of Infectious Disease-Related Public Health Emergencies on Suicide, Suicidal Behavior, and Suicidal Thoughts. Crisis 2020;1–14. https://doi.org/10.1027/0227-5910/a000753.
[50] Reger MA, Stanley IH, Joiner TE. Suicide Mortality and Coronavirus Disease 2019-A Perfect Storm? JAMA Psychiatry 2020. https://doi.org/10.1001/jamapsychiatry.2020.1060.
[51] Czeisler MÉ, Lane RI, Petrosky E, et al. Mental health, substance use, and suicidal ideation during the COVID-19 pandemic—United States, June 24–30, 2020. Morbidity Mortality Weekly Rep 2020;69(32):1049.
[52] Leske S, Kõlves K, Crompton D, et al. Real-time suicide mortality data from police reports in Queensland, Australia, during the COVID-19 pandemic: an interrupted time-series analysis. Lancet Psychiatry 2020;0(0). https://doi.org/10.1016/S2215-0366(20)30435-1.
[53] Bryan CJ, Bryan AO, Baker JC. Associations among state-level physical distancing measures and suicidal thoughts and behaviors among U.S. adults during the early COVID-19 pandemic. Suicide Life Threat Behav 2020. https://doi.org/10.1111/sltb.12653.
[54] John A, Okolie C, Eyles E, et al. The impact of the COVID-19 pandemic on self-harm and suicidal behaviour: a living systematic review. F1000Research. 2020;9:1097.
[55] Goyal K, Chauhan P, Chhikara K, et al. Fear of COVID 2019: First suicidal case in India ! Asian J Psychiatry 2020;49:101989.
[56] Mamun MA, Griffiths MD. First COVID-19 suicide case in Bangladesh due to fear of COVID-19 and xenophobia: Possible suicide prevention strategies. Asian J Psychiatry 2020;51:102073.
[57] Rogers JP, Chesney E, Oliver D, et al. Psychiatric and neuropsychiatric presentations associated with severe coronavirus infections: a systematic review and meta-

analysis with comparison to the COVID-19 pandemic. Lancet Psychiatry 2020;7(7):611–27.

[58] Mawhinney JA, Wilcock C, Haboubi H, et al. Neurotropism of SARS-CoV-2: COVID-19 presenting with an acute manic episode. BMJ Case Rep 2020;13(6): e236123.

[59] Lu S, Wei N, Jiang J, et al. First report of manic-like symptoms in a COVID-19 patient with no previous history of a psychiatric disorder. J Affect Disord 2020;277: 337–40.

[60] Lee SA, Mathis AA, Jobe MC, et al. Clinically significant fear and anxiety of COVID-19: A psychometric examination of the Coronavirus Anxiety Scale. Psychiatry Res 2020;290:113112.

[61] Shanafelt T, Ripp J, Trockel M. Understanding and addressing sources of anxiety among health care professionals during the COVID-19 pandemic. JAMA 2020; 323(21):2133–4.

[62] Asmundson GJG, Taylor S. How health anxiety influences responses to viral outbreaks like COVID-19: What all decision-makers, health authorities, and health care professionals need to know. J Anxiety Disord 2020;71:102211.

[63] Bo H-X, Li W, Yang Y, et al. Posttraumatic stress symptoms and attitude toward crisis mental health services among clinically stable patients with COVID-19 in China. Psychol Med 2020;1–2. https://doi.org/10.1017/S0033291720000999.

[64] Pappa S, Ntella V, Giannakas T, et al. Prevalence of depression, anxiety, and insomnia among healthcare workers during the COVID-19 pandemic: A systematic review and meta-analysis. Brain Behav Immun 2020; 88:901–7.

[65] Matías-Guiu J, Gomez-Pinedo U, Montero-Escribano P, et al. Should we expect neurological symptoms in the SARS-CoV-2 epidemic? Neurol Barc Spain 2020;35(3): 170–5.

[66] Desforges M, Le Coupanec A, Dubeau P, et al. Human coronaviruses and other respiratory viruses: underestimated opportunistic pathogens of the central nervous system? Viruses 2019;12(1):14.

[67] Sinha P, Matthay MA, Calfee CS. Is a "Cytokine Storm" Relevant to COVID-19? JAMA *Intern Med* 2020;180(9): 1152–4.

[68] Chen W-W, Zhang X, Huang W-J. Role of neuroinflammation in neurodegenerative diseases (Review). Mol Med Rep 2016;13(4):3391–6.

[69] Meyer JH, Cervenka S, Kim M-J, et al. Neuroinflammation in psychiatric disorders: PET imaging and promising new targets. Lancet Psychiatry 2020;7(12): 1064–74.

[70] Hong S, Banks WA. Role of the immune system in HIV-associated neuroinflammation and neurocognitive implications. Brain Behav Immun 2015;45:1–12.

[71] Berciano J. Axonal degeneration in Guillain-Barré syndrome: a reappraisal. J Neurol 2020. https://doi.org/10.1007/s00415-020-10034-y.

[72] Rose NR. Negative selection, epitope mimicry and autoimmunity. Curr Opin Immunol 2017;49:51–5.

[73] Wohleb ES, McKim DB, Sheridan JF, et al. Monocyte trafficking to the brain with stress and inflammation: a novel axis of immune-to-brain communication that influences mood and behavior. Front Neurosci 2014; 8:447.

[74] Commissioner O of the. COVID-19 Frequently Asked Questions. FDA. 2020. Available at: https://www.fda.gov/emergency-preparedness-and-response/coronavirus-disease-2019-covid-19/covid-19-frequently-asked-questions. Accessed December 4, 2020.

[75] Commissioner O of the. FDA Issues Emergency Use Authorization for Convalescent Plasma as Potential Promising COVID–19 Treatment, Another Achievement in Administration's Fight Against Pandemic. FDA. 2020. Available at: https://www.fda.gov/news-events/press-announcements/fda-issues-emergency-use-authorization-convalescent-plasma-potential-promising-covid-19-treatment. Accessed December 4, 2020.

[76] Therapeutic Management. COVID-19 Treatment Guidelines. Available at: https://www.covid19treatmentguidelines.nih.gov/therapeutic-management/. Accessed December 4, 2020.

[77] Malgie J, Schoones JW, Pijls BG. Decreased mortality in COVID-19 patients treated with Tocilizumab: a rapid systematic review and meta-analysis of observational studies. Clin Infect Dis 2020. https://doi.org/10.1093/cid/ciaa1445.

[78] Sanders JM, Monogue ML, Jodlowski TZ, et al. Pharmacologic Treatments for Coronavirus Disease 2019 (COVID-19): A Review. JAMA 2020;323(18): 1824–36.

[79] Lenze EJ, Mattar C, Zorumski CF, et al. Fluvoxamine vs Placebo and Clinical Deterioration in Outpatients With Symptomatic COVID-19: A Randomized Clinical Trial. JAMA 2020;324(22):2292–300.

[80] Eastman RT, Roth JS, Brimacombe KR, et al. Remdesivir: A Review of Its Discovery and Development Leading to Emergency Use Authorization for Treatment of COVID-19. ACS Cent Sci 2020. https://doi.org/10.1021/acscentsci.0c00489.

[81] eua-fact-sheet-for-hcps.pdf. Available at: https://www.gilead.com/-/media/files/pdfs/remdesivir/eua-fact-sheet-for-hcps.pdf. Accessed December 4, 2020.

[82] Grein J, Ohmagari N, Shin D, et al. Compassionate Use of Remdesivir for Patients with Severe Covid-19. N Engl J Med 2020;382(24):2327–36.

[83] Beigel JH, Tomashek KM, Dodd LE. Remdesivir for the Treatment of Covid-19 - Preliminary Report. Reply *N Engl J Med* 2020;383(10):994.

[84] Gulati G, Kelly BD. Does remdesivir have any neuropsychiatric adverse effects? Ir J Psychol Med 2020;1–2. https://doi.org/10.1017/ipm.2020.67.

[85] Lewis DA, Smith RE. Steroid-induced psychiatric syndromes. A report of 14 cases and a review of the literature. J Affect Disord 1983;5(4):319–32.

[86] Warrington TP, Bostwick JM. Psychiatric adverse effects of corticosteroids. Mayo Clin Proc 2006;81(10):1361–7.

[87] Delamarre L, Gollion C, Grouteau G, et al. COVID-19-associated acute necrotising encephalopathy successfully treated with steroids and polyvalent immunoglobulin with unusual IgG targeting the cerebral fibre network. J Neurol Neurosurg Psychiatry 2020;91(9):1004–6.

[88] Wani WA, Jameel E, Baig U, et al. Ferroquine and its derivatives: new generation of antimalarial agents. Eur J Med Chem 2015;101:534–51.

[89] Garcia P, Revet A, Yrondi A, et al. Psychiatric Disorders and Hydroxychloroquine for Coronavirus Disease 2019 (COVID-19): A VigiBase Study. Drug Saf 2020;43(12):1315–22.

[90] Lan S-H, Lai C-C, Huang H-T, et al. Tocilizumab for severe COVID-19: a systematic review and meta-analysis. Int J Antimicrob Agents 2020;56(3):106103.

[91] Koike T, Harigai M, Inokuma S, et al. Effectiveness and safety of tocilizumab: postmarketing surveillance of 7901 patients with rheumatoid arthritis in Japan. J Rheumatol 2014;41(1):15–23.

[92] Miller BJ, Dias JK, Lemos HP, et al. An open-label, pilot trial of adjunctive tocilizumab in schizophrenia. J Clin Psychiatry 2016;77(2):275–6.

[93] Dubey S, Biswas P, Ghosh R, et al. Psychosocial impact of COVID-19. Diabetes Metab Syndr 2020;14(5):779–88.

[94] Scavone C, Brusco S, Bertini M, et al. Current pharmacological treatments for COVID-19: What's next? Br J Pharmacol 2020;177(21):4813–24.

[95] Menninger K. Psychoses associated with influenza: i. general data: statistical analysis. JAMA 1919;72(4):235–41.

[96] Krebs FC, Ross H, McAllister J, et al. HIV-1-associated central nervous system dysfunction. Adv Pharmacol San Diego Calif 2000;49:315–85.

[97] Johnson RT. Emerging viral infections of the nervous system. J Neurovirol 2003;9(2):140–7.

[98] Das T, Jaffar-Bandjee MC, Hoarau JJ, et al. Chikungunya fever: CNS infection and pathologies of a re-emerging arbovirus. Prog Neurobiol 2010;91(2):121–9.

[99] Chen B-S, Lee H-C, Lee K-M, et al. Enterovirus and Encephalitis. Front Microbiol 2020;11:261.

[100] Lee DTS, Wing YK, Leung HCM, et al. Factors Associated with Psychosis among Patients with Severe Acute Respiratory Syndrome: A Case-Control Study. Clin Infect Dis 2004;39(8):1247–9.

[101] Druss BG. Addressing the COVID-19 Pandemic in Populations With Serious Mental Illness. JAMA Psychiatry 2020;77(9):891–2.

[102] Xiang Y-T, Zhao Y-J, Liu Z-H, et al. The COVID-19 outbreak and psychiatric hospitals in China: managing challenges through mental health service reform. Int J Biol Sci 2020;16(10):1741–4.

[103] Li W, Yang Y, Liu Z-H, et al. Progression of Mental Health Services during the COVID-19 Outbreak in China. Int J Biol Sci 2020;16(10):1732–8.

[104] Wright JH, Caudill R. Remote Treatment Delivery in Response to the COVID-19 Pandemic. Psychother Psychosom 2020;89(3):130–2.

[105] Spivak S, Spivak A, Cullen B, et al. Telepsychiatry Use in U.S. Mental Health Facilities, 2010-2017. Psychiatr Serv Wash DC 2020;71(2):121–7.

[106] Greenhalgh T, Wherton J, Shaw S, et al. Video consultations for covid-19. BMJ 2020;368:m998.

Advances in Psychiatry and Behavioral Health 1 (2021) 173–183

ADVANCES IN PSYCHIATRY AND BEHAVIORAL HEALTH

The Use of Repetitive Transcranial Magnetic Stimulation in Depression and Other Psychiatric Disorders; the Knowns and the Unknowns

Mandana Modirrousta, MD, PhD, FRCPC[a,b,*], Benjamin P. Meek, BSc, MA[b], Mohamed Abo Aoun, BSc[b]

[a]Rady Faculty of Health Sciences, University of Manitoba, Winnipeg, Manitoba, Canada; [b]St. Boniface Hospital Albrechtsen Research Centre, Winnipeg, Manitoba, Canada

KEYWORDS

• TMS • Neuromodulation • Depression • Psychiatric disorders • Treatment

KEY POINTS

- The clinical use of rTMS for the treatment of depression is well established, yet protocols continue to evolve in search of improved efficacy.
- A variety of factors related to symptomatology, patient characteristics, and treatment delivery influence safety and efficacy considerations.
- While there is promising evidence in support of rTMS for the treatment of a variety of neuropsychiatric conditions, further research is required to establish consensus recommendations for its use in each condition.

INTRODUCTION

The use of neuromodulation in treating psychiatric disorders dates back to the 1930s and the development of electroconvulsive therapy (ECT) [1]. By the 1980s, a noninvasive method of neuromodulation called transcranial magnetic stimulation (TMS) had been devised and was soon being tested for its clinical utility [2,3]. A TMS machine can stimulate neurons in a particular region of the brain by running electricity through a coil to generate an alternating magnetic field. When placed against the scalp, this magnetic field passes through the skull and induces electrical activity in underlying neurons [4]. The magnetic pulses produced by a TMS machine can be applied repetitively (rTMS) in order to produce long-lasting changes in neural activity, and the frequency and pattern of pulse application can be adjusted to alter the effects of TMS on cortical activity, that is, inhibition versus excitation [5].

rTMS was first investigated for the treatment of depression when Hoflich and colleagues reported two such cases in 1993 [3]. Since then, depression has continued to be the principal focus for rTMS intervention, and parameters for its safe and effective application have been established [6]. In 2008, the FDA approved the first rTMS device for the treatment of depression [7]. Numerous randomized controlled trials (RCTs) have demonstrated the efficacy of rTMS when compared to a placebo condition in adult populations, and meta-analyses have reinforced these conclusions [8]. As a result, expert clinical groups have endorsed level A evidence—definite efficacy—in favor of rTMS therapy for depression [7,9–11].

*Corresponding author. St. Boniface Hospital, M4-McEwen Building, 409 Taché Avenue, Winnipeg, Manitoba R2H2A6, Canada. *E-mail address:* mmodirrousta@sbgh.mb.ca

https://doi.org/10.1016/j.ypsc.2021.05.002
2667-3827/21/

Similar to other treatment modalities, a variety of factors play a role in the eventual response to rTMS in patients with depression. In this review, we discuss characteristics of patients, disease presentation, and treatment administration that may alter clinical efficacy, and we provide a practice approach when considering this treatment for psychiatric populations.

PATIENT FACTORS

Patient factors are characteristics related to an individual which should be considered in the choice of a treatment.

Certain demographic variables, such as age and gender, may play a role in rTMS treatment efficacy. Female gender is considered a positive predictor of response, as studies with a higher proportion of female patients show better outcomes [12]. With regard to age, most studies have only included working-age adults and overlooked patients at either end of the age spectrum [13,14]. However, preliminary evidence indicates that rTMS can be used effectively to alleviate depressive symptoms in adolescents [15,16], with some authors recently suggesting that rTMS may even be more effective for depression in adolescents than adults [17]. Risks of rTMS do not seem to be any different for children than for adults [18], and rTMS does not appear to negatively impact neurocognitive development [14]. Results from geriatric studies have been less consistent; some RCTs have found no difference between active and sham stimulation in older populations [19,20], whereas more recent studies have indicated good rTMS efficacy in older adults [21,22]. Using age as covariate in adult studies has also provided mixed results; while some studies have not found any correlation between age and treatment outcome [23], others have concluded that older age is associated with poorer response [24,25]. There are several factors unique to an older population, such as brain atrophy and certain comorbidities, which might necessitate the adoption of different rTMS parameters—higher rTMS stimulation intensity or more treatments—to achieve an optimal response [13,26].

Baseline neuropsychiatric characteristics and comorbidities have been investigated for their potential influence or predictive utility regarding rTMS. For instance, higher persistence scores measured by the Temperament and Character Inventory are associated with better treatment outcomes [27]. Patients with better cognitive control, verbal learning, and cognitive flexibility also appear to respond better to rTMS [28,29]. Intriguingly, numerous studies have reported improved cognitive functions along with reduced depressive symptoms following rTMS therapy [28,30]. Recent evidence suggests no significant difference in remission rates between patients with or without comorbid anxiety disorders [31], although there is some indication that comorbid anxiety is associated with high symptom severity and poor treatment response [32].

Brain-state dynamics prior to treatment and their potential interference with rTMS efficacy is also an area of great interest. It has been shown that altering baseline neural activity using rTMS can have a significant influence on the effects of subsequent rTMS stimulation. For example, "priming" a region of the brain with excitatory rTMS can interfere with or even abolish the effects of subsequent inhibitory rTMS [33]. Pretreatment neuronal activity can be influenced by a variety of factors, such as substance use (eg, caffeine intake), stress, sleep patterns, or menstrual cycle [6,34,35], making these factors a consideration for both efficacy and patient safety. A small-sample study observed that while caffeine intake doesn't alter motor threshold (MT), it may reduce long-term potentiation induced by rTMS, which could have an effect on the durability of rTMS response [36]. While it has been documented that sleep deprivation increases cortical excitability [37,38], there are inconsistent results regarding the effect of sleep deprivation on MT [39,40]. The full impact of these factors on rTMS safety and efficacy are yet to be fully explored.

Individual differences in cortical functional connectivity may also play a role in treatment response. For instance, better response rates to rTMS over dorsolateral prefrontal cortex (DLPFC) have been observed in patients with stronger pretreatment functional connectivity between DLPFC and striatum [41], as well as hyperconnectivity between the subgenual cingulate (SgC) and superior medial frontal gyrus [42], between SgC and ventro- and dorso-medial prefrontal cortex, and between DLPFC and posterior parietal cortex (PPC) [43]. Whereas lower baseline connectivity between SgC and insula and amygdala, as well as between dorsomedial prefrontal cortex (DMPFC) and thalamus and amygdala are associated with better outcomes when targeting DMPFC [44]. Higher pretreatment activity in anterior cingulate cortex (ACC) has also been positively correlated with better treatment response [45]. Further, changes in functional connectivity following a single session of rTMS may act as a predictor of treatment response [46]. These kind of observations are important for a number of reasons: (i) for understanding the mechanisms by which rTMS exerts its effects, (ii) for classifying subgroups of patients who are more likely to respond to treatment, and (iii) for personalizing treatments by selecting appropriate stimulation targets depending on a patient's neural connectivity [41,47,48].

Other investigated biological characteristics that have been linked to treatment outcome include heart rate and heart rate variability [49,50], brain-derived neurotrophic factor, cortisol, thyroid hormones (eg, TSH, fT3, and fT4) [51], and a number of neuroimmunoendocrine markers (eg, LH, FSH, estradiol, progesterone, and DHEA; for a review, see [52]). Although there are some interesting preliminary findings, further research is needed to elucidate these relationships.

DISEASE FACTORS

Disease factors are the presence or absence of specific symptoms related to a disease, or disease characteristics such as severity or duration.

In depression, treatment refractoriness, high severity, psychotic symptoms, and failure to respond to previous ECT are considered poor prognostic factors for rTMS treatment [24,53–55]. In contrast, shorter duration of the current depression episode, recurrent rather than a single episode, and previous response to rTMS have been linked to a greater likelihood of treatment response [29,53,55]. Data regarding the utility of symptom profiles in selecting the best candidates for rTMS therapy have yielded inconsistent results. A recent study by Rostami and colleagues showed that patients with affective symptoms—sadness, feelings of guilt, loss-of-interest, or pessimism—benefit more from rTMS compared to those with somatic symptoms, such as fatigue or pain [25]. However, a previous study reported an opposite pattern: depressed mood and guilty feelings being negative predictors, with psychomotor retardation—a somatic symptom—being a positive predictor of response [56]. Interestingly, Siddiqi and colleagues suggest that patients with dysphoric symptoms, such as sadness and anhedonia, may respond best to DLPFC stimulation, whereas anxiety and somatic symptoms may respond best to DMPFC stimulation [27]. Although encouraging, changing the stimulation target according to depressive symptomatology requires further prospective and validating study designs before being adopted in clinical settings.

TREATMENT-SPECIFIC FACTORS

Treatment-specific factors relate to the different parameters of a treatment that can be adjusted and/or measured in order to optimize treatment outcome. In rTMS therapy, factors such as the total number or frequency of pulses, the intensity of stimulation, and the brain region being targeted are important determinants of treatment outcome. Consensus recommendations for safe application as well as clinical guidelines for rTMS therapy in depression have been developed by experts from across the world [6,7,57].

Frequency

The frequency of pulses is a key factor in rTMS therapy as it determines the neurophysiological effect of treatment. As previously mentioned, the pattern of magnetic pulses can be adjusted to alter the effects of rTMS on cortical activity. Conventional rTMS is often divided into two categories: low-frequency (LF; 1 Hz) and high-frequency (HF; 5–20 Hz) stimulation, with LF decreasing and HF increasing cortical excitability [5]. A patterned stimulation protocol called theta-burst stimulation (TBS), which uses triplets of pulses at 50 Hz and is thought to better imitate neuronal firing patterns, has recently gained popularity due to its ability to exert similar neurologic effects with a much shorter treatment session [58]. Frequency is also an important safety consideration, as HF protocols can carry the risk of inducing a seizure [6]. In order to reduce the risk of this rare adverse event, safety guidelines outline the recommended reduction in the number of sequential pulses (ie, length of a stimulation train) with increasing stimulation frequencies [6,59].

Number of Pulses

Three thousand pulses is the generally recommended session maximum for HF stimulation with a standard figure-of-eight coil, and this number is closer to 2000 for deeper penetrating H-coils [7]. For TBS protocols, the number of pulses in each session is generally lower, ranging from 300 to 1800 (Table 1) [60,61]. Careful consideration should be given when adjusting these numbers, as data from electrophysiological studies provide evidence that too many pulses per session can alter brain dynamics and potentially reverse the intended effects of stimulation. For example, Gamboa and colleagues found that doubling the length of conventional TBS protocols results in a reversal of the cortical excitability effect compared to what is typically expected, that is, intermittent TBS (iTBS), which normally produces a facilitatory effect, becomes inhibitory with longer application, and continuous TBS (cTBS), which is normally inhibitory, has the opposite effect [62]. These findings highlight the importance of understanding the physiologic effects of various rTMS parameters when considering treatment efficacy and patient safety.

TABLE 1
Current rTMS Protocols in the Treatment of Depression

Protocol (Level of Evidence)	Frequency (Hz)	Stimulation Intensity (% MT)	Stimulation Location	Pulses/ Session[a]	Sessions/ day[b]	Total Sessions[c]
HF (level A) [11]	10–20	110–120	Left DLPFC	1200–3000	1–10	20–30
LF (level B) [11]	1	110–120	Right DLPFC	600–1200	1–10	20–30
Bilateral HF + LF (level B) [11]	HF + LF	110–120	Left + right DLPFC	600–1800 on each side	1–10	20–30
iTBS (not inferior to HF) [111]	Intermittent trains (2 s on, 10 s off) of 50 Hz triplets repeated at 5 Hz	80[d]	Left DLPFC	600–1800	1–10	20–30
cTBS (level C) [11]	Continuous 50 Hz triplets repeated at 5 Hz	80	Right DLPFC	600–1800	1–10	20–30
Bilateral iTBS + cTBS (level B) [11]	iTBS + cTBS	80	Left + right DLPFC	600–1800 on each side	1–10	20–30

Abbreviations: cTBS, continuous theta burst stimulation; DLPFC, dorsolateral prefrontal cortex; HF, high frequency; iTBS, intermittent theta burst stimulation; LF, low frequency; MT, motor threshold.
[a] Numbers of pulses/session varies between studies.
[b] Accelerated treatment protocols using multiple sessions/day are largely investigational at this time.
[c] Some patients may benefit from additional sessions beyond 30.
[d] Noninferiority trial treated at 120% MT [111].

The total number of pulses over a full course of treatment generally depends on the total number of sessions a patient receives. There is some debate regarding the relative influence of the total number of pulses versus the number of treatment sessions, with some evidence suggesting that the number of individual treatment sessions may actually have a larger effect on treatment outcome than the total number of pulses delivered [63].

Stimulation Intensity

Stimulation intensity is generally calculated based upon an individual's resting MT. A recent pooled analysis of multiple rTMS trials revealed a significantly greater response rate in trials which use suprathreshold, 110% or 120%, output compared to those using 100% MT [55]. Accordingly, conventional LF or HF rTMS protocols now commonly set stimulator output at 110% or 120% MT [7]. Lower stimulation intensities (80% or 90% MT) are generally employed with TBS protocols in order to reduce the chance of seizure induction [6].

Stimulation Target

An important treatment factor that varies depending on the underlying psychiatric disorder is the region of the brain selected for stimulation. Target selection must incorporate two primary considerations: (i) the presumed underlying neuropathology and (ii) the physical limitations of the rTMS coil used for treatment. Depression has been associated with abnormalities of functional connectivity in a number of brain networks, specifically the default mode network, the central executive network, and the salience network (for more detail, see [48]). These networks connect various cortical and subcortical regions that could theoretically be stimulated to modulate network activity. The most common target for rTMS depression treatment is the DLPFC due to its anatomic proximity to the brain surface and its functional connectivity with other key regions within depression networks [48,64].

The aforementioned level A evidence for the efficacy of rTMS therapy for depression generally refers to the use of HF stimulation over the left DLPFC [7,9–11]. LF rTMS applied to the right DLPFC and bilateral protocols employing both HF right- and LF left-sided treatment are also used for depression. Although some studies have reported no difference in response when comparing these protocols, the evidence for their use is not quite as strong as HF left-DLPFC stimulation [11]. Similar recommendations are provided for the use of bilateral right-sided continuous TBS and left-sided intermittent TBS (see Table 1). The use of rTMS coils that can stimulate deeper brain regions has opened the door for the targeting of other cortical regions involved in depression pathophysiology such as DMPFC, frontopolar cortex, ventromedial prefrontal cortex, and ventrolateral prefrontal cortex [47,65].

New evidence supports the idea of multiple neurophysiological subtypes of depression [66]. The ability to target different cortical regions allows for the exciting possibility of personalized treatments, in which different patients may benefit from different stimulation targets [66,67]. For instance, deep TMS may preferentially benefit patients with a higher depression severity [68], and bilateral rTMS stimulation may be more effective at reducing suicidal ideation [69].

Beyond target selection, accurate placement of the rTMS coil over the stimulation site during treatment is an important consideration. A widely employed method in depression trials is the "5cm-rule," in which the location of the DLPFC is estimated by measuring anterior along the scalp from the hand region of the motor cortex [7]. However, there is evidence that this method may not be sufficiently accurate and that a more lateral and anterior location may result in better treatment outcomes [70–72]. Other techniques—employing EEG coordinate systems or MRI-guided "neuro-navigation"—may have the potential to more reliably target the desired stimulation site [73–75]. Indeed, functional MRI-guided techniques may allow for even greater precision in site selection based on individual brain activity. For instance, a recent study found that patients who had failed a course of rTMS using standard target-localization techniques responded to a second course of rTMS using MRI-guided targeting based on resting-state functional connectivity analysis [76].

Duration of Treatment

Some studies indicate that response rates plateau around the 26th to 28th treatment sessions [77,78]. However, late responders or patients with severe depression may benefit from receiving additional sessions [77,79]. While rTMS effects can be durable, lasting at least 12 months in many cases [80], relapse is fairly common, with as many as three-quarters of responders relapsing by 6 months posttreatment [81]. The pool of controlled studies examining maintenance protocols is currently too limited to reach consensus recommendations on best practice [7,9], but it is well established that some form of maintenance offers marked benefit to patients, with the ability to prolong remission for many years [82].

More recently, "accelerated" treatment protocols, in which multiple (2–10) sessions are administered each day, have been studied [83]. Preliminary observations suggest that twice-daily treatments are no less effective than a traditional once-daily schedule and can elicit more rapid symptom improvements [63,84]. More aggressive protocols involving 10 iTBS sessions per day guided by resting-state functional MRI connectivity analysis have demonstrated remarkable remission rates (>90%) without negative cognitive side effects or notable safety concerns [85].

Accelerated protocols may result in altered response trajectories, such as continued symptom improvement beyond the final treatment session [86,87]. In contrast, it has been suggested that highly accelerated protocols may result in rapid improvements but also rapid rates of relapse [88]. Nonetheless, these observations highlight the importance of adequate follow-up assessments in determining both treatment response and the durability of clinical improvement. While previous studies have so far demonstrated that a very large number of daily high-frequency pulses can be administered with no serious adverse events and minimal side effects [85,89,90], safety considerations should be kept in mind. especially with regards to patient populations who may be at a higher risk for induced seizures.

Side Effects

The three most common side effect of rTMS are transient headaches, fatigue, and discomfort at the site of stimulation or nearby face regions [7,91,92], which tend to diminish over the course of treatment [9,92,93]. Other less common side effects can include syncope, hearing damage, or the induction of mania/hypomania, where syncope is likely a vasodepressor response to anxiety or discomfort associated with rTMS, and hearing concerns can largely be mitigated through the use of ear protection during treatment [6,7]. Seizure is a rare side effect of rTMS with an estimate prevalence of 1 in 30,000 [78]. The risk of seizure can be largely reduced by selecting stimulation parameters in accordance with safety guidelines and by careful screening of patients for seizure risk factors [94].

Pre-TMS Evaluation

Prior to treatment, factors that may increase seizure-risk or compromise treatment efficacy should be assessed.

Consensus review guidelines highlight the following factors in pre-TMS evaluation [5–7,95]:

1. Personal or family history of epilepsy or seizures;
2. Past stroke or head injury with neurologic sequelae;
3. Concurrent use of medications or substances that significantly affect seizure threshold (eg, bupropion increases seizure risk, whereas anticonvulsants may interfere with rTMS effect);
4. Presence of unstable medical conditions or conditions that might lower seizure threshold (eg, increased intracranial pressure, withdrawal from substances of abuse, etc.);
5. Presence of ferromagnetic implanted medical devices (pacemakers, cochlear implants, etc.) or metal objects in the head or neck area, which are considered rTMS contraindications.

rTMS IN OTHER PSYCHIATRIC DISORDERS

By modulating cortical activity in a noninvasive and relatively focal manner, rTMS has the potential to be successfully administered in other psychiatric disorders. Here, we briefly describe some of the findings from rTMS studies in other disorders; a more comprehensive review on this topic can be found in articles by Lefaucheur and colleagues [11,96].

Obsessive Compulsive Disorder (OCD)

Dysfunction of the orbitofrontal-striatal-pallido-thalamic circuit is the hallmark of OCD pathology [97]. Several studies have investigated the efficacy of both HF and LF rTMS over the DLPFC. While HF studies have reported mixed results, LF stimulation to the right DLPFC appears more promising [11,98]. There is also evidence for clinical improvement using LF stimulation targeting supplementary motor area (SMA) and pre-SMA [99], as well as HF deep rTMS targeting medial prefrontal cortex and ACC [100].

Schizophrenia

Studies have generally reported improvements in auditory hallucinations following LF rTMS and cTBS of the left temporoparietal junction [101]. Positive predictive factors include young age, female gender, and smaller scalp-to-cortex distance [102,103]. For negative symptoms, meta-analyses report improvements following HF stimulation over the left DLPFC [104], and there is also preliminary evidence in favor of cerebellar modulation [105].

Substance Use Disorder

Promising, though variable, results have been seen for the use of rTMS to reduce cravings and consumption with regards to alcohol, tobacco, methamphetamine, and cocaine in patients with substance use disorder, with right and left DLPFC being the most prevalent stimulation targets [106].

Eating Disorders

HF stimulation of the DMPFC with a double cone coil in bulimia nervosa has produced decreases in weekly binge/purge frequency by more than 50%, and the response has been shown to be associated with a measurable improvement in frontostriatal connectivity [107]. Fewer studies are available for anorexia nervosa, with one study using HF stimulation to the left DLPFC reporting improvements in mood without changes in weight gain [108].

Anxiety Disorders

A small number of studies have reported improvements in anxiety symptoms, emotion regulation, and sleep quality in patients with anxiety disorders following rTMS, primarily targeting right and left DLPFC but also the right PPC [11,109].

Posttraumatic Stress Disorder (PTSD)

Several rTMS protocols have been studied in the treatment of PTSD. Among them, HF stimulation to the right DLPFC has demonstrated the best results in reducing anxiety and in producing long-lasting improvement in other PTSD symptoms [110].

Overall, early data regarding the use of rTMS in these psychiatric disorders are promising but generally not sufficient to recommend its routine use in clinical settings. Further research is needed to reproduce the results of preliminary pilot studies and elucidate the most effective treatment paradigms.

SUMMARY

Through its ability to focally stimulate a variety of different brain networks, rTMS—a noninvasive neuromodulation tool—holds potential for the treatment of many neuropsychiatric disorders without major side effects. However, despite having been used for more than two decades, its approved application is currently still limited to the treatment of depression. Furthermore, determining the best candidates to receive rTMS for depression and rTMS protocols that will provide the most efficient and durable recovery are only now beginning to be elucidated. Given the dramatic increase in rTMS research over the past decade with thousands of manuscripts now being published each year, new knowledge and recommendations regarding the clinical application of rTMS are sure to evolve rapidly in the near future. It will behoove clinicians to stay abreast of this rapidly advancing field.

CLINICS CARE POINTS

Dos and don'ts for the clinical consideration of rTMS therapy in psychiatric disorders

Do:

- Identify the main psychiatric disorder;
- Identify comorbidities;
- Review current medications: are they potentially unsafe or could they interfere with rTMS efficacy?
- Review the level of rTMS evidence for this psychiatric disorder;
- Check for rTMS contraindications;
- Evaluate the likelihood of response based on patient- and disease-related factors;
- Identify the best evidence-based rTMS protocol;
- Provide informed consent: discuss potential risks and side-effects;
- Evaluate the availability of a recent brain MRI or the feasibility of attaining one (if performing MRI-guided rTMS);
- Conduct a pre-rTMS symptom assessment using standardized scales;
- Monitor side effects;
- Assess response status during and at the end of treatment using standardized scales;
- Determine if additional rTMS is appropriate;
- Provide follow-up visits to monitor for signs of relapse and the need for maintenance treatment.

Don't:

- Change medications during treatment;
- Introduce a new treatment during rTMS (eg, psychotherapy);
- Offer rTMS if there is little evidence of efficacy for that particular disorder;
- Treat people with ferromagnetic objects in the head or neck area;
- Use rTMS if there is an ongoing unstable medical condition or a high risk of seizure.

DISCLOSURE

The authors have nothing to disclose.

REFERENCES

[1] Cerletti U, Bini L. L'Elettroshock. Arc/i Gen Neurol Psichiatr Psicoanal 1938;19:266.

[2] Barker AT, Freeston IL, Jalinous R, et al. Non-invasive stimulation of motor pathways within the brain using timevarying magnetic fields. Electroencephalogr Clin Neurophysiol 1985;61:S245.

[3] Hoflich G, Kasper S, Hufnagel A, et al. Application of transcranial magnetic stimulation in treatment of drug-resistant major depression: a report of two cases. Hum Psychopharmacol 1993;8:361–5.

[4] Hasey GM. Transcranial magnetic stimulation: using a law of physics to treat psychopathology. J Psychiatry Neurosci 1999;24(2):97–101.

[5] Fitzgerald PB, Daskalakis ZF. Repetitive transcranial magnetic stimulation treatment for depressive disorders a practical guide. 1st edition. Berlin: Springer Berlin Heidelberg; 2013.

[6] Rossi S, Hallett M, Rossini PM, et al. Safety, ethical considerations, and application guidelines for the use of transcranial magnetic stimulation in clinical practice and research. Clin Neurophysiol 2009;120(12):2008–39.

[7] McClintock SM, Reti IM, Carpenter LL, et al. Consensus Recommendations for the Clinical Application of Repetitive Transcranial Magnetic Stimulation (rTMS) in the Treatment of Depression. J Clin Psychiatry 2018;79(1):16cs10905.

[8] Health Quality Ontario. Repetitive Transcranial Magnetic Stimulation for Treatment-Resistant Depression: A Systematic Review and Meta-Analysis of Randomized Controlled Trials. Ont Health Technol Assess Ser 2016;16(5):1–66.

[9] Milev RV, Giacobbe P, Kennedy SH, et al. CANMAT Depression Work Group. Canadian Network for Mood and Anxiety Treatments (CANMAT) 2016 Clinical Guidelines for the Management of Adults with Major Depressive Disorder: Section 4. Neurostimulation Treatments. Can J Psychiatry 2016;61(9):561–75.

[10] Perera T, George MS, Grammer G, et al. The Clinical TMS Society Consensus Review and Treatment Recommendations for TMS Therapy for Major Depressive Disorder. Brain Stimul 2016;9(3):336–46.

[11] Lefaucheur JP, Aleman A, Baeken C, et al. Evidence-based guidelines on the therapeutic use of repetitive transcranial magnetic stimulation (rTMS): An update (2014-2018). Clin Neurophysiol 2020;131(2):474–528.

[12] Kedzior KK, Azorina V, Reitz SK. More female patients and fewer stimuli per session are associated with the short-term antidepressant properties of repetitive transcranial magnetic stimulation (rTMS): a meta-

analysis of 54 sham-controlled studies published between 1997–2013. Neuropsychiatr Dis Treat 2014; 10:727–56.

[13] Sabesan P, Lankappa S, Khalifa N, et al. Transcranial magnetic stimulation for geriatric depression: Promises and pitfalls. World J Psychiatry 2015;5(2):170–81.

[14] Malone LA, Sun LR. Transcranial Magnetic Stimulation for the Treatment of Pediatric Neurological Disorders. Curr Treat Options Neurol 2019;21(11):58.

[15] Donaldson AE, Gordon MS, Melvin GA, et al. Addressing the needs of adolescents with treatment resistant depressive disorders: a systematic review of rTMS. Brain Stimul 2014;7:7–12.

[16] MacMaster FP, Croarkin PE, Wilkes TC, et al. Repetitive transcranial magnetic stimulation in youth with treatment resistant major depression. Front Psychiatry 2019;10:170.

[17] Zhang T, Zhu J, Xu L, et al. Addon rTMS for the acute treatment of depressive symptoms is probably more effective in adolescents than in adults: evidence fromreal-world clinical practice. Brain Stimul 2019;12: 103–9.

[18] Allen CH, Kluger BM, Buard I. Safety of Transcranial Magnetic Stimulation in Children: A Systematic Review of the Literature. Pediatr Neurol 2017;68:3–17.

[19] Manes F, Jorge R, Morcuende M, et al. A controlled study of repetitive transcranial magnetic stimulation as a treatment of depression in the elderly. Int Psychogeriatr 2001;13:225–31.

[20] Mosimann UP, Schmitt W, Greenberg BD, et al. Repetitive transcranial magnetic stimulation: a putative add-on treatment for major depression in elderly patients. Psychiatry Res 2004;126:123–33.

[21] Jorge RE, Moser DJ, Acion L, et al. Treatment of vascular depression using repetitive transcranial magnetic stimulation. Arch Gen Psychiatry 2008;65:268–76.

[22] Leblhuber F, Steiner K, Fuchs D. Treatment of patients with geriatric depression with repetitive transcranial magnetic stimulation. J Neural Transm (Vienna) 2019; 126(8):1105–10.

[23] Herrmann LL, Ebmeier KP. Factors modifying the efficacy of transcranial magnetic stimulation in the treatment of depression: a review. J Clin Psychiatry 2006; 67:1870–6.

[24] Beuzon G, Timour Q, Saoud M. Predictors of response to repetitive transcranial magnetic stimulation (rTMS) in the treatment of major depressive disorder. Encéphale 2017;43:3–9.

[25] Rostami R, Kazemi R, Nitsche MA, et al. Clinical and demographic predictors of response to rTMS treatment in unipolar and bipolar depressive disorders. Clin Neurophysiol 2017;128(10):1961–70.

[26] Galvez V, Ho KA, Alonzo A, et al. Neuromodulation therapies for geriatric depression. Curr Psychiatry Rep 2015;17(7):59.

[27] Siddiqi SH, Chockalingam R, Cloninger CR, et al. Use of the Temperament and Character Inventory to Predict Response to Repetitive Transcranial Magnetic Stimulation for Major Depression. J Psychiatr Pract 2016; 22(3):193–202.

[28] Abo Aoun M, Meek BP, Modirrousta M. Cognitive profiles in major depressive disorder: Comparing remitters and non-remitters to rTMS treatment. Psychiatry Res 2019;279:55–61.

[29] Kaur M, Naismith SL, Lagopoulos J, et al. Sleep-wake, cognitive and clinical correlates of treatment outcome with repetitive transcranial magnetic stimulation for young adults with depression. Psychiatry Res 2019; 271:335–42.

[30] Martin DM, McClintock SM, Forster JJ, et al. Cognitive enhancing effects of rTMS administered to the prefrontal cortex in patients with depression: A systematic review and meta-analysis of individual task effects. Depress Anxiety 2017;34(11):1029–39.

[31] Clarke E, Clarke P, Gill S, et al. Efficacy of repetitive transcranial magnetic stimulation in the treatment of depression with comorbid anxiety disorders. J Affect Disord 2019;252:435–9.

[32] Dold M, Bartova L, Souery D, et al. Clinical characteristics and treatment outcomes of patients with major depressive disorder and comorbid anxiety disorders - results from a European multicenter study. J Psychiatr Res 2017;91:1–13.

[33] Tallabs FA, Hammond-Tooke GD. Theta priming of 1-Hz rTMS in healthy volunteers: effects on motor inhibition. J Clin Neurophysiol 2013;30(1):79–85.

[34] Inghilleri M, Conte A, Currà A, et al. Ovarian hormones and cortical excitability. An rTMS study in humans. Clin Neurophysiol 2005;115:1063–8.

[35] Zhang W, Llera A, Hashemi MM, et al. Discriminating stress from rest based on resting-state connectivity of the human brain: A supervised machine learning study. Hum Brain Mapp 2020;41(11):3089–99.

[36] Hanajima R, Tanaka N, Tsutsumi R, et al. Effect of caffeine on long-term potentiation-like effects induced by quadripulse transcranial magnetic stimulation. Exp Brain Res 2019;237(3):647–51.

[37] Badawy RA, Curatolo JM, Newton M, et al. Sleep deprivation increases cortical excitability in epilepsy: syndrome-specific effects. Neurology 2006;67(6): 1018–22.

[38] Placidi F, Zannino S, Albanese M, et al. Increased cortical excitability after selective REM sleep deprivation in healthy humans: a transcranial magnetic stimulation study. Sleep Med 2013;14(3):288–92.

[39] Manganotti P, Palermo A, Patuzzo S, et al. Decrease in motor cortical excitability in human subjects after sleep deprivation. Neurosci Lett 2001;304(3):153–6.

[40] Kreuzer P, Langguth B, Popp R, et al. Reduced intracortical inhibition after sleep deprivation: a transcranial magnetic stimulation study. Neurosci Lett 2011;493(3): 63–6.

[41] Avissar M, Powell F, Ilieva I, et al. Functional connectivity of the left DLPFC to striatum predicts treatment

response of depression to TMS. Brain Stimul 2017;10: 919–25.
[42] Baeken C, Marinazzo D, Wu G-R, et al. Accelerated HF-rTMS in treatment-resistant unipolar depression: Insights from subgenual anterior cingulate functional connectivity. World J Biol Psychiatry 2014;15:286–97.
[43] Liston C, Chen AC, Zebley BD, et al. Default mode network mechanisms of transcranial magnetic stimulation in depression. Biol Psychiatry 2014;76(7):517–26.
[44] Salomons TV, Dunlop K, Kennedy SH, et al. Resting state cortico-thalamic-striatal connectivity predicts response to dorsomedial prefrontal rTMS in major depressive disorder. Neuropsychopharmacology 2014; 39(2):488–98.
[45] Langguth B, Wiegand R, Kharraz A, et al. Pre-treatment anterior cingulate activity as a predictor of antidepressant response to repetitive transcranial magnetic stimulation (rTMS). Neuro Endocrinol Lett 2007;28(5): 633–8.
[46] Corlier J, Wilson A, Hunter AM, et al. Changes in Functional Connectivity Predict Outcome of Repetitive Transcranial Magnetic Stimulation Treatment of Major Depressive Disorder. Cereb Cortex 2019;29(12): 4958–67.
[47] Downar J, Daskalakis ZJ. New targets for rTMS in depression: a review of convergent evidence. Brain Stimul 2013;6(3):231–40.
[48] Anderson RJ, Hoy KE, Daskalakis ZJ, et al. Repetitive transcranial magnetic stimulation for treatment resistant depression: Re-establishing connections. Clin Neurophysiol 2016;127(11):3394–405.
[49] Makovac E, Thayer JF, Ottaviani C. A meta-analysis of non-invasive brain stimulation and autonomic functioning: Implications for brain-heart pathways to cardiovascular disease. Neurosci Biobehav Rev 2017; 74(Pt B):330–41.
[50] Iseger TA, Arns M, Downar J, et al. Cardiovascular differences between sham and active iTBS related to treatment response in MDD. Brain Stimulation 2020;13(1): 167–74.
[51] Kito S, Hasegawa T, Fujita K, et al. Changes in hypothalamic-pituitary-thyroid axis following successful treatment with low-frequency right prefrontal transcranial magnetic stimulation in treatment-resistant depression. Psychiatry Res 2010;175(1–2):74–7.
[52] Fidalgo TM, Morales-Quezada JL, Muzy GS, et al. Biological markers in noninvasive brain stimulation trials in major depressive disorder: a systematic review. J ECT 2014;30(1):47–61.
[53] Dumas R, Padovani R, Richieri R, et al. Stimulation magnétique transcrânienne répétée dans la prise en charge des épisodes dépressifs majeurs : facteurs prédictifs de réponse thérapeutique. Encephale 2012;38(4): 360–8.
[54] Grammer GG, Kuhle AR, Clark CC, et al. Severity of depression predicts remission rates using transcranial magnetic stimulation. Front Psychiatry 2015;6:114.
[55] Fitzgerald PB, Hoy KE, Anderson RJ, et al. A study of the pattern of response to rTMS treatment in depression. Depress Anxiety 2016;33:746–53.
[56] Brakemeier EL, Luborzewski A, Danker-Hopfe H, et al. Positive predictors for antidepressive response to prefrontal repetitive transcranial magnetic stimulation (rTMS). J Psychiatr Res 2007;41(5):395–403.
[57] Wassermann EM. Risk and safety of repetitive transcranial magnetic stimulation: report and suggested guidelines from the International Workshop on the Safety of Repetitive Transcranial Magnetic Stimulation, June 5-7, 1996. Electroencephalogr Clin Neurophysiol 1998;108(1):1–16.
[58] Huang YZ, Edwards MJ, Rounis E, et al. Theta burst stimulation of the human motor cortex. Neuron 2005;45(2):201–6.
[59] Chen R, Gerloff C, Classen J, et al. Safety of different inter-train intervals for repetitive transcranial magnetic stimulation and recommendations for safe ranges of stimulation parameters. Electroencephalogr Clin Neurophysiol 1997;105:415–21.
[60] Chung SW, Hoy KE, Fitzgerald PB. Theta-burst stimulation: a new form of TMS treatment for depression? Depress Anxiety 2015;32(3):182–92.
[61] Suppa A, Huang YZ, Funke K, et al. Ten Years of Theta Burst Stimulation in Humans: Established Knowledge, Unknowns and Prospects. Brain Stimul 2016;9(3): 323–35.
[62] Gamboa OL, Antal A, Moliadze V, et al. Simply longer is not better: reversal of theta burst after-effect with prolonged stimulation. Exp Brain Res 2010;204(2):181–7.
[63] Schulze L, Feffer K, Lozano C, et al. Number of pulses or number of sessions? An open-label study of trajectories of improvement for once-vs. twice-daily dorsomedial prefrontal rTMS in major depression. Brain Stimul 2018;11(2):327–36.
[64] Helm K, Viol K, Weiger TM, et al. Neuronal connectivity in major depressive disorder: a systematic review. Neuropsychiatr Dis Treat 2018;14:2715–37.
[65] Kreuzer PM, Downar J, de Ridder D, et al. A Comprehensive Review of Dorsomedial Prefrontal Cortex rTMS Utilizing a Double Cone Coil. Neuromodulation 2019;22(8):851–66.
[66] Drysdale AT, Grosenick L, Downar J, et al. Resting-state connectivity biomarkers define neurophysiological subtypes of depression. Nat Med 2017;23(1):28–38.
[67] Siddiqi SH, Taylor SF, Cooke D, et al. Distinct Symptom-Specific Treatment Targets for Circuit-Based Neuromodulation. Am J Psychiatry 2020;177(5): 435–46.
[68] Feffer K, Lapidus KAB, Braw Y, et al. Factors associated with response after deep transcranial magnetic stimulation in a real-world clinical setting: Results from the first 40 cases of treatment-resistant depression. Eur Psychiatry 2017;44:61–7.
[69] Weissman CR, Blumberger DM, Brown PE, et al. Bilateral Repetitive Transcranial Magnetic Stimulation

Decreases Suicidal Ideation in Depression. J Clin Psychiatry 2018;79(3):17m11692.

[70] Herbsman T, Avery D, Ramsey D, et al. More lateral and anterior prefrontal coil location is associated with better repetitive transcranial magnetic stimulation antidepressant response. Biol Psychiatry 2009; 66(5):509–15.

[71] Ahdab R, Ayache SS, Brugières P, et al. Comparison of "standard" and "navigated" procedures of TMS coil positioning over motor, premotor and prefrontal targets in patients with chronic pain and depression. Neurophysiol Clin 2010;40(1):27–36.

[72] Johnson KA, Baig M, Ramsey D, et al. Prefrontal rTMS for treating depression: location and intensity results from the OPT-TMS multi-site clinical trial. Brain Stimul 2013;6(2):108–17.

[73] Peleman K, Van Schuerbeek P, Luypaert R, et al. Using 3D-MRI to localize the dorsolateral prefrontal cortex in TMS research. World J Biol Psychiatry 2010;11(2 Pt 2):425–30.

[74] Fitzgerald PB, Hoy K, McQueen S, et al. A randomized trial of rTMS targeted with MRI based neuro-navigation in treatment-resistant depression. Neuropsychopharmacology 2009;34(5):1255–62.

[75] Mir-Moghtadaei A, Caballero R, Fried P, et al. Concordance Between BeamF3 and MRI-neuronavigated Target Sites for Repetitive Transcranial Magnetic Stimulation of the Left Dorsolateral Prefrontal Cortex. Brain Stimul 2015;8(5):965–73.

[76] Moreno-Ortega M, Kangarlu A, Lee S, et al. Parcel-guided rTMS for depression. Transl Psychiatry 2020; 10(1):283.

[77] McDonald WM, Durkalski V, Ball ER, et al. Improving the antidepressant efficacy of transcranial magnetic stimulation: maximizing the number of stimulations and treatment location in treatment-resistant depression. Depress Anxiety 2011;28(11):973–80.

[78] Carpenter LL, Janicak PG, Aaronson ST, et al. Transcranial magnetic stimulation (TMS) for major depression: a multisite, naturalistic, observational study of acute treatment outcomes in clinical practice. Depress Anxiety 2012;29(7):587–96.

[79] Avery DH, Isenberg KE, Sampson SM, et al. TMS in the acute treatment of major depression: clinical response in an open-label extension trial. J Clin Psychiatry 2008;69(3):441–51.

[80] Dunner DL, Aaronson ST, Sackeim HA, et al. A multisite, naturalistic, observational study of transcranial magnetic stimulation for patients with pharmacoresistant major depressive disorder: durability of benefit over a 1-year follow-up period. J Clin Psychiatry 2014; 75(12):1394–401.

[81] Cohen RB, Boggio PS, Fregni F. Risk factors for relapse after remission with repetitive transcranial magnetic stimulation for the treatment of depression. Depress Anxiety 2009;26:682–8.

[82] Rachid F. Maintenance repetitive transcranial magnetic stimulation (rTMS) for relapse prevention in with depression: A review. Psychiatry Res 2018;262:363–72.

[83] Sonmez AI, Camsari DD, Nandakumar AL, et al. Accelerated TMS for Depression: A systematic review and meta-analysis. Psychiatry Res 2019;273:770–81.

[84] Modirrousta M, Meek BP, Wikstrom SL. Efficacy of twice-daily vs once-daily sessions of repetitive transcranial magnetic stimulation in the treatment of major depressive disorder: a retrospective study. Neuropsychiatr Dis Treat 2018;14:309–16.

[85] Cole EJ, Stimpson KH, Bentzley BS, et al. Stanford Accelerated Intelligent Neuromodulation Therapy for Treatment-Resistant Depression. Am J Psychiatry 2020;177(8):716–26.

[86] Holtzheimer PE 3rd, McDonald WM, Mufti M, et al. Accelerated repetitive transcranial magnetic stimulation for treatment-resistant depression. Depress Anxiety 2010;27(10):960–3.

[87] Duprat R, Desmyter S, Rudi de R, et al. Accelerated intermittent theta burst stimulation treatment in medication-resistant major depression: A fast road to remission? J Affect Disord 2016;200:6–14.

[88] Caulfield KA. Is accelerated, high-dose theta burst stimulation a panacea for treatment-resistant depression? J Neurophysiol 2020;123(1):1–3.

[89] Anderson B, Mishory A, Nahas Z, et al. Tolerability and safety of high daily doses of repetitive transcranial magnetic stimulation in healthy young men. J ECT 2006; 22(1):49–53.

[90] George MS, Raman R, Benedek DM, et al. A two-site pilot randomized 3 day trial of high dose left prefrontal repetitive transcranial magnetic stimulation (rTMS) for suicidal inpatients. Brain Stimul 2014;7(3):421–31.

[91] Loo CK, McFarquhar TF, Mitchell PB. A review of the safety of repetitive transcranial magnetic stimulation as a clinical treatment for depression. Int J Neuropsychopharmacol 2008;11(1):131–47.

[92] Humaira A, Gao S, Wu L, et al. Side effects of trajectories in rTMS treatment for depression: 10 Hz vs. intermittent theta-burst stimulation. Brain Stimul 2019; 12(2):478.

[93] Borckardt JJ, Nahas ZH, Teal J, et al. The painfulness of active, but not sham, transcranial magnetic stimulation decreases rapidly over time: results from the double-blind phase of the OPT-TMS Trial. Brain Stimul 2013; 6(6):925–8.

[94] Lerner AJ, Wassermann EM, Tamir DI. Seizures from transcranial magnetic stimulation 2012-2016: Results of a survey of active laboratories and clinics. Clin Neurophysiol 2019;130(8):1409–16.

[95] Hunter AM, Minzenberg MJ, Cook IA, et al. Concomitant medication use and clinical outcome of repetitive Transcranial Magnetic Stimulation (rTMS) treatment of Major Depressive Disorder. Brain Behav 2019;9(5): e01275.

[96] Lefaucheur JP, André-Obadia N, Antal A, et al. Evidence-based guidelines on the therapeutic use of repetitive transcranial magnetic stimulation (rTMS). Clin Neurophysiol 2014;125(11):2150–206.
[97] Del Casale A, Kotzalidis GD, Rapinesi C, et al. Functional neuroimaging in obsessive-compulsive disorder. Neuropsychobiology 2011;64(2):61–85.
[98] Rapinesi C, Kotzalidis GD, Ferracuti S, et al. Brain Stimulation in Obsessive-Compulsive Disorder (OCD): A Systematic Review. Curr Neuropharmacol 2019;17(8): 787–807.
[99] Rehn S, Eslick GD, Brakoulias V. A Meta-Analysis of the Effectiveness of Different Cortical Targets Used in Repetitive Transcranial Magnetic Stimulation (rTMS) for the Treatment of Obsessive-Compulsive Disorder (OCD). Psychiatr Q 2018;89(3):645–65.
[100] Carmi L, Tendler A, Bystritsky A, et al. Efficacy and Safety of Deep Transcranial Magnetic Stimulation for Obsessive-Compulsive Disorder: A Prospective Multicenter Randomized Double-Blind Placebo-Controlled Trial. Am J Psychiatry 2019;176(11):931–8.
[101] Nathou C, Etard O, Dollfus S. Auditory verbal hallucinations in schizophrenia: current perspectives in brain stimulation treatments. Neuropsychiatr Dis Treat 2019;15:2105–17.
[102] Nathou C, Simon G, Dollfus S, et al. Cortical Anatomical Variations and Efficacy of rTMS in the Treatment of Auditory Hallucinations. Brain Stimul 2015;8(6): 1162–7.
[103] Koops S, Slotema CW, Kos C, et al. Predicting response to rTMS for auditory hallucinations: Younger patients and females do better. Schizophr Res 2018;195:583–4.
[104] Aleman A, Enriquez-Geppert S, Knegtering H, et al. Moderate effects of noninvasive brain stimulation of the frontal cortex for improving negative symptoms in schizophrenia: Meta-analysis of controlled trials. Neurosci Biobehav Rev 2018;89:111–8.
[105] Escelsior A, Belvederi Murri M, Calcagno P, et al. Effectiveness of Cerebellar Circuitry Modulation in Schizophrenia: A Systematic Review. J Nerv Ment Dis 2019; 207(11):977–86.
[106] Coles AS, Kozak K, George TP. A review of brain stimulation methods to treat substance use disorders. Am J Addict 2018;27(2):71–91.
[107] Dunlop K, Woodside B, Lam E, et al. Increases in frontostriatal connectivity are associated with response to dorsomedial repetitive transcranial magnetic stimulation in refractory binge/purge behaviors. Neuroimage Clin 2015;8:611–8.
[108] Dalton B, Bartholdy S, McClelland J, et al. Randomised controlled feasibility trial of real versus sham repetitive transcranial magnetic stimulation treatment in adults with severe and enduring anorexia nervosa: the TIARA study. BMJ Open 2018;8(7):e021531.
[109] Rodrigues PA, Zaninotto AL, Neville IS, et al. Transcranial magnetic stimulation for the treatment of anxiety disorder. Neuropsychiatr Dis Treat 2019;15:2743–61.
[110] Kan RLD, Zhang BBB, Zhang JJQ, et al. Non-invasive brain stimulation for posttraumatic stress disorder: a systematic review and meta-analysis. Transl Psychiatry 2020;10(1):168.
[111] Blumberger DM, Vila-Rodriguez F, Thorpe KE, et al. Effectiveness of theta burst versus high-frequency repetitive transcranial magnetic stimulation in patients with depression (THREE-D): a randomised non-inferiority trial. Lancet 2018;391(10131):1683–92.

Advances in Psychiatry and Behavioral Health 1 (2021) 185–203

ADVANCES IN PSYCHIATRY AND BEHAVIORAL HEALTH

Advances in Depression Management

Multifunctional Antidepressant Medications

Michael Ingram, MD[a], Gerald Maguire, MD[a], Stephen M. Stahl, MD, PhD, Dsc (Hon)[a,b,c,d,*]

[a]Department of Psychiatry, University of California Riverside; [b]Department of Psychiatry, University of California San Diego; [c]Department of Psychiatry, University of Cambridge; [d]Neuroscience Education Institute

KEYWORDS

• Antidepressants • Monoamines • Multifunctional • Combination treatments • Treatment resistance

KEY POINTS

- Combining drugs that target multiple monoaminergic sites has become the standard treatment for patients who do not respond to targeting single monoaminergic sites such as the serotonin transporter.
- One therapeutic strategy for treatment-resistant depression is to combine agents that target multiple monoamine transporters such as those for serotonin (SERT), norepinephrine (NET), and dopamine (DAT).
- Another strategy is to combine agents that target both monoamine transporters and monoamine receptors.
- Future use of this strategy may take this combination targeting approach earlier in the sequence of options for treatment resistance or even at the initiation of treatment for best possible outcomes.

INTRODUCTION

As our understanding of the neurobiology of psychiatric illness continues to evolve, so does the armamentarium of psychopharmacological treatments [1,2]. Unfortunately, the suboptimal efficacy of currently available antidepressants has left many providers and patients discouraged. It is a sobering statistic that up to one-third of patients in a real clinical practice setting never fill their first antidepressant prescription [3]. This wary attitude isn't helped by the results from the STAR*D trial in which only one-third of patients remitted on their first antidepressant treatment [4]. Even more disheartening is that roughly one-third of patients don't achieve remission of their symptoms after a year of treatment with adequate trials of 4 different antidepressants [1,4–7]. Yet, despite these discouraging statistics, physicians continue to prescribe these antidepressants because they can be lifesaving for many individuals. It takes only a short time in clinical practice to appreciate the powerful therapeutic potential of currently available antidepressants in many patients.

The traditional approach to treating depression has been to prescribe monotherapies in sequence, an approach congruent with currently recommended treatment guidelines [1,5–7]. However, given the lack of robust responses to monotherapy in many patients, the paradigm has rapidly shifted to using multiple antidepressants with different mechanisms—or using a single antidepressant with multiple mechanisms—earlier in treatment to achieve more robust responses [1,2,5–18]. If a serotonin selective reuptake inhibitor (SSRI) only gets us half way [5,8], perhaps adding another antidepressant targeting a different neurotransmitter system or even a completely different mechanism of action [11,16] would work synergistically to propel depressed patients out of the abyss—a concept akin to the treatment of multidrug-resistant tuberculosis, human immunodeficiency virus (HIV), and refractory hypertension.

*Corresponding author. Department of Psychiatry, University of California Riverside. *E-mail address:* smstahl@neiglobal.com

https://doi.org/10.1016/j.ypsc.2021.05.001
2667-3827/21/

Anecdotal experience [1,5–7,19] further legitimizes the powerful therapeutic effects of combining single-action and multiple-action agents despite the dearth of clinical trial data supporting these practices.

It would be naïve and overly simplistic to conceptualize a complex and multifactorial behavioral disorder like depression as a dysfunction in one neurotransmitter system or neural circuit. After all, the brain is an incomprehensibly intricate network of billions of neurons with trillions of connections with different functions depending on numerous variables—a network we are only beginning to understand. A more realistic conceptualization of depression, and likely many other behavioral disorders, is that depression is the final common pathway resulting from a dynamic interplay of various genes and environmental insults leading to aberrant activity in multiple systems and neural circuits [1,5,7].

Peculiar changes in gene expression and the resulting dysfunction of numerous neurotransmitter systems and circuits may be a more accurate view of how depression manifests [1,5,7]. The fine tuning of serotonergic, dopaminergic, and noradrenergic systems to varying degrees may be enough to solve the puzzle of depression in some patients but not in others. With this working framework, we turn now to a review of the various mechanisms for treating depression followed by a discussion of the potential positive and negative effects of combining different mechanisms using one or more medications to achieve an antidepressant response.

MULTIFUNCTIONAL ANTIDEPRESSANT MECHANISMS

Monoamine reuptake inhibition

Monoamine neurotransmitters such as serotonin, norepinephrine, and dopamine represent a small fraction of all neurotransmitters in the brain but have very important roles in the modulation and regulation of neurotransmission in a variety of neurocircuits. Monoamines released from presynaptic nerve terminals must be rapidly removed from the synaptic cleft to prepare for the next impulse. The rapid removal of monoamine neurotransmitters from the synaptic cleft occurs via multiple mechanisms, which include active transport back into the presynaptic nerve terminal by monoamine transporters, passive diffusion, and enzymatic degradation [5].

Monoamine transporters located at the presynaptic nerve terminals are named after the specific monoamine they remove from the synaptic cleft. However, the specificity of monoamine transporters is variable (ie, multiple monoamines can be taken up by a single monoamine transporter). For example, norepinephrine transporters (NETs) show specificity for both norepinephrine and dopamine, which may be important for the removal of both norepinephrine and dopamine in regions of the brain such as the prefrontal cortex, where dopamine transporters are expressed at relatively low levels [5]. Blocking monoamine transporters selectively or in combination leads to accumulation of these neurotransmitters in the synaptic cleft and theoretically contributes, in part, to both the therapeutic and adverse effects of many psychotropic medications (eg, antidepressants [1,5–7]).

As described below, varying degrees and combinations of serotonin, norepinephrine, and dopamine reuptake inhibition, for example, SSRIs, serotonin norepinephrine reuptake inhibitors (SNRI), norepinephrine reuptake inhibitors (NRIs), and norepinephrine dopamine reuptake inhibitors (NDRIs) in certain brain regions may provide additive or even synergistic effects—a rational argument for antidepressant polypharmacy in patients unresponsive to a single mechanism or the use of "multimodal" antidepressants with multiple mechanisms built in to a single molecule [1,2,5–7,10,15–18].

Combining types of monoamine reuptake inhibition for multifunctional treatment of depression

Serotonin reuptake inhibition

The monoamine hypothesis of depression states that monoamines such as serotonin and norepinephrine may be deficient at both the somatodendritic region and in the synaptic cleft of serotonin-producing neurons [5] (Fig. 1A). Psychotropic medications like the widely used selective serotonin reuptake inhibitors (SSRIs) selectively block serotonin transporters (SERTs) at both the somatodendritic region (Fig. 1B, C) and the nerve terminal region (Fig. 1D), resulting in the accumulation of serotonin in those areas [5,8]. Interestingly, serotonin levels rise to a greater degree at the somatodendritic end of serotonin neurons in the midbrain raphe nuclei (see Fig. 1B) than the nerve terminal regions when antidepressants like SSRIs are initiated [5]. Even more perplexing is the observation that medications like SSRIs that selectively block SERTs do not immediately produce improvements in mood. These findings suggest that elevation of serotonin at both the somatodendritic and synaptic cleft is only a piece of the desired antidepressant response [5].

The neurotransmitter receptor hypothesis of depression may explain the delayed onset of mood changes observed with many antidepressants [5,7]. The receptor hypothesis of depression proposes that monoamine

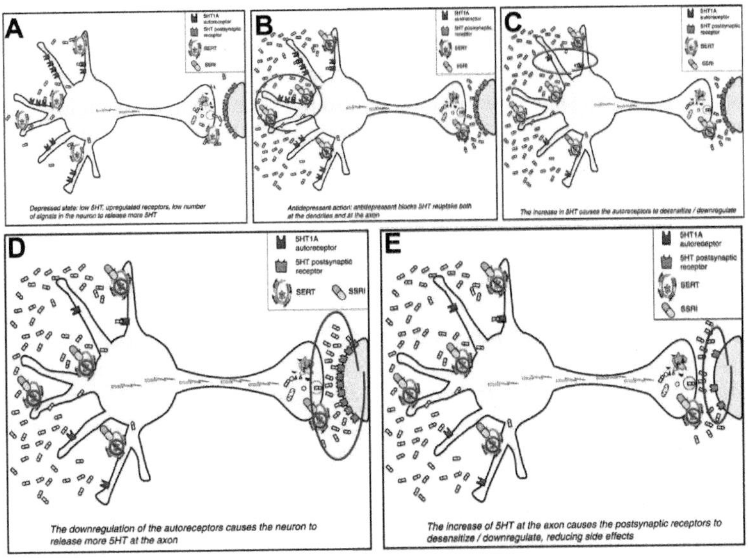

FIG. 1 (*A*) Mechanism of action of selective serotonin reuptake inhibitors (SSRIs), part 1. Depicted here is a serotonin (5HT) neuron in a depressed patient. In depression, the 5HT neuron is conceptualized as having a relative deficiency of the neurotransmitter 5HT. Also, the number of 5HT receptors is upregulated, including presynaptic 5HT1A autoreceptors as well as postsynaptic 5HT receptors. (*B*) Mechanism of action of selective serotonin reuptake inhibitors (SSRIs), part 2. When an SSRI is administered, it immediately blocks the serotonin reuptake pump [see icon of an SSRI drug capsule blocking the reuptake pump, or serotonin transporter (SERT)]. However, this causes serotonin to increase initially only in the somatodendritic area of the serotonin neuron (left) and not very much in the axon terminals (right). (*C*) Mechanism of action of selective serotonin reuptake inhibitors (SSRIs), part 3. The consequence of serotonin increasing in the somatodendritic area of the serotonin (5HT) neuron, as depicted in Figs. 7–14, is that the somatodendritic 5HT1A autoreceptors desensitize or downregulate (*red circle*). (*D*). Mechanism of action of selective serotonin reuptake inhibitors (SSRIs), part 4. Once the somatodendritic receptors downregulate, as depicted in Figs. 7–15, there is no longer inhibition of impulse flow in the serotonin (5HT) neuron. Thus, neuronal impulse flow is turned on. The consequence of this is release of 5HT in the axon terminal (*red circle*). However, this increase is delayed as compared with the increase of 5HT in the somatodendritic areas of the 5HT neuron, depicted in Figs. 7–14. This delay is the result of the time it takes for somatodendritic 5HT to downregulate the 5HT1A autoreceptors and turn on neuronal impulse flow in the 5HT neuron. This delay may explain why antidepressants do not relieve depression immediately. It is also the reason why the mechanism of action of antidepressants may be linked to increasing neuronal impulse flow in 5HT neurons, with 5HT levels increasing at axon terminals before an SSRI can exert its antidepressant effects. (*E*) Mechanism of action of selective serotonin reuptake inhibitors (SSRIs), part 5. Finally, once the SSRIs have blocked the reuptake pump [or serotonin transporter (SERT) in Figs. 7–14], increased somatodendritic serotonin (5HT) (see Figs. 7–14), desensitized somatodendritic 5HT1A autoreceptors (see Figs. 7–15), turned on neuronal impulse flow (see Figs. 7–16), and increased release of 5HT from axon terminals (Figs. 7–16), the final step (shown here) may be the desensitization of postsynaptic 5HT receptors. This desensitization may mediate the reduction of side effects of SSRIs as tolerance develops.

receptors such as postsynaptic serotonin receptors and presynaptic somatodendritic $5HT_{1A}$ autoreceptors may be upregulated in the depressed brain (see Fig. 1A) [5]. Recall that somatodendritic $5HT_{1A}$ autoreceptors, when stimulated by serotonin, decrease the firing rate of serotonin neurons. Therefore, overexpression of $5HT_{1A}$ receptors may account for the dysregulated firing patterns of neurons in certain areas of the depressed brain, ultimately affecting information processing and the development of specific symptoms, depending upon which regions are affected (see Fig. 1A).

Acute administration of medications that block serotonin transporters (SERTs) leads to immediate increases in serotonin levels at the somatodendritic region more so than the nerve terminal region [5] (see Fig. 1B). Repeated perturbation of $5HT_{1A}$ autoreceptors by elevated serotonin levels at the somatodendritic region may lead to the desensitization and downregulation of $5HT_{1A}$ autoreceptors and the disinhibition of serotonin firing (see Fig. 1C). The increased firing rate of serotonin neurons due to downregulation of somatodendritic $5HT_{1A}$ autoreceptors in combination with the potent inhibition of serotonin transporters at the nerve terminal may lead to robust increases in serotonin levels in the synaptic cleft of the nerve terminal regions (see Fig. 1D) and may account for the initial side effects observed when initiating serotonin reuptake inhibitors (anxiety, nausea, and jitteriness). The delayed therapeutic effect of antidepressants may be explained, in part, by the slow downregulation of postsynaptic serotonin receptors due to persistently elevated serotonin levels in the synaptic cleft as a result of serotonin reuptake inhibition (Fig. 1E) [5].

Combining serotonin and norepinephrine reuptake inhibition

Norepinephrine is a catecholamine synthesized from tyrosine and stored in synaptic vesicles located at the nerve terminal of norepinephrine neurons (Fig. 2) [5]. Once released, norepinephrine acts on postsynaptic receptors to mediate changes in signal transduction and eventually postsynaptic gene expression [5]. Like serotonin, norepinephrine is rapidly removed from the synaptic cleft by passive diffusion, active reuptake by presynaptic norepinephrine transporters (NETs) (Fig. 3), or enzymatic degradation by metabolizing enzymes such as monoamine oxidase (MAO) and catechol-*O*-methyltransferase (COMT) (Fig. 4) [5,7].

Most of the norepinephrine neurons which project to numerous cortical and subcortical regions originate in a region of the pons called the locus coeruleus [1,5,7]. However, there are also descending noradrenergic (and serotonergic) neurons which also originate in brainstem nuclei and synapse in the dorsal horn of the spinal cord to where they appear to modulate afferent pain signals from the periphery [7,15]. Blockade of norepinephrine transporters results in the accumulation of norepinephrine in the synaptic cleft, similar to the increased serotonin seen with blockade of the serotonin transporter (SERT) described above.

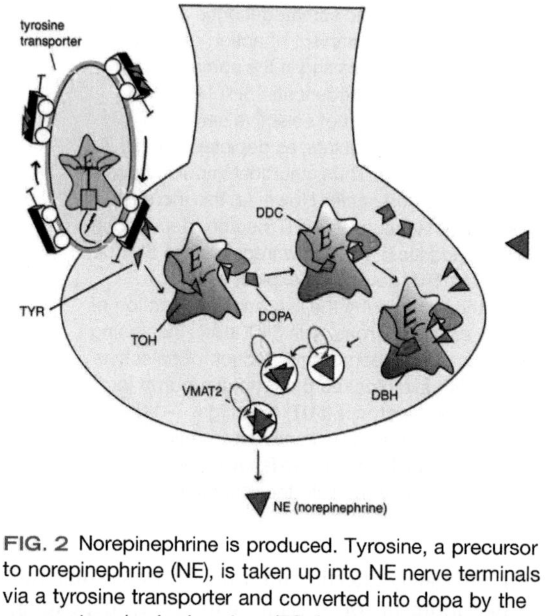

FIG. 2 Norepinephrine is produced. Tyrosine, a precursor to norepinephrine (NE), is taken up into NE nerve terminals via a tyrosine transporter and converted into dopa by the enzyme tyrosine hydroxylase (TOH). Dopa is then converted into dopamine (DA) by the enzyme dopa decarboxylase (DDC). Finally, DA is converted into NE by dopamine beta hydroxylase (DBH). After synthesis, NE is packaged into synaptic vesicles via the vesicular monoamine transporter (VMAT2) and stored there until its release into the synapse during neurotransmission.

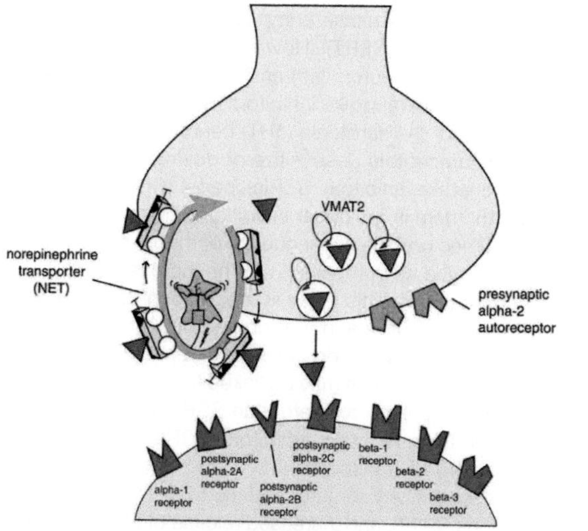

FIG. 3 Norepinephrine receptors. Shown here are receptors for norepinephrine that regulate its neurotransmission. The norepinephrine transporter (NET) exists presynaptically and is responsible for clearing excess norepinephrine out of the synapse. The vesicular monoamine transporter (VMAT2) takes norepinephrine up into synaptic vesicles and stores it for future neurotransmission. There is also a presynaptic alpha 2 autoreceptor, which regulates release of norepinephrine from the presynaptic neuron. In addition, there are several postsynaptic receptors. These include alpha 1, alpha 2A, alpha 2B, alpha 2C, beta 1, beta 2, and beta 3 receptors.

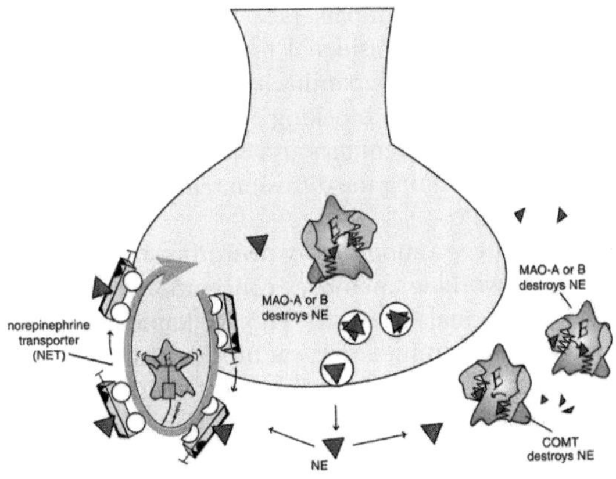

FIG. 4 Norepinephrine's action is terminated. Norepinephrine's action can be terminated through multiple mechanisms. Dopamine can be transported out of the synaptic cleft and back into the presynaptic neuron via the norepinephrine transporter (NET), where it may be repackaged for future use. Alternatively, norepinephrine may be broken down extracellularly via the enzyme catechol-O-methyl-transferase (COMT). Other enzymes that break down norepinephrine are monoamine oxidase A (MAO-A) and monoamine oxidase B (MAO-B), which are present in mitochondria both within the presynaptic neuron and in other cells, including neurons and glia.

Inhibiting NET in various brain circuits in certain individuals may restore the dysregulated or "deficient" noradrenergic neurotransmission in regions associated with specific depressive symptoms such as fatigue, difficulty concentrating, and amotivation [5,10–14]. Noradrenergic modulation of afferent pain signals in the dorsal horn of the spinal cord may partially explain the proven efficacy of some tricyclic antidepressants and duloxetine, a serotonin norepinephrine reuptake inhibitor, for alleviating pain with or without depression [5,14].

If boosting serotonergic neurotransmission in various brain areas alleviates depressive symptoms in some individuals, then one wonders whether boosting both serotonin and norepinephrine neurotransmission would be even better (Fig. 5), which explains the reasoning behind developing drugs that inhibit both serotonin and norepinephrine transporters, also called the serotonin norepinephrine reuptake inhibitors (SNRIs). To date, clinical trials have not demonstrated superior efficacy of SNRIs over SSRIs, but anecdotal reports and existing trends have suggested that SNRIs may be more effective agents [10–12,14].

Combining norepinephrine and dopamine reuptake inhibition

Initially, there was debate whether norepinephrine (NE) or serotonin (5HT) was the more important deficiency in the monoamine hypothesis of depression, and dopamine was relatively neglected. Now the monoamine theory suggests that boosting any or all of the 3 monoamines (serotonin, norepinephrine, dopamine) could have therapeutic benefits in depression.

As mentioned previously, norepinephrine transporters (NETs) are widely expressed in the prefrontal cortex and have specificity for dopamine as well as norepinephrine (Fig. 6A) [5]. When dopamine is released in the prefrontal cortex, there are few dopamine transporters (DATs) for the reuptake of dopamine

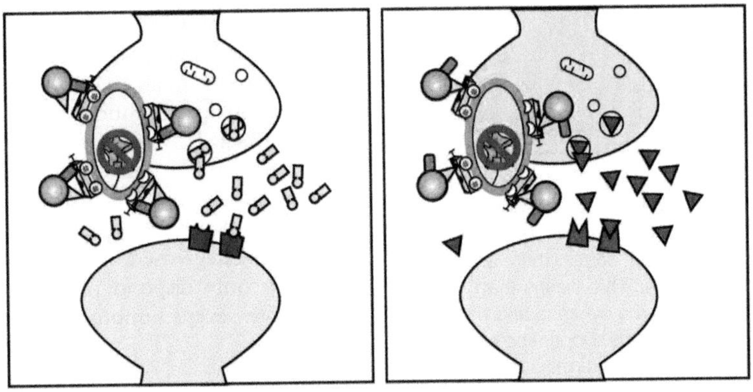

FIG. 5 SNRI actions. The dual actions of the serotonin norepinephrine reuptake inhibitors (SNRIs) are shown. Both the serotonin reuptake inhibitor (SRI) portion of the SNRI molecule (*left panel*) and the norepinephrine reuptake inhibitor (NRI) portion of the SNRI molecule (*right panel*) are inserted into their respective reuptake pumps. Consequently, both pumps are blocked, and the drug mediates an antidepressant effect.

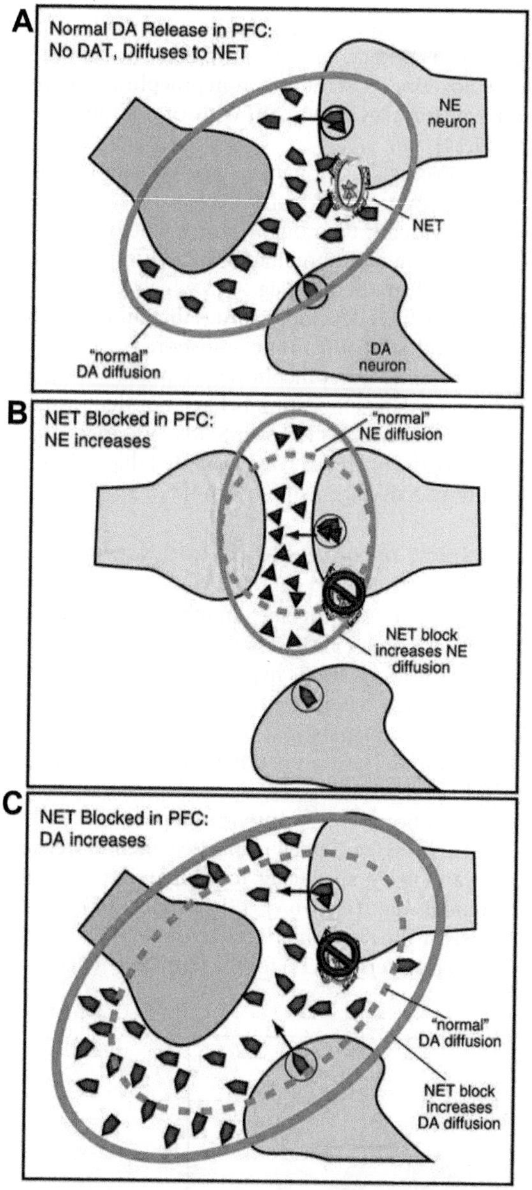

FIG. 6 Norepinephrine transporter blockade and dopamine in the prefrontal cortex. (*A*) Although there are abundant serotonin transporters (SERTs) and norepinephrine transporters (NETs) in the prefrontal cortex, there are very few dopamine transporters (DATs). This means that dopamine can diffuse away from the synapse and therefore exert its actions within a larger radius. Dopamine's actions are terminated at norepinephrine axon terminals, because DA is taken up by NET. (*B*) NET blockade in the prefrontal cortex leads to an increase in synaptic norepinephrine, thus increasing norepinephrine's diffusion radius. (*C*) Because NET takes up dopamine as well as norepinephrine, NET blockade also leads to an increase in synaptic dopamine, further increasing its diffusion radius. Thus, agents that block NET increase norepinephrine throughout the brain and both norepinephrine and dopamine in the prefrontal cortex.

into presynaptic terminals (see Fig. 6A) [5]. Consequently, NETs are considered the primary mechanism for the reuptake of dopamine that has diffused away from its synapse and blocking NETs in the prefrontal cortex indirectly potentiates dopaminergic neurotransmission by expanding the diffusion radius of dopamine (see Fig. 6A) [5].

Dopamine is a modulatory neurotransmitter associated with working memory, concentration, salience, and motivational behaviors [1,5,7]. Rapid elevations in synaptic dopamine levels via blockade of dopamine transporters (DATs) or increased dopamine release in the nucleus accumbens contributes to the pleasurable and reinforcing aspects of most drugs of abuse [1,5,7]. However, decreased dopaminergic tone in the prefrontal circuits and nucleus accumbens could theoretically explain the fatigue, amotivation, concentration deficits, and anhedonia seen in many depressed patients [1,5,7]. It appears the solution would be a medication that enhances dopaminergic transmission just enough in the nucleus accumbens and prefrontal circuits to relieve depressive symptoms without the euphoric and reinforcing effects of too much dopamine (Fig. 6B, C). Antidepressants such as venlafaxine (SNRI) [12,14], bupropion (NDRI) [13], and atomoxetine (NRI) [5] enhance dopaminergic transmission indirectly in the frontal cortex by the mechanism described above without the euphoria or reinforcing effects. These antidepressants may be best suited for patients feeling lethargic, unmotivated, and anhedonic.

Adding an SNRI or SSRI with an NDRI: A triple-action combination

If targeting 2 monoamine neurotransmitters is better than 1, then maybe 3 is best. Triple-action antidepressant therapy by modulating all 3 monoamines (5HT, DA, and NE) would be predicted to occur by combining either an SSRI with an NDRI, perhaps the most popular combination in US antidepressant psychopharmacology (Fig. 7A), or by combining an SNRI with an NDRI (Fig. 7B), providing even more noradrenergic and dopaminergic action [7,10,13–16]. The combination of sertraline, an SSRI, and bupropion, an NDRI, is a common strategy used by many clinicians for individuals who only respond partially to one agent, who have more severe symptoms, or who would benefit

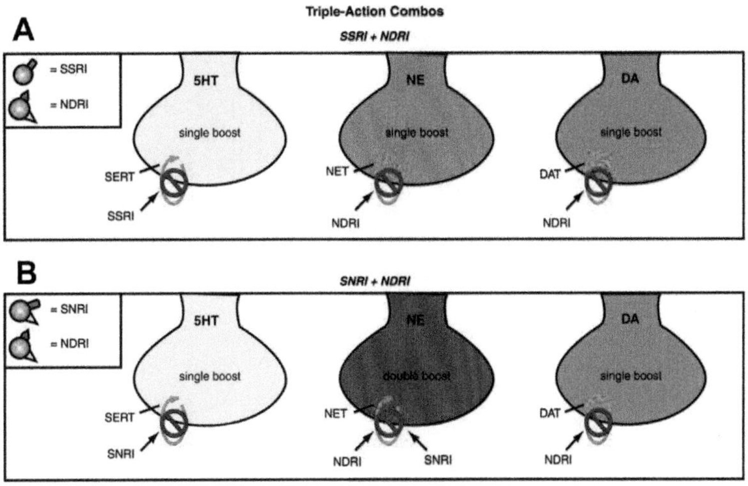

FIG. 7 (*A*). SSRI plus NDRI. Selective serotonin reuptake inhibitor (SSRI) plus a norepinephrine dopamine reuptake inhibitor (NDRI) leads to a single boost for serotonin (5HT), norepinephrine (NE), and dopamine (DA). (*B*). SNRI plus NDRI. Serotonin norepinephrine reuptake inhibitor (SNRI) plus a norepinephrine dopamine reuptake inhibitor (NDRI) leads to a single boost for serotonin (5HT), a double boost for norepinephrine (NE), and a single boost for dopamine (DA).

from the additional dopaminergic and noradrenergic boost to help alleviate fatigue, poor concentration, or even the sexual side effects of serotonergic antidepressants.

Arousal combinations: SNRI + stimulant

The frequent complaints of residual fatigue, loss of energy, low motivation, decreased libido, and poor concentration may be approached by combining either a stimulant or modafinil with an SNRI to recruit triple monoamine action with the focus on enhancing dopaminergic neurotransmission (Fig. 8) [1,5–7]. The long-acting stimulant lisdexamfetamine, which links the amino acid lysine to the stimulant D-amphetamine, slows the delivery and potentially reduces the abuse liability of D-amphetamine after oral administration [6].

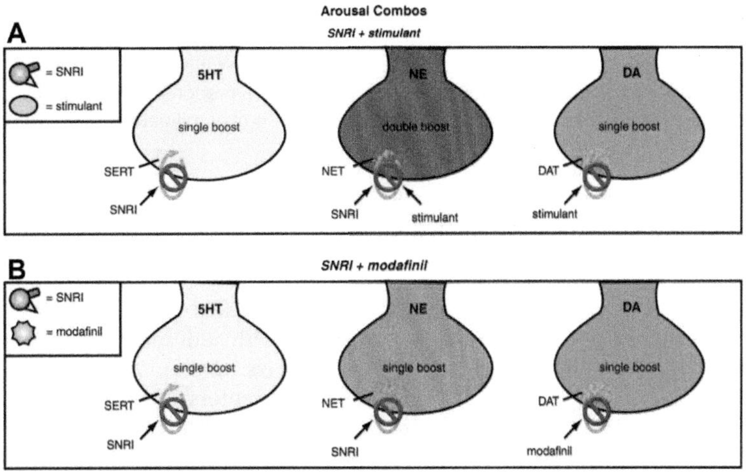

FIG. 8 (*A*) SNRI plus stimulant. Here serotonin (5HT) and dopamine (DA) are single-boosted and norepinephrine (NE) is double-boosted. (*B*) SNRI plus modafinil. Here serotonin (5HT) and norepinephrine (NE) are single-boosted by the serotonin norepinephrine reuptake inhibitor (SNRI), while dopamine (DA) is single-boosted by modafinil.

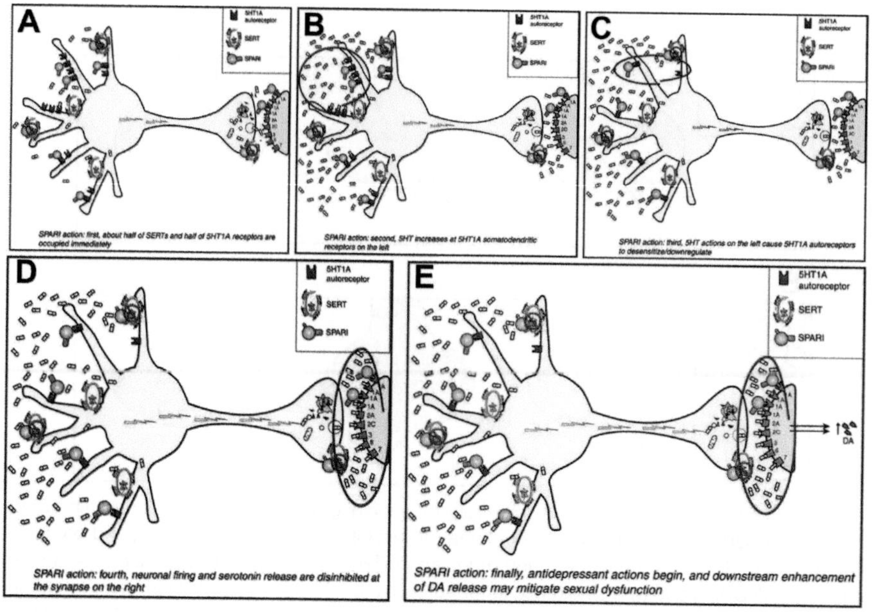

FIG. 9 (*A*) Mechanism of action of serotonin partial agonist reuptake inhibitors (SPARIs), part 1. When an SPARI is administered, about half of serotonin transporters (SERTs) and half of serotonin 1A (5HT1A) receptors are occupied immediately. (*B*) Mechanism of action of serotonin partial agonist reuptake inhibitors (SPARIs), part 2. Blockade of the serotonin transporter (SERT) causes serotonin to increase initially in the somatodendritic area of the serotonin neuron (*left*). (*C*) Mechanism of action of serotonin partial agonist reuptake inhibitors (SPARIs), part 3. The consequence of serotonin increasing in the somatodendritic area of the serotonin (5HT) neuron, as depicted in Fig. 7-26, is that the somatodendritic 5HT1A autoreceptors desensitize or downregulate (*red circle*). (*D*) Mechanism of action of serotonin partial agonist reuptake inhibitors (SPARIs), part 4. Once the somatodendritic receptors downregulate, as depicted in Fig. 7-27, there is no longer inhibition of impulse flow in the serotonin (5HT) neuron. Thus, neuronal impulse flow is turned on. The consequence of this is release of 5HT in the axon terminal (*red circle*). (*E*) Mechanism of action of serotonin partial agonist reuptake inhibitors (SPARIs), part 5. Finally, once the SPARIs have blocked the serotonin transporter (SERT) (*B*), increased somatodendritic serotonin (5HT) (*C*), desensitized somatodendritic 5HT1A autoreceptors (Fig. 7-27), turned on neuronal impulse flow (*D*), and increased release of 5HT from axon terminals (*E*), the final step (shown here, *red circle*) may be the desensitization of postsynaptic 5HT receptors. This timeframe correlates with antidepressant action. In addition, the predominance of 5HT1A actions may lead to downstream enhancement of dopamine (DA) release, which may mitigate sexual dysfunction.

Given its simple once-daily dosing schedule, long half-life, and reduced abuse potential, lisdexamfetamine is a good choice for adults and adolescents with attention deficit hyperactivity disorder or perhaps as an augmenting agent for patients with treatment-resistant depression [1,5,6].

Combining serotonin reuptake inhibition with agonist or antagonist actions at multiple serotonin receptor subtypes

Serotonin receptors

Before discussing the various combinations of serotonin reuptake inhibition and serotonin receptor agonism and antagonism, we will briefly review the serotonin receptors relevant to psychopharmacology. Approximately 14 different serotonin receptors have been identified to date, which are classified as $5HT_{1-7}$ with additional subtypes within each numeric class (Figs. 9–14). All serotonin receptors, except $5HT_3$ receptors, are G-protein-coupled receptors (GPCRs); $5HT_{1A}$ receptors were mentioned previously. $5HT_{1B/D}$ receptors are primarily autoreceptors located on the presynaptic nerve terminals of serotonin neurons and decrease the amount of serotonin released with each nerve impulse, providing a negative feedback mechanism for serotonin release.

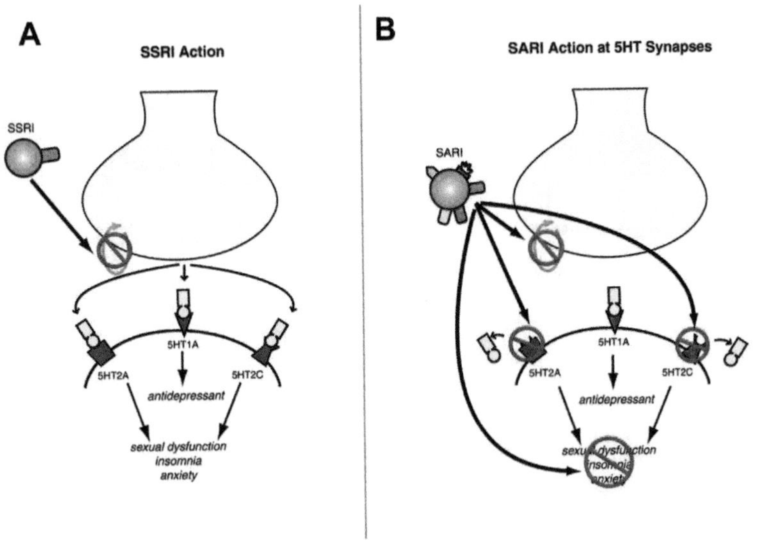

FIG. 10 SSRI versus SARI. (*Left*) Inhibition of the serotonin transporter (SERT) by a selective serotonin reuptake inhibitor (SSRI) at the presynaptic neuron increases serotonin at all receptors, with 5HT1A-mediated antidepressant actions but also 5HT2A- and 5HT2C-mediated sexual dysfunction, insomnia, and anxiety. (*Right*) SERT inhibition by a serotonin 2A antagonist/reuptake inhibitor (SARI) at the presynaptic neuron increases serotonin at 5HT1A receptors, where it leads to antidepressant actions. However, SARI action also blocks serotonin actions at 5HT2A and 5HT2C receptors, thus failing to cause sexual dysfunction, insomnia, or anxiety. In fact, these blocking actions at 5HT2A and 5HT2C receptors can improve insomnia and anxiety, and theoretically can exert antidepressant actions of their own.

$5HT_{1B/D}$ agonists, such as sumatriptan, are widely used to treat migraines [1,5,7].

$5HT_{2A}$ receptors are almost exclusively postsynaptic and are thought to be involved in the hallucinogenic properties of drugs such as LSD and the hallucinatory phenomena commonly associated with Parkinson disease [1,5,20]. $5HT_{2A}$ receptors are important in the regulation of dopamine release in the striatum where antagonism of these receptors hypothetically mitigates the risk of extrapyramidal side effects associated with antipsychotics [5].

$5HT_{2C}$ receptors are widespread in the central nervous system, particularly the choroid plexus, the hypothalamus, and the cerebral cortex. When $5HT_{2C}$ receptors are knocked out in rodent models or antagonized pharmacologically in humans, there appears to be significant weight gain [1,5,14]. In addition, $5HT_{2C}$ receptors located on GABA interneurons in the brainstem modulate the release of norepinephrine and dopamine in the prefrontal cortex (PFC), and will be discussed later.

Interestingly, both $5HT_{2A}$ and $5HT_{2C}$ receptors have been implicated in the common side effects associated with initiating SSRIs such as sexual dysfunction, insomnia, and anxiety [1,5,7]. Not surprisingly, antidepressants with both $5HT_{2A}$ and $5HT_{2C}$ antagonism such as mirtazapine [9], trazodone [15] and nefazodone are associated with less insomnia, anxiety, and sexual dysfunction than SSRIs and SNRIs (see Fig. 10).

$5HT_3$ receptors are postsynaptic ionotropic receptors that regulate GABA interneurons in various brain areas which, in turn, regulate other neurotransmitter systems such as glutamate, acetylcholine, norepinephrine, dopamine, histamine, and serotonin itself [5]. Mechanisms relevant to antidepressants will be discussed in the relevant sections below.

$5HT_3$ receptors are also highly expressed both in the circumventricular organs and peripherally in the gut, where they regulate the vomiting reflex and bowel motility, respectively [5]. Antiemetics like ondansetron are thought to work via $5HT_3$ antagonism to relieve nausea associated with medications or chemotherapeutic agents. $5HT_3$ antagonism theoretically reduces the nausea and gastrointestinal side effects associated with initiating serotonergic antidepressants.

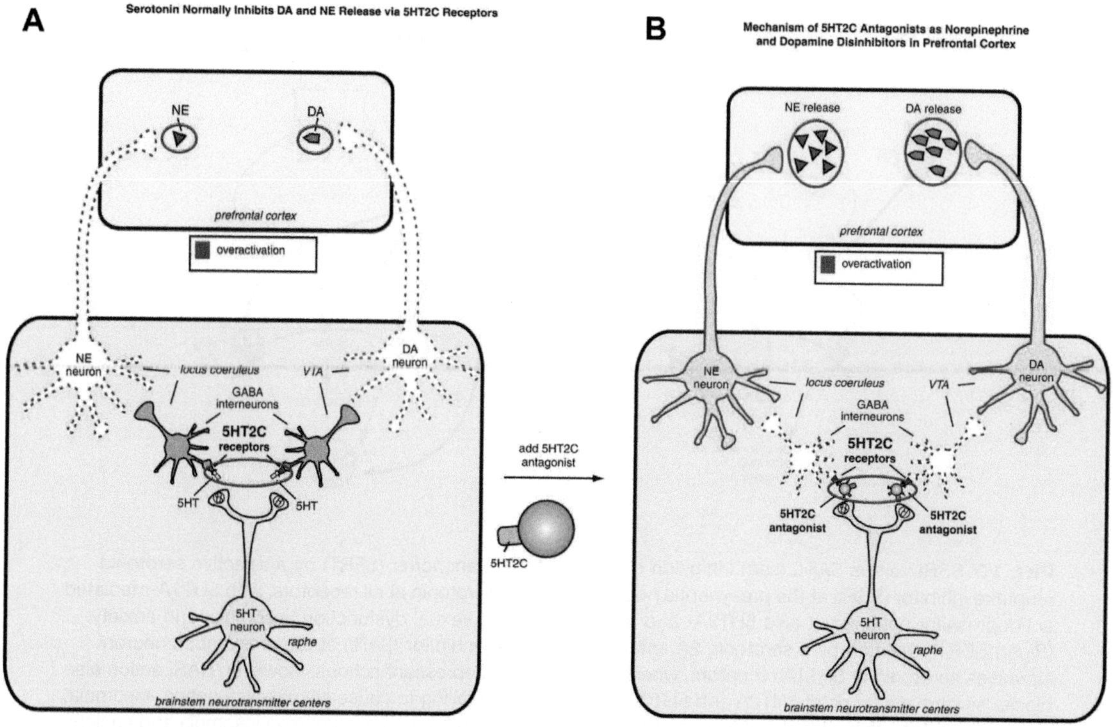

FIG. 11 (*A*) Serotonin inhibits norepinephrine and dopamine release. Normally, serotonin binding at 5HT2C receptors on gamma-aminobutyric acid (GABA) interneurons (*bottom red circle*) inhibits norepinephrine and dopamine release in the prefrontal cortex (*top red circle*). (*B*) 5HT2C antagonists disinhibit norepinephrine and dopamine release. When a 5HT2C antagonist binds to 5HT2C receptors on GABA interneurons (*bottom red circle*), it prevents serotonin from binding there and thus prevents inhibition of norepinephrine and dopamine release in the prefrontal cortex; in other words, it disinhibits their release (*top red circle*).

Lastly, $5HT_7$ receptors, like $5HT_{2C}$ receptors, are expressed on GABA interneurons in the brainstem and cortex, where they modulate serotonin and glutamate release in the prefrontal cortex. Antagonism of $5HT_7$ receptors may have antidepressant effects as discussed below [5].

Combining serotonin reuptake inhibition with serotonin 1A partial agonism (SPARI)

The combination of serotonin reuptake inhibition and serotonin $5HT_{1A}$ partial agonism has been used by many clinicians to boost antidepressant response and mitigate side effects [1,5,7,8,10,11,17]. Recall that $5HT_{1A}$ autoreceptors located at the somatodendritic end of serotonin neurons act as a negative feedback mechanism for serotonin release by inhibiting the firing rate of serotonin neurons. As discussed earlier, repeated stimulation of somatodendritic $5HT_{1A}$ autoreceptors on serotonin neurons in the dorsal raphe nucleus leads to desensitization and downregulation of these receptors, resulting in increased serotonin neuronal impulse flow and serotonin release. Stimulation of postsynaptic $5HT_{1A}$ receptors in the cortex and raphe nucleus has downstream effects enhancing dopamine release and may hypothetically explain the decreased sexual side effects seen with medications that stimulate postsynaptic $5HT_{1A}$ receptors [13].

By combining $5HT_{1A}$ partial agonism with SERT inhibition, one can appreciate the hypothetical additive or synergistic enhancement of serotonin release by hastening the downregulation of $5HT_{1A}$ autoreceptors (see Fig. 9). This combination, in theory, would lead to a faster and more robust response than either action alone.

Adding the $5HT_{1A}$ partial agonist properties of buspirone to an SSRI or SNRI to mitigate side effects and/or to boost the antidepressant effects in patients unresponsive to monotherapy has become common practice [1,4], leading to the development of medications such as vilazodone [18] and vortioxetine [2] with both actions in one medication. Many atypical antipsychotics such as aripiprazole, brexpiprazole, cariprazine, and quetiapine

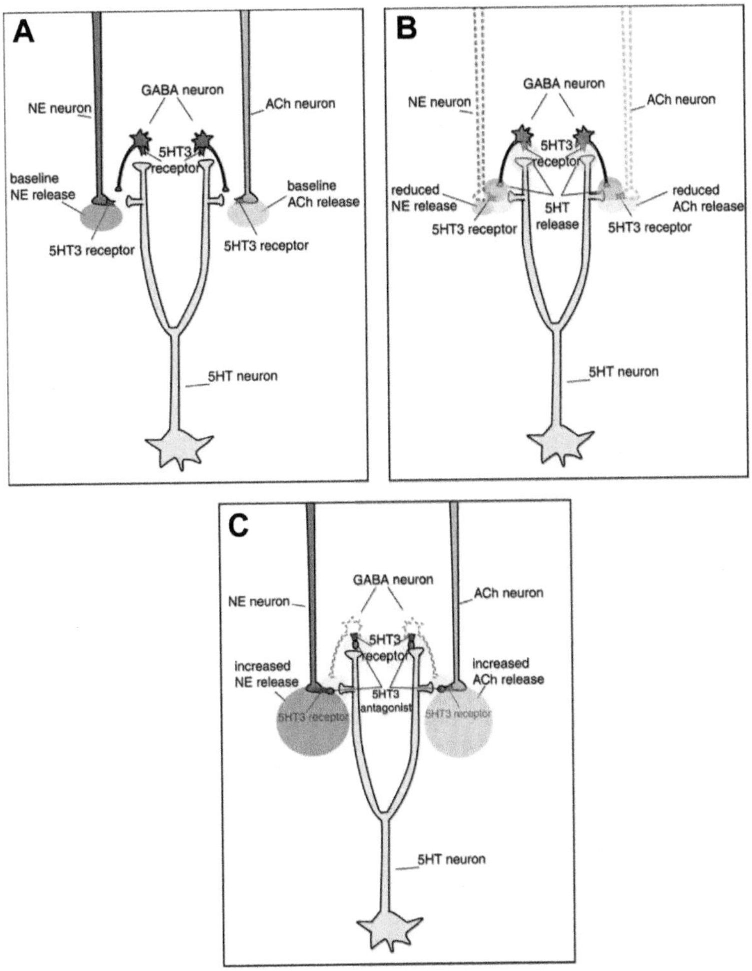

FIG. 12 5HT3 antagonists increase norepinephrine and acetylcholine release. (*A*) Serotonergic neurons synapse with noradrenergic neurons, cholinergic neurons, and GABA-ergic interneurons, all of which contain serotonin 3 (5HT3) receptors. (*B*) When serotonin is released, it binds to 5HT3 receptors on GABA-ergic neurons, which release GABA onto noradrenergic and cholinergic neurons, thus reducing release of norepinephrine and acetylcholine, respectively. In addition, serotonin may bind to 5HT3 receptors on noradrenergic and cholinergic neurons, further reducing release of those neurotransmitters. (*C*) A 5HT3 antagonist binding at GABA-ergic neurons inhibits GABA release, which in turn disinhibits (or turns on) noradrenergic and cholinergic neurons, leading to release of norepinephrine and acetylcholine, respectively. Likewise, a 5HT3 antagonist binding directly at noradrenergic and cholinergic neurons prevents serotonin from binding there and inhibiting release of their neurotransmitters.

have prominent $5HT_{1A}$ partial agonist actions among their many pharmacologic properties [1,5–7] and are commonly used as augmentation agents in depressed patients unresponsive to an SSRI or SNRI. Finally, one of the newer antidepressants vortioxetine [2,5] combines $5HT_{1A}$ agonism with 5HT reuptake inhibition in addition to several other actions at serotonin receptors which are discussed below [1,5,6].

Combining serotonin reuptake inhibition with serotonin receptor antagonism

Combining serotonin reuptake inhibition with 5HT2A and/or 5HT2C antagonism

When $5HT_{2C}$ receptors located on GABA interneurons in the brainstem are stimulated by serotonin they stimulate GABA interneurons acting on norepinephrine and dopamine neurons in the locus coeruleus and ventral

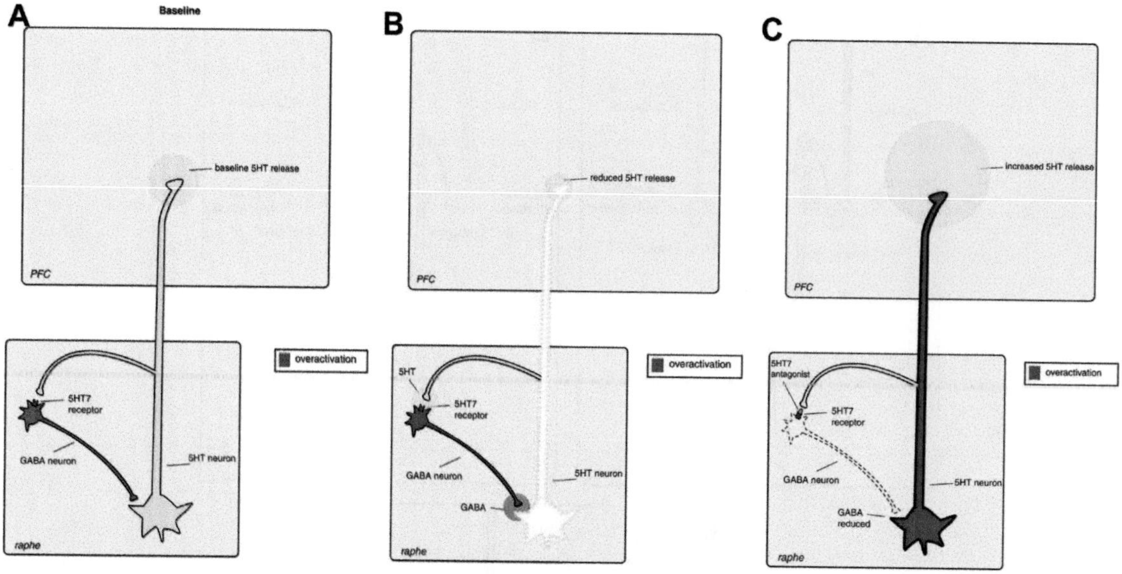

FIG. 13 (*A*) Function of 5HT7 receptors in the raphe nucleus. Shown here is a serotonergic neuron projecting from the raphe nucleus to the prefrontal cortex, where it releases serotonin. The release of serotonin is regulated in part by GABA-ergic neurons within the raphe nucleus that contains 5HT7 receptors. (*B*) Stimulation of 5HT7 receptors in the raphe reduces serotonin release. When serotonin binds to 5HT7 receptors on GABA-ergic interneurons within the raphe nucleus, this activates the GABA neuron (indicated by the red color of the neuron) to release GABA. GABA then inhibits serotonergic projections from the raphe nucleus to the prefrontal cortex, thus reducing serotonin release there (indicated by the dotted outline of the serotonin neuron). (*C*) Blockade of 5HT7 receptors in the raphe nucleus increases serotonin release. If 5HT7 receptors on GABA-ergic interneurons in the raphe nucleus are blocked, then GABA release is inhibited (indicated by the dotted outline of the GABA neuron). Without the presence of GABA, the serotonergic projection from the raphe nucleus to the prefrontal cortex can become overactivated (indicated by the red color of the neuron), leading to increased serotonin release in the prefrontal cortex.

tegmental area, respectively, which subsequently inhibits norepinephrine and dopamine projections to the prefrontal cortex (see Fig. 11A) [5,7]. By inhibiting $5HT_{2C}$ receptors, both norepinephrine and dopamine neurons projecting to the prefrontal cortex are disinhibited and increase their monoamines there (see Fig. 11B) [5]. This may lead to beneficial changes in mood and may partially explain the antidepressant mechanism of $5HT_{2C}$ antagonists. The addition of an SSRI/SNRI to a 5HT2A/5HT2C antagonist may have additive or synergistic antidepressant effects when an SSRI or SNRI alone is not enough [5,9,11,15–18]. However, as discussed previously, $5HT_{2C}$ receptors are also located in the hypothalamus, where antagonism has been associated with weight gain. The propensity toward weight gain with $5HT_{2C}$ antagonists may be beneficial for elderly cachectic patients and/or intolerable for those concerned about weight gain.

Some antidepressants such as trazodone [15] have both SERT inhibition and $5HT_{2A}/5HT_{2C}$ antagonism properties built in (see Fig. 10B) [5]. The combination of SERT inhibition with $5HT_{2A}/5HT_{2C}$ antagonism may provide some protection from, or treatment of, the initial side effects seen with SSRI/SNRIs, as discussed above, and potentiate the antidepressant effect of serotonin reuptake inhibition either additively or synergistically [5,15].

It is worth mentioning that pimavanserin, a selective $5HT_{2A}$ and $5HT_{2C}$ antagonist approved for psychosis associated with Parkinson disease [5,20] has preliminary evidence of efficacy in treatment-resistant depression (Acadia Pharmaceuticals, personal communication) [1,5,6]. Pimavanserin's antidepressant actions can be hypothetically explained by the increased dopaminergic and noradrenergic tone in the prefrontal cortex associated with blockade of

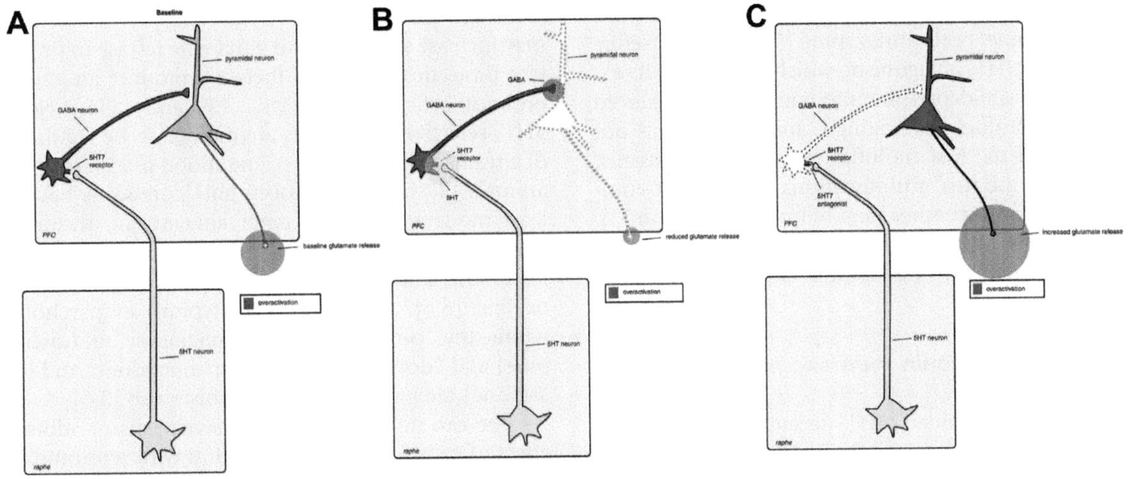

FIG. 14 (*A*) Function of 5HT7 receptors in the prefrontal cortex. A major function of 5HT7 receptors may be to regulate serotonin–glutamate interactions. Serotonergic projections from the raphe nucleus to the prefrontal cortex synapse with GABA-ergic interneurons that contain 5HT7 receptors. The GABA-ergic neurons, in turn, synapse with glutamatergic pyramidal neurons. (*B*) Stimulation of 5HT7 receptor in the prefrontal cortex reduces glutamate release from pyramidal neurons. Serotonin binds to 5HT7 receptors on GABA interneurons in the prefrontal cortex. This stimulates GABA release (indicated by the red color of the neuron), which in turn inhibits glutamate release (indicated by the dotted outline of the glutamatergic neuron). (*C*) Blockade of 5HT7 receptors in the prefrontal cortex increases glutamate release from pyramidal neurons. If 5HT7 receptors on GABA-ergic interneurons in the prefrontal cortex are blocked, then GABA release is inhibited (indicated by the dotted outline of the GABA neuron). Without the presence of GABA, glutamatergic pyramidal neurons in the prefrontal cortex can become overactivated (indicated by the red color of the neuron), leading to increased glutamate release.

$5HT_{2A}$ and $5HT_{2C}$ receptors [5]. The $5HT_{2A}$ antagonist properties of pimavanserin have been thought to decrease the hallucinations and paranoia commonly seen in patients with Parkinson disease, as well as patients with dementia-related psychosis, without the risk of exacerbating extrapyramidal symptoms, a common problem with the use of currently available antipsychotics [5,20].

Combining serotonin reuptake inhibition with $5HT_3$ antagonism

Stimulation of $5HT_3$ receptors on GABA interneurons results in decreased release of acetylcholine and norepinephrine in the prefrontal cortex (see Fig. 12A, B) [5]. Therefore, inhibiting $5HT_3$ receptors increases acetylcholine and norepinephrine release in the prefrontal cortex, which may have antidepressant effects (see Fig. 12C). Perhaps $5HT_3$ receptor antagonism is much more important than previously thought given the positive results seen with the new medication vortioxetine [2], a medication with multimodal mechanisms

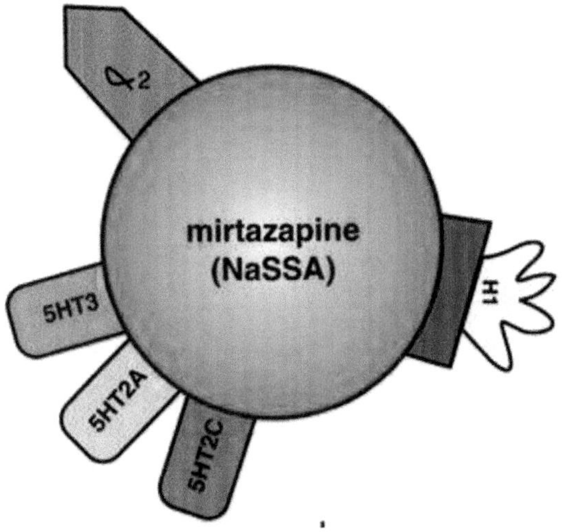

FIG. 15 Mirtazapine. Mirtazapine is sometimes called a noradrenergic and specific serotonergic antidepressant (NaSSA). Its primary therapeutic action is alpha 2 antagonism. It also blocks 3 serotonin (5HT) receptors: 5HT2A, 5HT2C, and 5HT3. Finally, it blocks histamine 1 (H1) receptors.

including potent $5HT_3$ and SERT inhibition as well as others. Of note, both mirtazapine [9] and vortioxetine have potent $5HT_3$ antagonism, which hypothetically explains their antidepressant mechanisms and reduced side effect profiles. Interestingly, mirtazapine was not only one of the first multifunctional antidepressants, it was also the first multifunctional agent with combined mechanisms other than reuptake inhibition [5]. Mirtazapine's mechanism of action will be discussed in more detail in the section on norepinephrine antagonism.

Combining serotonin reuptake inhibition with $5HT_7$ antagonism

As previously explained, $5HT_7$ receptors are expressed on GABA interneurons in the brainstem and cortex, where they stimulate GABA interneurons that project onto, and inhibit, serotonin and glutamate neurons (see Figs. 13 and 14) [5]. Blocking $5HT_7$ receptors may increase serotonin and glutamate release in important projection areas and therefore produce an antidepressant effect (see Figs. 13 and 14). Novel $5HT_7$-selective antagonists are thought to be regulators of circadian rhythms, sleep, and mood in experimental animals [5,7]. Several proven antidepressants have at least moderate $5HT_7$ receptor antagonism, including amoxapine, desipramine, imipramine, mianserin, fluoxetine, and the experimental antidepressant vortioxetine [5,6]. Several of the atypical antipsychotics within the "pines" (clozapine, quetiapine, and asenapine) and "dones" (risperidone, paliperidone, and lurasidone) are potent $5HT_7$ antagonists also [5,6].

One can now appreciate the synergistic or additive effect of combining SERT inhibition with serotonin receptor antagonism, which supports the combined use of some medications and the growing interest in

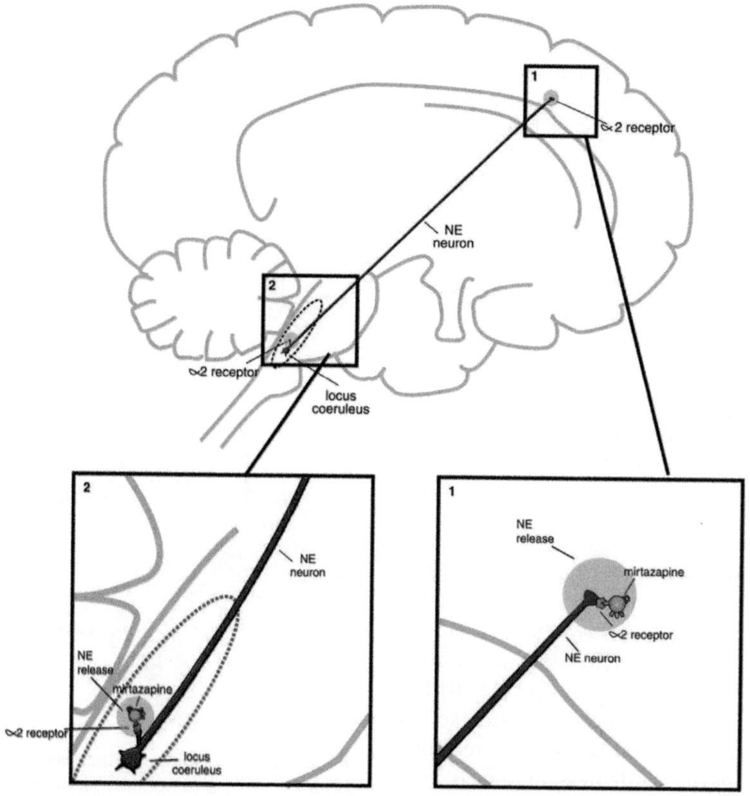

FIG. 16 Alpha 2 antagonism increases norepinephrine release in raphe and cortex. Alpha 2 adrenergic receptors are presynaptic autoreceptors and thus are the "brakes" on noradrenergic neurons. Alpha 2 antagonists (eg, mirtazapine) can therefore increase norepinephrine release by binding to these receptors in the locus coeruleus (*A*) and in the cortex (*B*).

developing medications with multiple mechanisms already "built into" the molecule.

Norepinephrine antagonism and mirtazapine

Mirtazapine is an alpha 2 noradrenergic antagonist, as well as an antagonist of 5HT2A, 5HT2, 5HT3, and H1 histamine receptors (Fig. 15) [5,6,9]. Antagonism of alpha 2 receptors is another mechanism for enhancing the release of monoamines to exert an antidepressant response. Norepinephrine turns off its own release by interacting with presynaptic alpha 2 autoreceptors on noradrenergic neurons [5]. Therefore, inhibiting alpha 2 receptors disinhibits noradrenergic neuronal impulse flow and enhances the release of norepinephrine in the raphe nucleus and cortex (Figs. 16 and 17).

In addition to regulating its own release, norepinephrine also regulates serotonin release by two primary mechanisms. The first involves activation of alpha 2 heteroreceptors on serotonin neurons, which inhibits the release of serotonin [5]. Blocking alpha 2 heteroreceptors in the raphe nucleus and cortex enhances serotonin release (see Fig. 17; Fig. 18). The second mechanism by which norepinephrine regulates serotonin release involves activation of alpha 1 receptors located on the somatodendritic end of serotonin neurons in the raphe nucleus which, when stimulated by norepinephrine, stimulates serotonin neuronal impulse flow and enhances release of serotonin in the cortex (Fig. 19) [5]. One can now see how blocking alpha 2 receptors will enhance norepinephrine release in the raphe nucleus, as described above, and therefore lead to enhanced stimulation of alpha 1 receptors with the effect of increasing serotonin release in the cortex (see Fig. 19).

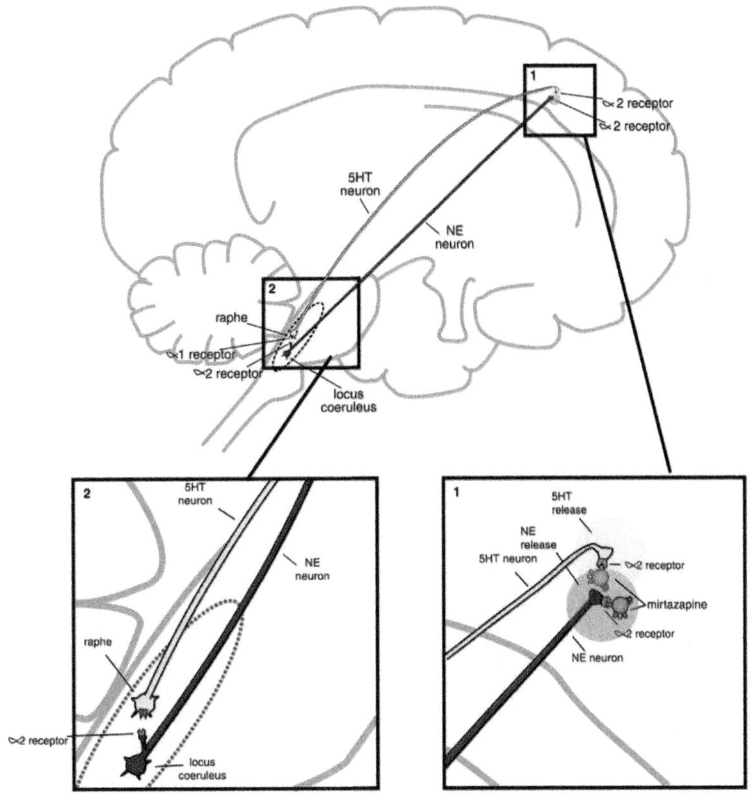

FIG. 17 Alpha 2 antagonism increases serotonin and norepinephrine release in the cortex. Both noradrenergic and serotonergic neurotransmission are illustrated to be enhanced by alpha 2 antagonists. The noradrenergic neuron is disinhibited in the cortex because an alpha 2 antagonist is blocking its presynaptic alpha 2 autoreceptors. This has the effect of "cutting the brake cables" for norepinephrine (NE) release. In addition, alpha 2 antagonists "cut the 5HT brake cable" when alpha 2 presynaptic heteroreceptors are blocked on the 5HT axon terminal, thus leading to enhanced serotonin release.

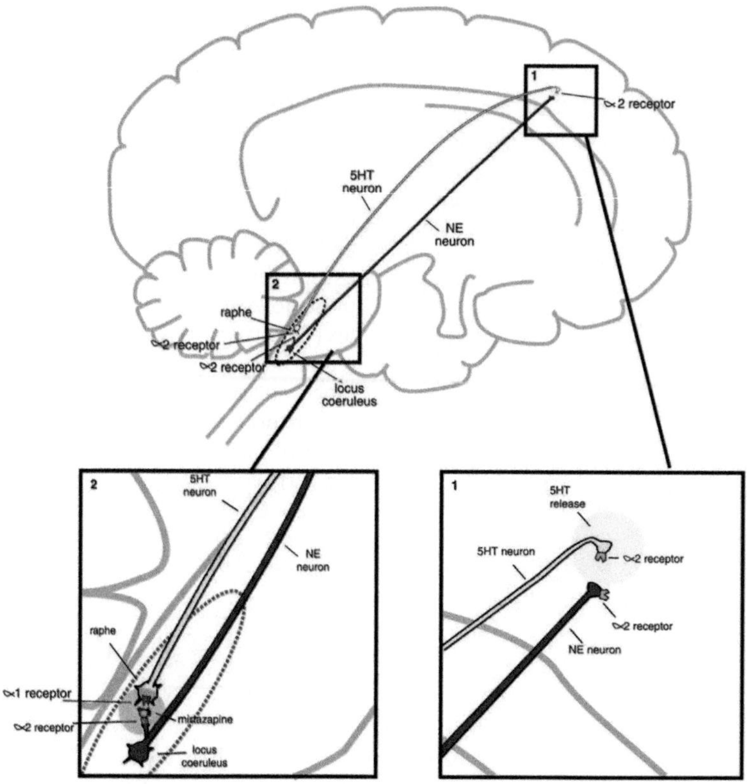

FIG. 18 Alpha 2 antagonism in raphe stimulates serotonin release in cortex. The noradrenergic neuron is disinhibited at its axon terminals in the brainstem because an alpha 2 antagonist is blocking its presynaptic alpha 2 autoreceptors (2). This has the effect of "cutting the brake cables" for norepinephrine (NE) release. Norepinephrine can then stimulate alpha 1 receptors on the serotonergic neuron, leading to serotonin release in the cortex (1).

Antagonism of alpha 2 receptors is thought to be one of the major antidepressant mechanisms of mirtazapine [9]. In addition to alpha 2 antagonism, mirtazapine also has actions at $5HT_3$, $5HT_{2A}$, $5HT_{2C}$, and H_1 receptors, all contributing to both its antidepressant effects and side effects (see Fig. 15) [5,6,9]. Mirtazapine is a unique antidepressant in that it does not have serotonin uptake inhibition properties. For this reason, mirtazapine is often added to SSRIs/SNRIs as an augmentation agent and/or to mitigate the initial side effects seen with SSRIs/SNRIs.

The combination of mirtazapine and an SNRI (such as venlafaxine) is colloquially termed "California rocket fuel" [5] and is a commonly used strategy to "propel" severely depressed patients out of their depressive states (Fig. 20). This potentially powerful combination utilizes the pharmacologic synergy obtained by adding the enhanced serotonin and norepinephrine release from inhibition of both serotonin and norepinephrine reuptake to the disinhibition of both serotonin and norepinephrine release by the alpha 2 antagonist actions of mirtazapine. It is possible that additional pro-dopaminergic actions result from the combination of norepinephrine reuptake inhibition from the SNRI in the prefrontal cortex and the disinhibition of dopamine release via $5HT_{2C}$ antagonism of mirtazapine.

Combinations of mirtazapine with various SSRIs and SNRIs have also been studied as potential initial treatments for unipolar major depression [1,5–7].

Should a combination of antidepressant mechanisms be the standard for treating unipolar depression?

Antidepressant monotherapy has been the traditional first-line treatment for unipolar major depressive disorder given the cost-effectiveness and available evidence for monotherapy treatment. However, increasing numbers of clinicians are finding monotherapy to be inadequate at relieving depressive symptoms in many patients. The STAR*D trial confirmed the overall inadequacy of monotherapy as only one-third of patients remitted on their first monotherapy treatment [4]. Even more discouraging was that one-third of patients never reached remission even after a year of treatment with adequate trials of 4 different antidepressants in sequence. These findings suggest that multiple trials of monotherapy in sequence may not be the best strategy for treating unipolar depression.

Perhaps an initial trial of monotherapy should be followed by selecting more aggressive treatment strategies early, such as using a combination of antidepressant mechanisms by switching to multimodal agents or augmenting monotherapy with agents like lithium, levothyroxine, trazodone, bupropion, or atypical antipsychotics [1,5,7,10,16,17]. The controversial question that remains to be answered is whether monotherapy really *is* the best initial treatment.

It is worth noting that multiple mechanisms do not always mean multiple agents. As discussed extensively in previous sections, antidepressants such as mirtazapine [9], vilazodone [18], trazodone [15], and vortioxetine [2] are multimodal agents targeting more than one neurotransmitter system and utilizing more than one mechanism. Although controversial, many experts believe SNRIs [14] and other multifunctional agents are more effective for depression than single-mechanism agents and should be utilized earlier in treatment. It is important to note that there is little clinical trial data supporting the superior efficacy of combining multiple antidepressant mechanisms, but equally important is the recognition that a lack of data does not necessarily equate to lack of efficacy. Many combinations of

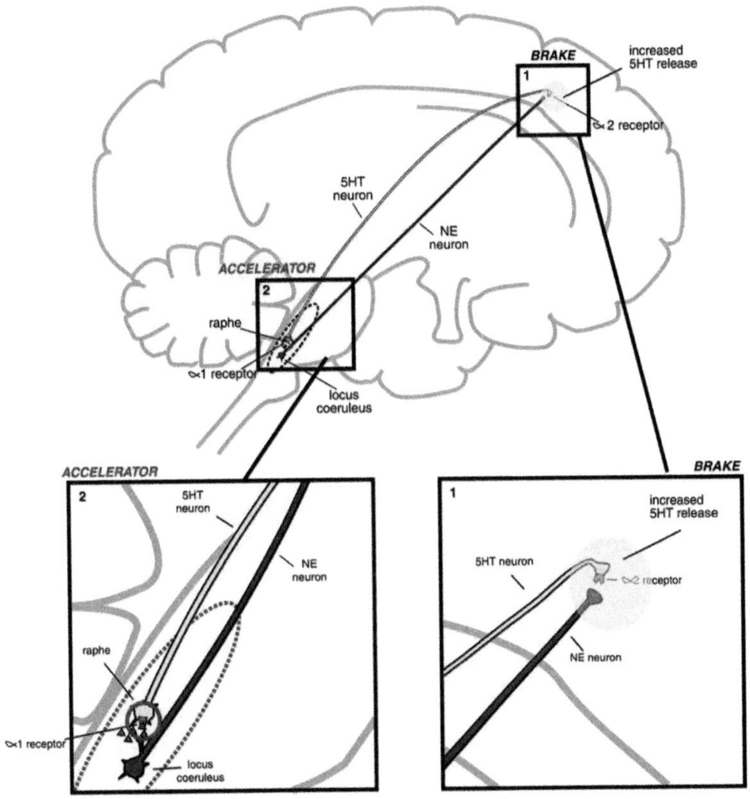

FIG. 19 Raphe alpha 1 receptors stimulate serotonin release. Alpha 1 adrenergic receptors are located in the somatodendritic regions of serotonin neurons. When these receptors are unoccupied by norepinephrine, some serotonin is released from the serotonin neuron. However, when norepinephrine binds to the alpha 1 receptor (2) this stimulates the serotonin neuron, accelerating release of serotonin (1).

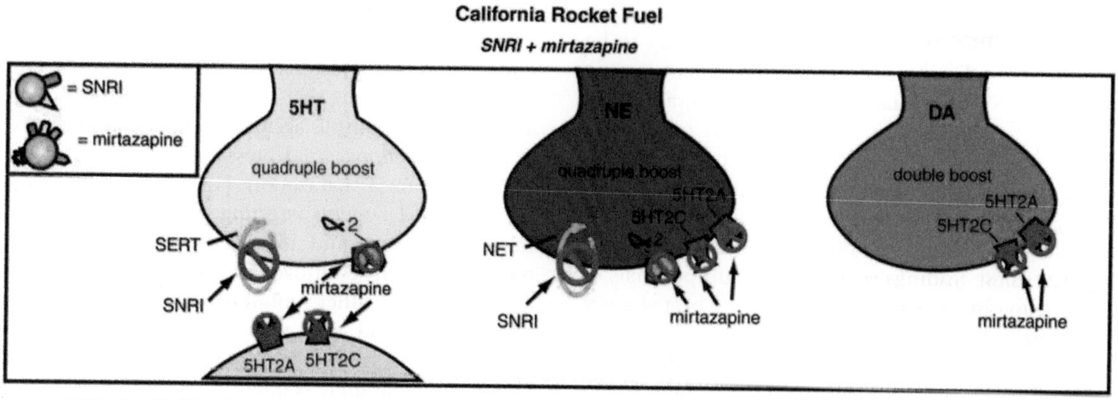

FIG. 20 California rocket fuel (SNRI plus mirtazapine). Serotonin norepinephrine reuptake inhibitor (SNRI) plus mirtazapine is a combination that has a great degree of theoretic synergy: norepinephrine reuptake blockade plus alpha 2 blockade, serotonin (5HT) reuptake plus 5HT2A and 5HT2C antagonism, and thus many 5HT actions plus norepinephrine (NE) actions. Specifically, 5HT is quadruple-boosted (with reuptake blockade, alpha 2 antagonism, 5HT2A antagonism, and 5HT2C antagonism), NE is quadruple-boosted (with reuptake blockade, alpha 2 antagonism, 5HT2A antagonism, and 5HT2C antagonism), and there may even be a double boost of dopamine (with 5HT2A and 5HT2C antagonism).

antidepressants have enjoyed widespread use with positive results and may be useful in some patients.

SUMMARY

While the future of antidepressant pharmacology remains to be determined, it is evident that a paradigm shift has occurred in recent years. Anecdotal evidence and clinical experience suggest superior efficacy associated with targeting multiple monoamine systems, which is further supported by the observation that many patients are prescribed more than one antidepressant or multimodal agents to achieve remission. And given the complex nature of depression pathophysiology, it isn't surprising that some patients do not respond to monoaminergic agents at all. For some, an SSRI does the trick. For others, a combination of multiple monoamine mechanisms is needed to achieve remission. And yet still for some others, none of the combinations seem to alleviate their symptoms at all. For those patients who fail to achieve remission with the above combinations, the logical final step would be to use interventional (ie, ECT, TMS, DBS) or pharmacologic treatments targeting systems other than the monoamines such as the glutamate system (ketamine/esketamine), the neurosteroid axis, or the endogenous opioid and cannabinoid systems.

DISCLOSURES

S.M. Stahl is an Adjunct Professor of Psychiatry at the University of California San Diego, Honorary Visiting Senior Fellow at the University of Cambridge, UK, and Director of Psychopharmacology for California Department of State Hospitals. Over the past 12 months (January–December 2020), Dr S.M. Stahl has served as a consultant to Acadia, Alkermes, Allergan, AbbVie, Arbor Pharmaceuticals, Axovant, Axsome, Celgene, Concert, Clearview, EMD Serono, Eisai Pharmaceuticals, Ferring, Impel NeuroPharma, Intra-Cellular Therapies, Ironshore Pharmaceuticals, Janssen, Karuna, Lilly, Lundbeck, Merck, Otsuka, Pfizer, Relmada, Sage Therapeutics, Servier, Shire, Sunovion, Takeda, Taliaz, Teva, Tonix, Tris Pharma, and Viforpharma; he is a board member of Genomind; he has served on speakers' bureaus for Acadia, Lundbeck, Otsuka, Perrigo, Servier, Sunovion, Takeda, Teva, and Vertex and he has received research and/or grant support from Acadia, Avanir, Braeburn Pharmaceuticals, Eli Lilly, Intra-Cellular Therapies, Ironshore, ISSWSH, Neurocrine, Otsuka, Shire, Sunovion, and TMS NeuroHealth Centers.

REFERENCES

[1] Goldberg J, Stahl SM. Practical psychopharmacology. New York: Cambridge University Press; 2021.
[2] Stahl SM. Modes and nodes explain the mechanism of action of vortioxetine, a multimodal agent (MMA): enhancing serotonin release by combining serotonin (5HT) transporter inhibition with actions at 5HT receptors (5HT1A, 5HT1B, 5HT1D, 5HT7 receptors); CNS Spectrums 20: 93 – 97 2015.

[3] Rossom Rebecca C. Antidepressant adherence across diverse populations and healthcare settings. Depress Anxiety 2016;33:765–74.
[4] Rush AJ, Trivedi MH, Wisniewski SR, et al. Acute and longer term outcomes in depressed outpatients requiring one or several treatment steps: a STAR*D report. Am J Psychiatry 2006;163:1905–17.
[5] Stahl SM. Stahls essential psychopharmacology: neuroscientific basis and practical applications. 5th edition. New York: Cambridge University Press; 2021.
[6] Stahl, S. M. Stahl's essential psychopharmacology: Prescriber's guide (7th ed.). New York, NY: Cambridge University Press.
[7] Schatzberg AF, Nemeroff CB. The American Psychiatric Association textbook of psychopharmacology. Arlington, VA: American Psychiatric Association Publishing; 2017.
[8] Stahl SM. Serotonergic mechanisms and the new antidepressants. Psychol Med 1993;23:281–5.
[9] Stimmel GL, Dopheide JA, Stahl SM. Mirtazapine: an antidepressant with selective alpha-2 adrenoceptor antagonist effects. Pharmacotherapy 1997;17(1):10–21.
[10] Stahl SM. Are two antidepressant mechanisms better than one? J Clin Psychiatry 1997;58(8):339–41.
[11] Stahl SM. Basic psychopharmacology of antidepressants (Part 1): Antidepressants have seven distinct mechanisms of action. J ofClinical Psychiatry 1998; 59(Suppl.4):514.
[12] Stahl SM, Entsuah AR, Rudolph RL. Comparative efficacy between venlafaxine and SSRIs: A pooled analysis of patients with depression. Biol Psychiatry 2002;52(12): 1166–74.
[13] Stahl SM, Pradko J. A review of the neuropharmacology of bupropion SR: A Dual NE and DA reuptake inhibitor. J Clin Psychiatry Prim Care Companion 2004;6(4): 159–66.
[14] Stahl SM, Grady MM, Moret C, et al. Serotonin and norepinephrine reuptake inhibitors (SNRIs): A review of their pharmacology, clinical efficacy and tolerability in comparison to other classes of antidepressant. CNS Spectrums,Sept 2005;10(9):732–47.
[15] Stahl SM. Mechanism of action of trazodone: a multifunctional drug. CNS Spectrums 2009;14(10):536–46.
[16] Stahl SM. Enhancing outcomes from major depression: using antidepressant combination therapies with multifunctional pharmacological mechanisms from the initiation of treatment, CNS Spectrums 15: 2 2010. p. 677–91.
[17] Schwartz TL, Stahl SM. Optimizing antidepressant management of depression: current status and future perspectives. In: Cryan FJ, Leonard BD, S. Karger AG, editors. Depression: From psychopathology to pharmacotherapy. The future of antidepressants. 2011. 2011. p. 254–67, Basel, Switzerland 2010.
[18] Schwartz TL, Siddiqui UA, Stahl SM. Vilazodone: A brief pharmacologic and clinical review of the novel SPARI (Serotonin Partial Agonist and Reuptake Inhibitor). Ther Adv Psychopharmacol 2011;1(3):81–7.
[19] Stahl SM. Essential psychopharmacology case studies. London: Cambridge University Press; 2011.
[20] Cummings J, Isaacson S, Mills R, et al. Pimavanserin for patients with Parkinson's disease psychosis: a randomised, placebo-controlled phase 3 trial. Lancet 2014; 383:533–40.

Education

Advances in Psychiatry and Behavioral Health 1 (2021) 205–217
ADVANCES IN PSYCHIATRY AND BEHAVIORAL HEALTH

Dementia After Traumatic Brain Injury

From Neural Mechanisms to Psychiatry

Vassilis E. Koliatsos, MD[a,b,c,d,*], Vani Rao, MD[c], Athanasios S. Alexandris, MBChB[a]
[a]Department of Pathology (Neuropathology), Johns Hopkins University School of Medicine; [b]Department of Neurology, Johns Hopkins University School of Medicine; [c]Department of Psychiatry and Behavioral Sciences, Johns Hopkins University School of Medicine; [d]Neuropsychiatry Program, Sheppard Pratt Health System

KEYWORDS
• Cognitive impairments • Brain contusions • Diffuse axonal injury • Chronic traumatic encephalopathy • Alzheimer's disease • Parkinson's disease • Frontal lobe syndrome • Depression

KEY POINTS

- Chronic traumatic brain injury (TBI) is a paradigmatic neuropsychiatric disease, and TBI-associated neuropsychiatric deficits are a major cause of disability and poor outcome.
- Cognitive impairments are common in chronic TBI and constitute a major part of its neuropsychiatric profile.
- Although chronic traumatic encephalopathy (CTE) is the most notorious remote consequence of TBI, especially repeat mild TBI, evidence linking CTE-type pathology and clinical symptoms is still evolving.
- The association of a history of moderate-severe TBI and more common types of age-associated dementias, including Alzheimer's disease, has been suggested by several studies but remains in question; this is a difficult problem, and there is a clear need for improved methodology.
- The most common cognitive impairments after TBI may be the direct consequences of contusions and diffuse axonal injury, with prominent executive dysfunction and other frontal-type deficits.
- When assessing and managing young athletes, clinicians should always consider common mood disorders and other causes of attentional/executive difficulties that have effective treatments and defer CTE formulations to future research.

THE PROBLEM AND ITS SIGNIFICANCE

Although known for a long time, the link between traumatic brain injury (TBI) and dementia has only recently come to focus after the widespread publicity of the increased prevalence of severe, chronic neuropsychiatric problems in veteran football players [1–3]. These problems almost universally include cognitive impairments, but, as shown with several retrospective analyses, they are also featured by early changes in mood, behavior, and personality traits years before cognitive and other neurologic impairments [4,5]. Such concerns have already expanded to other amateur and professional sports besides football and have become a major health concern, primarily because of the large number of young people engaging in amateur collision and contact sports in the United States. Similar concerns have been raised for warfighters suffering repeat concussions in the Iraq and Afghanistan war theaters [6]. These issues have raised important public health, research, and clinical dilemmas that we will briefly go over in this review.

The role of TBI in dementia is also important because it may add yet another cause of secondary

*Corresponding author E-mail addresses: koliat@jhmi.edu; vkoliatsos@sheppardpratt.org

https://doi.org/10.1016/j.ypsc.2021.05.018
2667-3827/21/

dementia to a long list of infections and inflammatory, hematologic, metabolic, and other potential causes (Table 1) that need to be considered in any comprehensive clinical dementia workup but also serve as important models of disease for exploring the pathogenesis of the more common neurodegenerative forms of dementia. For a while, TBI has been considered a potential cause of Alzheimer's disease (AD) [7] (see *Section 5*), and it is also a leading cause of cognitive impairments in children and young adults [8,9].

Any discussion of the relationship between trauma and dementia brings up additional questions. First, what type of dementia and what type of brain trauma are we talking about? If we accept, for the purpose of this review, that the potential outcome is neurodegenerative, what is the neurodegenerative disease whose incidence is potentially affected by a history of trauma? Second, what type(s) of TBI might be responsible? Third, what is the exact nature of the relationship? TBI could be a necessary and sufficient cause (a *true* cause), could be necessary but not sufficient (causative factor), could be a modifying factor that might accelerate or shape pathogenesis triggered by a third cause, or could be, in fact, the outcome of dementia (Fig. 1). Here we will discuss the types of TBI causing cognitive impairments, the types of enduring cognitive impairments linked to TBI, and some important mechanisms of processing from TBI to neurodegeneration and thus to dementia. We will also outline some methodological problems in research and the associated clinical dilemmas.

THE TYPOLOGY OF CHRONIC TRAUMATIC BRAIN INJURY

Traumatic Brain Injury: Transient Versus Chronic Disease

TBI is a common problem. In the United States alone, it is estimated that there are close to 3 million new cases of TBI requiring medical attention annually [10]. TBI is not a disease per se but a calamity that first causes primary lesions and then triggers secondary events responsible for transient or chronic diseases. These morbidities are conventionally classified by cause, specific pathology, and clinical severity or outcome. We have argued that TBI-related disease is best conceptualized with the classical clinicopathological method that links bedside

TABLE 1
Nondegenerative dementias

• Infectious ○ HIV ○ Syphilis ○ Prion disease (Creutzfeldt-Jakob) ○ Viral encephalitis (eg, herpes simplex 1) ○ Lyme's disease ○ Whipple's disease • Inflammatory/autoimmune ○ Hashimoto's ○ Primary and secondary central nervous system (CNS) vasculitis ○ Sarcoid ○ systemic lupus erythematosus (SLE) • Demyelinating ○ Multiple sclerosis • Vascular ○ Stroke (multiple infarcts) ○ Binswanger's disease ○ Post-coronary artery bypass graft (CABG) ○ Cerebral amyloid angiopathy ○ CADASIL (Cerebral autosomal dominant arteriopathy with subcortical infarcts and leukoencephalopathy)	• Toxic ○ Alcohol ○ Heavy metals • Metabolic ○ Hypothyroidism ○ Vitamin B12 deficiency (subacute combined degeneration) ○ Thiamine deficiency (Wernicke-Korsakoff encephalopathy) ○ Niacin deficiency (pellagra) ○ Hepatic encephalopathy ○ Uremia ○ Cushing's syndrome • Neoplasm-related ○ Tumor (certain locations) ○ Paraneoplastic limbic encephalitis ○ Brain radiation ○ Chemotherapy • Normal pressure hydrocephalus • Chronic TBI

Major groups and types of nonneurodegenerative dementias. For many of them, there are effective interventions at the level of prevention or treatment.

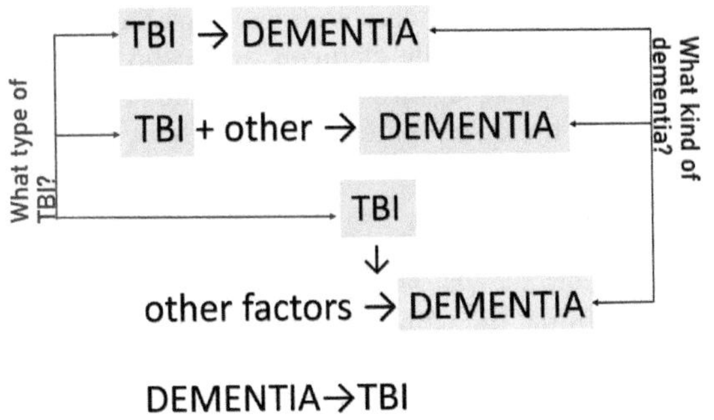

FIG. 1 A sketch of the types of causal relationships between TBI and dementia and related key questions.

clinical observations and prognoses to findings from the examination of patient tissues and then the formulation of pathologic hypotheses and testing them in models [11–13]. Although the complexity of TBI does not allow for straightforward correlations between clinical symptoms/signs and pathology, hypotheses, or models, the clinicopathological method can serve to outline key issues, point out remaining challenges in research and clinical practice, and track progress.

Mild TBI or concussion, a very common problem in the community, is typically a transient illness with good prognosis. On the other hand, moderate to severe TBI very often leads to chronic TBI and causes significant disability because of permanent damage to brain circuitry and possibly progressive disease. Moderate to severe TBI may be caused by focal contusions due to low-impact falls, diffuse axonal injury (DAI) associated with rotational acceleration forces in the course of motor vehicle accidents or high-impact falls, TBI due to repeat concussions, for example, from boxing or other collision/contact sports, and blast injury to brain, an old problem that has resurfaced in the wake of recent US conflicts in Iraq and Afghanistan.

Focal Contusions

Low-impact blunt TBI causes focal damage to brain and meninges, including hematomas and parenchymal contusions. Penetrating TBI is also, in part, an extensive focal TBI depending on the ballistics of the projectile and interface phenomena involving the skull and the meninges. Contusions are common lesions caused by falls, strike-by or strike-against events, and motor vehicle accidents and occur at both the site of impact (coup) and the diametrically opposite site (contrecoup). Striking the immobile head with blunt force, for example, with a weapon, causes skull fractures and coup lesions at the site of the impact, whereas the striking of a firm fixed surface by the moving head predominantly causes contrecoup lesions regardless of impact location. Contrecoup injuries tend to occur at ventral frontal and temporopolar locations for complex mechanical and perhaps also vascular reasons [12,13]. By virtue of their anatomic distribution at the frontotemporal olfactory paralimbic zone, contrecoup lesions typically cause complex "frontal" symptomatology with prominent behavioral and social impairments [12,13]. Focal neurologic signs may be absent.

Acceleration Injuries: Diffuse Axonal Injury

In contrast to brain contusions that primarily damage neuronal perikarya, traumatic (diffuse) axonal injury (DAI) is a primary axonal perturbation that occurs as a result of rotational acceleration of the head in the course of motor vehicle crashes and high-impact falls [14]. DAI leads to multifocal axonal disruption accompanied by focal microhemorrhages and, in severe cases, gross shearing lesions in large white matter tracts, especially corpus callosum, and at the gray-white matter junction in the form of gliding contusions [12,13]. With considerable variance in severity, DAI is a common denominator in all types of TBI, from concussions to blast and chronic traumatic encephalopathy (CTE). The human brain may be especially prone to DAI because of the disproportionate abundance of white matter but perhaps also the complex three-dimensional organization of intertwined white matter tracts [15]. DAI has been more difficult to study than contusions, perhaps because of a wider range of severity, variance in anatomic distribution, and the historical use of low-resolution imaging such as CT and conventional MRI. In classical cases, DAI is a frontal pathology much like contusions but involves the white matter and is predominantly medial-dorsal, whereas contusions involve gray matter and are ventral [16,17]. Most, but not all, studies have linked DAI with poor outcomes [18,19] and with a whole host of neuropsychiatric symptoms in the cognitive/executive, behavioral, and affective domains, with similarities to symptoms associated with contusions (see *Section 4*). There may be associated motor, cerebellar, and other focal symptoms and signs.

Repetitive Mild Traumatic Brain Injury and Chronic Traumatic Encephalopathy

Repeat concussions, associated with specific life styles or medical problems such as chronic involvement with collision and contact sports, partner or child abuse (exposure to repeat violence), epilepsy (falls), and autism (head banging), may have a cumulative effect on the brain. This problem distinguishes repetitive concussions from single concussions that typically have good prognosis. It has been argued that "subconcussive" injuries may also add to the outcome. In other words, the key factor in prognosis may be the total burden of life style, rather than the number of individual traceable concussive events.

Repeat concussions are associated with two main clinical presentations: One is postconcussive syndrome (see *Section 4*). The other is CTE, a progressive neurodegenerative disease featured by tau and 43-kDa transactive response DNA-binding protein (TDP-43) inclusions, and neuronal cell loss in neocortex and the limbic system. TBI-related neurodegeneration had been first described in boxers under the name "punch drunk" and "dementia pugilistica" before called CTE in the late 1950s [20–22]. In the era of immunohistochemistry, the problem has been redefined as a form of tau proteinopathy associated not just with boxing but with all collision and contact sports, especially American football [1,2]. Tau inclusions in neurons and astrocytes, especially around arterioles at the depths of the sulci, are the hallmark of the condition. These features distinguish CTE from classical degenerative tauopathies such as AD, frontotemporal lobar degeneration (FTLD), and progressive supranuclear palsy (PSP), although the boundaries are not clear and recently established diagnostic criteria may require revision [23]. It is thought that the disease begins in frontal cortex and then progresses caudally.

CTE has been touted as a neuropsychiatric disease with severe mood and behavioral symptoms even in the early stages [4,5]. However, despite considerable efforts by some investigators to define clinicopathological correlations and stages of progression based on the gold standard of Braak staging in AD [4], the natural course of CTE remains elusive. This task requires prospective studies with equal chance of including cases with relatively good outcomes [24]. Our present understanding of the problem is retrospective, predominantly from brains of boxers and increasingly also brains of professional football players many of whom died from suicide or unusual accidents, raising concerns of a sampling bias in the direction of overincluding cases with behavioral/cognitive impairments. In addition, in the brains of older athletes, distinction from other more common forms of age-associated degeneration is not easy, and the clinical significance of CTE-type pathology is not always clear [25].

Blast Injury to Brain

Blast TBI is a complex injury [12]. Besides the presumed primary effects of overpressure caused by the shock wave, there are secondary injuries from the forceful mobilization of mobile elements and debris that are shot shrapnel-like against the victim and tertiary injuries from the displacement of the body by the blast wind causing contrecoup contusions and DAI from rotational acceleration. There may also be quaternary injuries including flash burns from the intense heat of the explosion as well as asphyxiation and respiratory damage from the inhalation of toxic substances. Although the secondary and tertiary components of blast TBI are identical to other types of TBI reviewed in this article, the neuropathology associated with the primary effect of blast has not been well characterized. Part of the problem is lack of sufficient high-quality autopsy material, especially from long-term survivors of blast injuries and the rarity of isolated primary blast events, except low-level exposure during professional training with explosives or shoulder-fired weapons. Recent work on the brains of veterans with a history of blast exposure has shown a characteristic arrangement of traumatic axonal lesions at a submillimeter distance from arterioles forming 3D honeycombs [26], a pathologic pattern consistent with vascular-mediated injury [27]. These configurations appear to be distinct from the large fronts of axonal undulations and bulbs seen in classical DAI and from axonal abnormalities seen in other types of TBI or in the case of opiate overdose [26]. As in the case of repeat concussions, blast TBI is associated with numerous psychiatric symptoms, but cause-and-effect assumptions are tainted by methodological challenges [13].

SELECT MECHANISMS OF DEGENERATION AFTER TRAUMATIC BRAIN INJURY

Traumatic Axonopathy and Disconnection—the Importance of the White Matter

Brain contusions appear to have limited impact on the viability of parts of the brain away from the site of contusion, with the exception of remote physiologic effects known as diaschisis [28]. On the other hand, DAI is associated with important secondary effects first on the viability of axons and then on populations of neurons with injured axons or damaged inputs that may undergo retrograde and orthograde (transsynaptic) degeneration [29,30]. The seriousness of this problem is reflected on the progressive reduction in brain size weeks to months after severe acceleration injury [13,31,32]. Advances in cellular and molecular neuropathology, primarily based on axotomy models and the biology of Wallerian degeneration, begin to shed light into the nature and time course of these secondary changes especially in the white matter, and help establish windows for potential interventions.

Impaired plasticity and disruption or disintegration of white matter is at the root of many common neuropsychiatric disorders including developmental conditions (Fragile X, autism spectrum disorders, hypoxia-ischemia in preterm infants), metabolic diseases such as subacute combined degeneration, infectious diseases such as progressive multifocal leukoencephalopathy, autoimmune diseases such as anti-N-Methyl-D-aspartate (NMDA) receptor encephalitis, and age-associated microvascular disease. However, nowhere else is the vulnerability of white matter in the human brain demonstrated as vividly as in the case of DAI, perhaps because of the biomechanical liability imparted by the sheer bulk but also complexity of white matter tracts [15].

Our previous modeling work has helped characterize the retrograde and transsynaptic effects of axonal injury on neuronal function and viability [33–35]. Although the cellular and molecular idiosyncrasies of perikaryal degeneration after injury have been better understood than axonal degeneration, developments in the last 2 decades have favored the white matter. As it stands today, besides protecting the white matter from known offenders, that is, managing risk factors for atherosclerotic vascular disease, treating vitamin deficiencies, and preventing falls and motor vehicle accidents, it is important to better understand the molecular and cellular biology of the axon, especially its vulnerability to Wallerian degeneration [15,36]. Wallerian degeneration is a complex molecular program of axonal self-destruction activated by a wide range of injurious insults, including perhaps milder insults that may otherwise leave axons structurally robust and potentially salvageable. Detailed studies on animal models and postmortem human brains indicate that this type of partial injury may be the main initial pathology in DAI. Recent discoveries in our laboratory and elsewhere on the role of MAPK stress cascade and NAD salvage pathways have revealed that the decision that commits axons to degeneration is temporally separated from the time of injury, allowing for a critical window that can be leveraged for potentially effective pharmacologic interventions and new therapeutic opportunities [15].

Protein Aggregation (Proteinopathy)

Proteinopathy, that is, the acquisition of abnormal conformations by brain proteins that makes them prone to aggregation, is increasingly recognized as a common problem among major neurodegenerative diseases and, for some investigators, the real cause of these conditions. In fact, neurodegenerative diseases are often classified by their corresponding aggregated proteins, for example, amyloid beta (Aβ) in AD ("amyloidosis"), synuclein in Parkinson's disease, Lewy body dementia and multiple systems atrophy ("synucleopathies"), TDP-43, tau and fused in sarcoma in FTLD and amyotrophic lateral sclerosis (ALS), TDP-43, superoxide dismutase 1 and ubiquitin in ALS, tau in PSP, and so forth. Still, there is quite a bit of overlap of cellular and molecular pathologies in various autopsy-defined neurodegenerative diseases, and tau aggregates are nearly ubiquitous [37].

If proteinopathies are at the root of corresponding neurodegenerative diseases, the question arises how such protein configurations lead to widespread neuronal death. One of the prevailing theories is the formation of prions, that is, the seeding of misfolded proteins into stable (fibrillar) conformational states that can also hetero-template by nucleating ("corrupting") normal proteins. In this manner, seeds increase in number and size, disrupt normal neuronal function, cause neuronal death, and spread from one part of the brain to another [38]. Based on such hypotheses, rare diseases such as Creutzfeldt-Jacob may be turning into models for common neurodegenerative conditions [39]. Proteinopathy can coexist with axonal injury and with blood-brain barrier deficits or neuroinflammation that is prevalent in TBI. It may also be caused by the latter, for example, via excess tau accumulation, aberrant hydrolysis by serum-born enzymes, or excessive phosphorylation of tau within neuronal perikarya [40].

CHRONIC TRAUMATIC BRAIN INJURY AS NEUROPSYCHIATRIC DISEASE

Clinical Presentations

For a comprehensive examination of neuropsychiatric disorders associated with TBI, we refer to more topical reviews [41]. Neuropsychiatric presentations associated with TBI, although generally related to the pathologic entities examined in *Part 2*, do not precisely correspond to cause or severity of TBI and the location or type of pathology. Contusions and DAI correlate better with specific neuropsychiatric syndromes than blast and repeat concussions. Overall, TBI survivors have substantially higher rates of psychiatric disorders than the general population [42], and these disturbances are leading causes of disability and poor quality of life in chronic TBI. As further explained in the next section, this relationship may be because CNS regions and circuits involved in emotional regulation, behavioral control, and high-order cognitive operations are all affected in TBI. It should be noted that TBI has a bidirectional correlation with psychiatric illness: TBI increases the rate of psychiatric morbidity, but psychiatric illness is also a risk factor for TBI. Therefore, assigning causality in psychiatric symptoms emerging after TBI is not always straightforward: In many cases, TBI is merely an index event. Of course, neuropathology cannot explain all the psychiatric problems experienced by TBI survivors: Many patients with a history of moderate-severe TBI experience a catastrophic illness with dramatic and often permanent changes in their lives. They are exposed to continued chronic stress with hospitalizations, endless medical visits and the need for chronic rehabilitation, and sometimes legal battles over compensation. Last but not least, they seek meaning in the new reality set after the injury, often preoccupied with who they were and what they were doing before TBI or what was going on at the time of the event.

Among several psychiatric problems and disorders after TBI, organic personality changes, mood disorders, and cognitive impairments are common and clinically challenging. The term "personality change" denotes stable changes in affective or behavioral disposition in the aftermath of moderate-severe TBI that usually falls into discrete categories featured by irritability/aggression, impulsivity/disinhibition, mood lability, and apathy [41,43,44]. As shown in the next section, frontal pathology is common. In some individuals, these changes may represent an accentuation of previous personality traits, and in others, the emergence of new traits. The relationship between TBI and mood disorders is known for a very long time [45]. Depression is the commonest TBI-associated mood disorder and includes conditions ranging from adjustment disorders with depressed mood to enduring depression sometimes associated with anhedonia, vegetative signs and symptoms, and executive dysfunction [46]. A prior history of mood disorders and poor social functioning are well-established risk factors. TBI-associated depression is often expressed outward as aggression [47]. Neuropathology favors anterior frontal locations [47,48]. Mania after TBI is less frequent and may be preferentially associated with pathology in the right hemisphere [49]. Cognitive impairments are discussed in detail in the final section of this review.

A special problem associated with mild TBI is the so-called postconcussive syndrome that affects 10% to 20% of concussion survivors. Although symptoms of concussion in the most patients disappear after a few days to weeks, postconcussive patients experience enduring problems including mood changes such as depression and irritability, cognitive symptoms such as decreased attention/concentration and often impaired memory, various degrees of executive dysfunction, and other symptoms such as headache, insomnia, dizziness/vertigo, tinnitus, light and noise sensitivity, fatigue, and problems with coordination. Some of these cases may have underlying DAI [41]. Persistence of postconcussive symptoms for several months may be a sign of mental illness (eg, major depression, posttraumatic stress disorder), adverse effects of medications, substance abuse, and possibly embellishment related to ongoing litigation.

Brain-Behavior Correlations

As indicated in Fig. 2, the brain regions more commonly affected in TBI are the frontotemporal paralimbic zone and associated neocortex and the central white matter that hosts several longitudinal, commissural, cortico-subcortical, and U-fiber systems associated with both local and long-range circuits including basal ganglionic-thalamocortical loops. The involvement of frontal/frontotemporal regions, cortical associative and commissural tracts, and basal ganglia-thalamocortical loops is crucial because the affected regions/pathways and associated networks underlie important behavioral, cognitive, and social functions. Functional MRI has been extensively used to demonstrate some of these secondary effects, but there is also some evidence from high-resolution structural imaging, that is, diffusion tensor imaging, despite a need to establish better baselines [50]. Functional studies of frontal circuits and large-scale networks have demonstrated alterations in basal ganglia-thalamocortical loops engaging the caudate and also impairments in the default mode and salience networks [51–54]. In the case of DAI, there seems to be some correspondence between structural disintegration of white matter tracts and functional disconnection of overlying circuits [55,56].

Much of the psychiatric morbidity associated with TBI, especially disinhibition, aggression, and executive dysfunction, falls under the rubric of "frontal lobe syndrome" [57]. The problem is known for almost two centuries and, in the English-speaking literature, was popularized in the classical case report of Harlow on Phineas Gage. With the revival of connectional neuroanatomy in the 1980s, especially the concept of cortico-subcortical circuits engaging basal ganglia and thalamus [58], the generic frontal lobe syndrome was further specified into distinct anatomo-functional entities based on parallel segregated circuits. One clinically useful schema recognizes the orbitofrontal lesion pattern

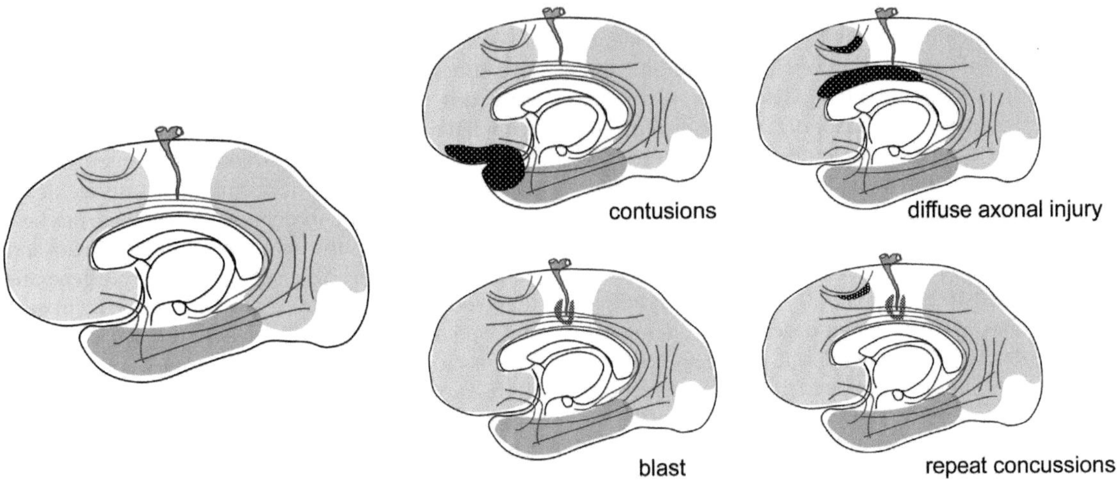

FIG. 2 This is a sketch of important anatomic elements involved in TBI-associated neuropathology. These include associative cortical areas in the frontal, parietal, and temporal lobes, local and associative white matter bundles, and medium-small size arteries supplying the brain. *Diagram on the left* shows main anatomy. *Diagrams on the right* show the involvement of the previous anatomic elements in the four main types of TBI-associated neuropathology namely contusions, DAI, blast, and repeat concussions: In contusion, there is focal damage in the frontal and temporal associative cortex. In DAI, there is multifocal involvement of both local and associative white matter tracts. Blast injury and repeat concussions involve perivascular injuries, and repeat concussions also affect gray matter at the depth of sulci. (*From* Koliatsos VE and Rao V: The behavioral neuroscience of traumatic brain injury in: Psychiatric Clinics: Neuropsychiatry [VE Koliatsos, editor] Elsevier, 2020.)

with behavioral disinhibition, the dorsolateral lesion pattern with executive dysfunction, and the anterior cingulate lesion pattern with apathy [13,59]. A recent cluster analysis has revealed four major trends in personality disturbances arising from frontal lobe lesions: dysregulation of both emotions and behavior, low emotion and energy (corresponding to apathy), distress/anxiety, and executive impairment that tends to be associated with all the other clusters [60]. This analysis elevates executive dysfunction as the central, if not the driving, problem in patients with frontal impairments.

Ever since Lishman's pioneer study on World War II patients with penetrating injuries [61], the right hemisphere has been suspected to have a special role in psychiatric morbidity after TBI. Although the relationship has not been sufficiently addressed in the existing literature, most patients with moderate-severe TBI followed up in the Neuropsychiatry Program at Sheppard Pratt have either right-selective or right-predominant lesions [62]. These patients present with a mixture of affective lability, anosognosia, inappropriate behaviors, aprosodia, deficits in pragmatics, and neglect. This syndrome is very much in keeping with the earlier conceptualizations of Heilman and colleagues [63] and is of great scientific and clinical interest.

COGNITIVE IMPAIRMENTS AND DEMENTIA AFTER TRAUMATIC BRAIN INJURY

Overview

Impairments in cognition are extremely common after moderate-severe TBI and are the best prognosticators of loss of independence and inability to return to work [41]. Severe injuries are associated with worse cognitive outcomes, but there are significant individual differences depending on preinjury functioning, intellect, and other individual factors. After an acute phase featured by alterations in level of consciousness and an ensuing delirious phase [64] that may last for weeks to months in moderate-severe injuries, stable cognitive impairments settle by 1 to 2 years after TBI. Such impairments involve nearly all cognitive domains including attention, memory, visual-spatial processing, language, social cognition, and executive functioning. The most common impairments are in the speed of information processing, attention, and working memory.

Patients usually complain about poor recall, but the underlying problems have more to do with impairments in speed of information processing, attention, and working memory. Frontal-type deficits in planning, cognitive flexibility, and reasoning also contribute to TBI-associated amnesia. Awareness deficits after TBI are also common, may be related to right hemisphere pathology, and profoundly impair the ability of the patient to engage with treatment and rehabilitative efforts [41].

As discussed in *Section 2*, TBI, especially repetitive mild TBI, has its own neurodegenerative dementia signature, that is, CTE, whose public health and clinical significance is further developed in the next section. There is also evidence, still debated, that moderate-severe and perhaps repeat mild TBI may be risk factors for late-onset neurodegenerative dementias including AD, Parkinson's disease (PD), and Lewy body dementia (LBD) [65–68] (*discussed in the following section*).

Neurodegenerative Disease Specific to Traumatic Brain Injury: the Problem of Athletic Concussions and Chronic Traumatic Encephalopathy

As stated in the beginning of this review, the main reason behind the current flurry of interest in CTE is the exposure of young Americans to athletic injuries in the course of contact and collision sports. Besides the 2000 or so active National Football League (NFL) members, there are over 5 million children and adolescents who play recreational football, over 1 million high school football players, and 70,000 college football players. As also noted in *Section 2*, neuropathological articles with retrospective exploration of medical histories of brain donors, mostly from retired NFL players, have emphasized the role of psychiatric symptoms in these subjects including mood disorders (especially depression), personality changes, and cognitive impairments that, in some cases, progress to dementia [4]. In most cases of young brains that came to autopsy, cause of death was suicide followed by self-inflicted accidents.

The proposed early occurrence of psychiatric illness in the course of CTE raises important clinical questions (Fig. 3). Psychiatric illness, especially depressive illness, is fairly common in the age range of young athletes, is prevalent, is often externalized especially in the male population, and often goes unreported because of the associated stigma. In addition, as explained in *Section 4*, major depression and its variants are common after TBI. If the early stages of CTE are featured by mood and behavioral symptoms, is the clinical presentation of depression in young athletes the manifestation of CTE or merely that of the common idiopathic depressive illness? On the other end of the age spectrum, how can one distinguish the symptoms associated with certain early-onset neurodegenerative disease, for example, the behavioral variant of frontotemporal dementia, and CTE? In the former case, are we dealing with a mere increase in depression risk that is to be expected with TBI? In the latter, are we faced with an accelerated incubation of early-onset neurodegeneration that would have happened anyway, especially in genetically predisposed individuals? On the neuropathology side, is tau accumulation, at least up to a point, a cause of disease or a marker of TBI exposure?

These questions have not been answered by current retrospective research, especially because most of this work is based on autopsy brains from patients with poor outcomes (depression, executive/impulse control problems, motor neuron disease) [13]. More work is needed to separate between CTE and other, more common, conditions, and this work requires prospective cohort studies aided by careful clinical characterization and, ideally, input by biomarkers. Unfortunately, despite substantial progress in molecular tau imaging, specific biomarkers are not available at this point [12,13]. One idea might be to use the prevalent and early neuropsychiatric symptoms as clinical "biomarkers," but there is only a dearth of neuropsychiatrists with TBI expertise in the United States, and the distinction between idiopathic and secondary ("organic") psychiatric illness is often subtle [13]. Still, such distinctions might be useful in prospective cohorts, and as many of us have stressed in professional meetings and panels, there is an urgent need for a greater presence of psychiatrists familiar with the topic.

A key question is why some athletes develop CTE and others not. Currently, the conventional wisdom is that the risk rises with concussive burden: in the case of boxing, the "bad" boxer who cannot protect himself from the punches of the opponent; in the case of football, either players who suffer the greatest number of hits including linebackers and linemen or players who endure the most severe blows such as running backs and quarterbacks. However, the severity of tauopathy may correlate with age the same or better than with severity of symptoms, indicating that the relationship between TBI burden and disease is complex [69,70]. Genetic and other predispositions such as prior history of concussions and other neurologic insults have not been addressed in the literature as of yet [13].

The previous ambiguities pose clinical dilemmas that have been addressed in a recent letter signed by

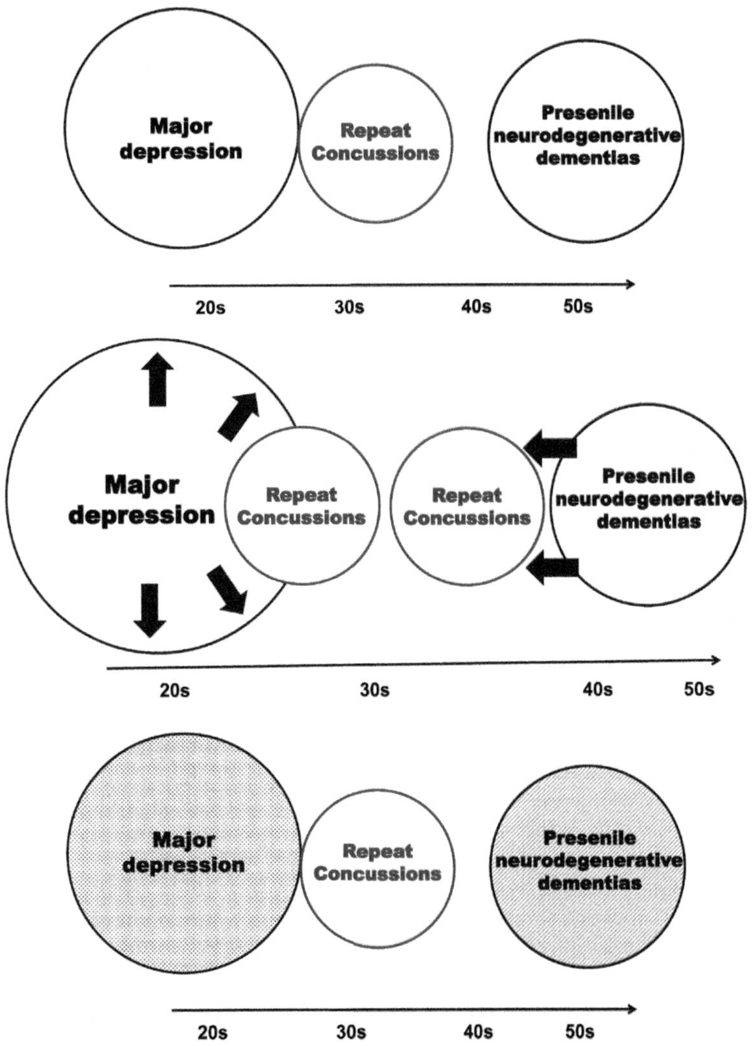

FIG. 3 The prominence of neuropsychiatric symptomatology in CTE and the debatable specificity of neuropathology raise important nosologic questions on the differentiation from common mood disorders and presenile dementias, especially of the frontotemporal type. *Top diagram* shows the sets of repeat concussions (*red*) and common mood disorders such as major depression (*purple*) and presenile neurodegenerative dementias (*blue*) along the age continuum. One possibility is that repetitive mild TBI increases the risk of other neuropsychiatric conditions in exposed patients including major depression (as TBI is known to do) or presenile neurodegenerative disorders (*middle diagram*). Another possibility is that repetitive mild TBI has a pathoplastic effect: Without increasing the incidence of major depression or accelerating a neurodegenerative process, it modifies depressive manifestations in the direction of aggressive or other acting out, or it adds a TBI-specific marker, for example, perivascular and deep sulcal pathology, to an independent neurodegenerative process (*bottom diagram*).

international experts in the field [24]. For example, if a psychiatrist examines a college football athlete player who presents with major depression (with or without alcohol or other substance abuse) and the patient asks if the mood change is the first stage in a disease that may eventually result in dementia, how does the clinician respond? Does he or she engage in discussion of prognosis? Moreover, how does the psychiatrist manage the patient? Based on the available evidence, our opinion is that the clinician should treat the patient as a case of common mood disorder with the appropriate recommended interventions, for example, antidepressants and cognitive-behavioral therapy. We would not engage in extensive discussion of CTE and focus, instead, on the favorable prognosis of a single mood episode. In our practice, we may state that such discussions are premature, and the likelihood that the presentation is related to CTE is extremely low. On the other hand, we bring up issues related to return to play or continued play and briefly discuss relevant recommendations from professional associations [71]. If the psychiatrist is not familiar with TBI or these recommendations, he or she may refer the patient for more expert advice.

Traumatic Brain Injury as a Risk Factor for Neurodegeneration Other Than Chronic Traumatic Encephalopathy

Earlier evidence that the amyloid precursor protein accumulates in injured axons in humans and animal models of TBI and some evidence that Aβ also accumulates inside and outside injured axons in the injured human brain [72,73] lends credence to multiple retrospective epidemiologic studies indicating that TBI increases risk for age-associated dementia [68,74–76] and that moderate-to-severe TBI increases AD × 2 [67,74,77,78]. However, Aβ deposits in the acute stage of TBI do not evolve into amyloid plaques [73]. In addition, the results of previous epidemiologic studies linking a history of TBI, especially moderate-severe TBI, and dementia or AD have come under scrutiny because they were based on self-reported history of TBI from subjects who are cognitively impaired and also on billing codes for ascertaining the presence of dementia or TBI. More recent studies have circumvented these problems either by including data from subjects with self-reported TBI while they were cognitively intact or by using more objective higher quality outcome measures, that is, pooled clinical and neuropathological data [65] or present-day clinical information aided by AD biomarkers [66].

One key study [65] used pooled clinical and neuropathologic data from 3 prospective community-based cohort studies on TBI and dementia (Religious Orders Study, the Memory and Aging Project, and the Adult Changes in Thought study, including 1589 autopsies) to indicate that TBI with loss of consciousness (LOC) was not associated with risk of AD-type neuropathology or AD dementia but showed association with Lewy body pathology, incidence of PD, and progression of parkinsonism. In addition, the study by Crane and colleagues found no role for APOE e4 genotype or gender in conferring AD risk [66]. Another study used Veterans Administration medical records to document a history of TBI, present-day clinical and neuropsychological data to ascertain the presence of dementia, and AD imaging biomarkers including structural (MRI) and molecular (florbetapir PET) to ascertain the presence of AD-type pathology [66]. This study found no effect of a prior history of TBI on cognition or biomarkers of AD. A more recent report based on data from the Health and Retirement Study also failed to find evidence of association between a history of TBI with the incidence of dementia or memory decline [79].

However, the problem of TBI as a causative factor for dementia remains open. For example, in a recent observational report using Denmark's comprehensive register systems with the impressive inclusion of 2.8 million people collectively exposed to 132,000 episodes of TBI during almost 4 decades (1977–2013) [80], the authors found significant increase of both all-cause dementia and AD risk; dementia risk was higher in the first 6 months after TBI and increased with number of TBI events. Another very large study [81] used data from Statistics Sweden and formed a retrospective, a case-control, and a sibling cohort to find that risk of dementia was 4 to 6 times higher in the first year after TBI, thereafter decreasing rapidly, yet remaining significant 3 decades later; risk was higher with severe or repetitive TBI. As commented in a recent review [82], the debate on the role of TBI in causing neurodegenerative disease continues because of the lack of an adequate characterization of TBI in existing studies and the insidious character of neurodegenerative disease. At any rate, the stronger association of dementia with TBI in the first year after TBI may argue for the role of the initial neuropathology (contusion, DAI, other) in causing severe cognitive impairments.

SUMMARY

Chronic TBI is a common medical problem resulting from brain contusions or DAI and perhaps also repeat concussions. Neuropsychiatric disorders are extremely common in chronic TBI, are a major cause of disability, and usually have a cognitive component. The neuropsychiatric profile of chronic TBI has recently come into sharp focus because of highly publicized cases of severe behavioral and cognitive problems in professional football players who fall under the rubric of CTE, a well-known but rare dementia previously restricted to boxers. Based on current hypotheses on CTE stages, the early phase of this condition is featured by depression and behavioral problems, making CTE a behavior-type dementia. Although this is a possibility, a clinician who is asked to assess such problems in young athletes should think of, and treat, common psychiatric disorders of this age range such as major depression. The later, presumably dementing, phase of CTE is not easy to differentiate from other common neurodegenerative dementias. Although prior exposure to TBI may have left a neuropathological signature in the brain, that is, perivascular and deep-sulcal tauopathy, the clinical significance of this is not entirely clear. Moderate-severe TBI may also be a risk factor for AD and AD-related dementias. Still, the most common cognitive impairments after TBI may be the direct consequences of frontal and associative pathologies featured by executive dysfunction and other frontal-type deficits.

ACKNOWLEDGMENT

This work was supported by NIA 3 P50 AG05146 and 1 R01 EY028039 from NIH and the Sidran Family Foundation.

REFERENCES

[1] Omalu BI, DeKosky ST, Minster RL, et al. Chronic traumatic encephalopathy in a National Football League player. Neurosurgery 2005;57(1):128–34 [discussion: 34].

[2] McKee AC, Cantu RC, Nowinski CJ, et al. Chronic traumatic encephalopathy in athletes: progressive tauopathy after repetitive head injury. J Neuropathol Exp Neurol 2009;68(7):709–35.

[3] Gregory S. The problem with football: how to make it safer: time magazine. 2010. Available at: http://content.time.com/time/subscriber/article/0,33009,1957459-2,00.html.

[4] McKee AC, Stern RA, Nowinski CJ, et al. The spectrum of disease in chronic traumatic encephalopathy. Brain 2013;136(Pt 1):43–64.

[5] Mahar I, Alosco ML, McKee AC. Psychiatric phenotypes in chronic traumatic encephalopathy. Neurosci Biobehav Rev 2017;83:622–30.

[6] McKee AC, Robinson ME. Military-related traumatic brain injury and neurodegeneration. Alzheimers Dement 2014;10(3 Suppl):S242–53.

[7] Academies IoMotN. Long-term consequences of traumatic brain injury. Gulf War and Health, vol. 7. Washington, DC: The National Academies Press; 2009.

[8] Babikian T, Merkley T, Savage RC, et al. Chronic Aspects of Pediatric Traumatic Brain Injury: Review of the Literature. J Neurotrauma 2015;32(23):1849–60.

[9] Rabinowitz AR, Li X, McCauley SR, et al. Prevalence and Predictors of Poor Recovery from Mild Traumatic Brain Injury. J Neurotrauma 2015;32(19):1488–96.

[10] Traumatic brain injury and concussion: Centers of disease control. 2019. Available at: https://www.cdc.gov/traumaticbraininjury/get_the_facts.html.

[11] Charcot JM, Harris R. Clinical lectures on diseases of the nervous system. London ; New York: Tavistock/Routledge; 1991 lxviii, xviii, 438.

[12] Koliatsos VE, Xu L, Ryu J, et al. A Modern Clinicopathological Approach to Traumatic Brain Injury. Conn's Translational Neurosci 2017;467–87.

[13] Koliatsos VE, Rao V. The Behavioral Neuroscience of Traumatic Brain Injury. Psychiatr Clin North Am 2020;43(2):305–30.

[14] Moe HK, Limandvik Myhr J, Moen KG, et al. Association of cause of injury and traumatic axonal injury: a clinical MRI study of moderate and severe traumatic brain injury. J Neurosurg 2019;1–9.

[15] Koliatsos VE, Alexandris AS. Wallerian degeneration as a therapeutic target in traumatic brain injury. Curr Opin Neurol 2019;32(6):786–95.

[16] Moenninghoff C, Kraff O, Maderwald S, et al. Diffuse axonal injury at ultra-high field MRI. PLoS One 2015;10(3):e0122329.

[17] Su E, Bell M. Diffuse axonal injury. In: Laskowitz D, Grant G, editors. Translational research in traumatic brain injury. Boca Raton (FL): Frontiers in Neuroscience; 2016.

[18] Ubukata S, Ueda K, Sugihara G, et al. Corpus Callosum Pathology as a Potential Surrogate Marker of Cognitive Impairment in Diffuse Axonal Injury. J Neuropsychiatry Clin Neurosci 2016;28(2):97–103.

[19] van Eijck MM, Schoonman GG, van der Naalt J, et al. Diffuse axonal injury after traumatic brain injury is a prognostic factor for functional outcome: a systematic review and meta-analysis. Brain Inj 2018;32(4):395–402.

[20] Corsellis JA, Bruton CJ, Freeman-Browne D. The aftermath of boxing. Psychol Med 1973;3(3):270–303.

[21] Critchley M. Medical aspects of boxing, particularly from a neurological standpoint. Br Med J 1957;1(5015):357–62.

[22] Martland HS. Punch drunk. J Am Med Assoc 1928;91:1103–7.

[23] McKee AC, Cairns NJ, Dickson DW, et al. The first NINDS/NIBIB consensus meeting to define neuropathological criteria for the diagnosis of chronic traumatic encephalopathy. Acta Neuropathol 2016;131(1):75–86.

[24] Stewart W, Allinson K, Al-Sarraj S, et al. Primum non nocere: a call for balance when reporting on CTE. Lancet Neurol 2019;18(3):231–3.

[25] Lee EB, Kinch K, Johnson VE, et al. Chronic traumatic encephalopathy is a common co-morbidity, but less frequent primary dementia in former soccer and rugby players. Acta Neuropathol 2019;138(3):389–99.

[26] Ryu J, Horkayne-Szakaly I, Xu L, et al. The problem of axonal injury in the brains of veterans with histories of blast exposure. Acta Neuropathol Commun 2014;2:153.

[27] Bauman RA, Ling G, Tong L, et al. An introductory characterization of a combat-casualty-care relevant swine model of closed head injury resulting from exposure to explosive blast. J Neurotrauma 2009;26(6):841–60.

[28] Carrera E, Tononi G. Diaschisis: past, present, future. Brain 2014;137(Pt 9):2408–22.
[29] Dinkin M. Trans-synaptic Retrograde Degeneration in the Human Visual System: Slow, Silent, and Real. Curr Neurol Neurosci Rep 2017;17(2):16.
[30] Ziogas N, Castillo M, Ryu J, et al. Retrograde Degeneration of Corticothalamic Circuits after Traumatic Contusions in Ventral Frontal Lobes. J Neurotrauma 2017; 34(13):A135–6.
[31] Stewan Feltrin F, Zaninotto AL, Guirado VMP, et al. Longitudinal changes in brain volumetry and cognitive functions after moderate and severe diffuse axonal injury. Brain Inj 2018;32(10):1208–17.
[32] Ubukata S, Oishi N, Sugihara G, et al. Transcallosal Fiber Disruption and its Relationship with Corresponding Gray Matter Alteration in Patients with Diffuse Axonal Injury. J Neurotrauma 2019;36(7):1106–14.
[33] Koliatsos VE, Crawford TO, Price DL. Axotomy induces nerve growth factor receptor immunoreactivity in spinal motor neurons. Brain Res 1991;549(2):297–304.
[34] Koliatsos VE, Dawson TM, Kecojevic A, et al. Cortical interneurons become activated by deafferentation and instruct the apoptosis of pyramidal neurons. Proc Natl Acad Sci U S A 2004;101(39):14264–9.
[35] Koliatsos VE, Price DL. Axotomy as an experimental model of neuronal injury and cell death. Brain Pathol 1996;6(4):447–65.
[36] Coleman MP, Hoke A. Programmed axon degeneration: from mouse to mechanism to medicine. Nat Rev Neurosci 2020;21(4):183–96.
[37] Robinson JL, Lee EB, Xie SX, et al. Neurodegenerative disease concomitant proteinopathies are prevalent, age-related and APOE4-associated. Brain 2018;141(7): 2181–93.
[38] Jucker M, Walker LC. Propagation and spread of pathogenic protein assemblies in neurodegenerative diseases. Nat Neurosci 2018;21(10):1341–9.
[39] Ayers JI, Paras NA, Prusiner SB. Expanding spectrum of prion diseases. Emerg Top Life Sci 2020;4(2):155–67.
[40] Koliatsos VE, Xu L. The Problem of Neurodegeneration in Cumulative Sports Concussions: Emphasis on Neurofibrillary Tangle Formation. In: Kobeissy FH, editor. Brain Neurotrauma: molecular, neuropsychological, and rehabilitation Aspects. Boca Raton (FL: Frontiers in Neuroengineering; 2015.
[41] Rao V, Koliatsos V, Ahmed F, et al. Neuropsychiatric disturbances associated with traumatic brain injury: a practical approach to evaluation and management. Semin Neurol 2015;35(1):64–82.
[42] Deb S, Lyons I, Koutzoukis C, et al. Rate of psychiatric illness 1 year after traumatic brain injury. Am J Psychiatry 1999;156(3):374–8.
[43] Stefan A, Mathe JF, group S. What are the disruptive symptoms of behavioral disorders after traumatic brain injury? A systematic review leading to recommendations for good practices. Ann Phys Rehabil Med 2016;59(1): 5–17.
[44] Starkstein SE, Pahissa J. Apathy following traumatic brain injury. Psychiatr Clin North Am 2014;37(1): 103–12.
[45] Meyer A. The anatomical facts and clinical varieties of traumatic insanity. Am J Insanity 1904;60(3):373–441.
[46] Jorge RE, Arciniegas DB. Mood disorders after TBI. Psychiatr Clin North Am 2014;37(1):13–29.
[47] Jorge RE, Robinson RG, Moser D, et al. Major depression following traumatic brain injury. Arch Gen Psychiatry 2004;61(1):42–50.
[48] Jorge RE, Robinson RG, Arndt SV, et al. Depression following traumatic brain injury: a 1 year longitudinal study. J Affect Disord 1993;27(4):233–43.
[49] Jorge RE, Robinson RG, Starkstein SE, et al. Secondary mania following traumatic brain injury. Am J Psychiatry 1993;150(6):916–21.
[50] Ljungqvist J, Nilsson D, Ljungberg M, et al. Longitudinal study of the diffusion tensor imaging properties of the corpus callosum in acute and chronic diffuse axonal injury. Brain Inj 2011;25(4):370–8.
[51] Bonnelle V, Ham TE, Leech R, et al. Salience network integrity predicts default mode network function after traumatic brain injury. Proc Natl Acad Sci U S A 2012; 109(12):4690–5.
[52] Bonnelle V, Leech R, Kinnunen KM, et al. Default mode network connectivity predicts sustained attention deficits after traumatic brain injury. J Neurosci 2011;31(38): 13442–51.
[53] De Simoni S, Grover PJ, Jenkins PO, et al. Disconnection between the default mode network and medial temporal lobes in post-traumatic amnesia. Brain 2016;139(Pt 12): 3137–50.
[54] De Simoni S, Jenkins PO, Bourke NJ, et al. Altered caudate connectivity is associated with executive dysfunction after traumatic brain injury. Brain 2018;141(1):148–64.
[55] Bigler ED. Traumatic brain injury, neuroimaging, and neurodegeneration. Front Hum Neurosci 2013;7:395.
[56] Hayes JP, Bigler ED, Verfaellie M. Traumatic Brain Injury as a Disorder of Brain Connectivity. J Int Neuropsychol Soc 2016;22(2):120–37.
[57] Stuss DT. Traumatic brain injury: relation to executive dysfunction and the frontal lobes. Curr Opin Neurol 2011;24(6):584–9.
[58] Alexander GE, DeLong MR, Strick PL. Parallel organization of functionally segregated circuits linking basal ganglia and cortex. Annu Rev Neurosci 1986;9:357–81.
[59] Cummings JL. Frontal-subcortical circuits and human behavior. Arch Neurol 1993;50(8):873–80.
[60] Barrash J, Stuss DT, Aksan N, et al. Frontal lobe syndrome"? Subtypes of acquired personality disturbances in patients with focal brain damage. Cortex 2018;106:65–80.
[61] Lishman WA. Brain damage in relation to psychiatric disability after head injury. Br J Psychiatry 1968; 114(509):373–410.
[62] Winkler AE, Koliatsos VE. Right Hemisphere Syndrome in the Real World of Traumatic Brain Injury: Three Longitudinal Cases Seen in the Neuropsychiatry Program at

Sheppard Pratt Health System. J Neuropsychiatry Clin Neurosci 2019;31(3):E27–8.
[63] Heilman KM, Bowers D, Valenstein E, et al. The right hemisphere: neuropsychological functions. J Neurosurg 1986;64(5):693–704.
[64] Sherer M, Nakase-Thompson R, Yablon SA, et al. Multidimensional assessment of acute confusion after traumatic brain injury. Arch Phys Med Rehabil 2005;86(5): 896–904.
[65] Crane PK, Gibbons LE, Dams-O'Connor K, et al. Association of Traumatic Brain Injury With Late-Life Neurodegenerative Conditions and Neuropathologic Findings. JAMA Neurol 2016;73(9):1062–9.
[66] Weiner MW, Crane PK, Montine TJ, et al. Traumatic brain injury may not increase the risk of Alzheimer disease. Neurology 2017;89(18):1923–5.
[67] Fleminger S, Oliver DL, Lovestone S, et al. Head injury as a risk factor for Alzheimer's disease: the evidence 10 years on; a partial replication. J Neurol Neurosurg Psychiatr 2003;74(7):857–62.
[68] Gardner RC, Langa KM, Yaffe K. Subjective and objective cognitive function among older adults with a history of traumatic brain injury: A population-based cohort study. Plos Med 2017;14(3):e1002246.
[69] Stein TD, Crary JF. Chronic Traumatic Encephalopathy and Neuropathological Comorbidities. Semin Neurol 2020;40(4):384–93.
[70] Kelley CM, Perez SE, Mufson EJ. Tau pathology in the medial temporal lobe of athletes with chronic traumatic encephalopathy: a chronic effects of neurotrauma consortium study. Acta Neuropathol Commun 2019;7(1): 207.
[71] Giza CC, Kutcher JS, Ashwal S, et al. Summary of evidence-based guideline update: evaluation and management of concussion in sports: report of the Guideline Development Subcommittee of the American Academy of Neurology. Neurology 2013;80(24):2250–7.
[72] Uryu K, Chen XH, Martinez D, et al. Multiple proteins implicated in neurodegenerative diseases accumulate in axons after brain trauma in humans. Exp Neurol 2007; 208(2):185–92.
[73] Chen XH, Johnson VE, Uryu K, et al. A lack of amyloid beta plaques despite persistent accumulation of amyloid beta in axons of long-term survivors of traumatic brain injury. Brain Pathol 2009;19(2):214–23.
[74] Plassman BL, Havlik RJ, Steffens DC, et al. Documented head injury in early adulthood and risk of Alzheimer's disease and other dementias. Neurology 2000;55(8): 1158–66.
[75] Wang HK, Lin SH, Sung PS, et al. Population based study on patients with traumatic brain injury suggests increased risk of dementia. J Neurol Neurosurg Psychiatr 2012;83(11):1080–5.
[76] Nordstrom P, Michaelsson K, Gustafson Y, et al. Traumatic brain injury and young onset dementia: a nationwide cohort study. Ann Neurol 2014;75(3):374–81.
[77] Guo Z, Cupples LA, Kurz A, et al. Head injury and the risk of AD in the MIRAGE study. Neurology 2000; 54(6):1316–23.
[78] Perry DC, Sturm VE, Peterson MJ, et al. Association of traumatic brain injury with subsequent neurological and psychiatric disease: a meta-analysis. J Neurosurg 2016;124(2):511–26.
[79] Grasset L, Glymour MM, Yaffe K, et al. Association of traumatic brain injury with dementia and memory decline in older adults in the United States. Alzheimers Dement 2020;16(6):853–61.
[80] Fann JR, Ribe AR, Pedersen HS, et al. Long-term risk of dementia among people with traumatic brain injury in Denmark: a population-based observational cohort study. Lancet Psychiatry 2018;5(5):424–31.
[81] Nordstrom A, Nordstrom P. Traumatic brain injury and the risk of dementia diagnosis: A nationwide cohort study. Plos Med 2018;15(1):e1002496.
[82] LoBue C, Cullum CM, Didehbani N, et al. Neurodegenerative Dementias After Traumatic Brain Injury. J Neuropsychiatry Clin Neurosci 2018;30(1):7–13.

Advances in Psychiatry and Behavioral Health 1 (2021) 219–228
ADVANCES IN PSYCHIATRY AND BEHAVIORAL HEALTH

Learning Psychiatry

Then and Now

Lisa MacLean, MD[a,*], Deepak Prabhakar, MD, MPH[b]
[a]Henry Ford Health System, One Ford Place, 1C, Detroit, MI 48202, USA; [b]Outpatient Services, Sheppard Pratt, 6501 North Charles Street, Baltimore, MD 21204, USA

KEYWORDS
• Clinician well-being • Education • Culture • Technology • Practice trends

KEY POINTS

- Understanding, measuring, teaching, and investing in trainee and faculty well-being creates learning environments that are caring and supportive.
- Mentoring and role modeling that is culturally sensitive, accepting, and shows healthy work-life integration helps to recruit and retain clinicians within psychiatry.
- Innovative training opportunities in multiple medical settings, an emphasis on neuroscience research, and advances in further understanding pain, trauma care, and suicide are critical to the future of psychiatry.

INTRODUCTION

Mental illness is a major public health problem across the world [1]. Furthermore, people with mental illness are among the most stigmatized, marginalized, and vulnerable members of society and suffer because of their illness [2]. In order to ensure that the psychiatric workforce remains sustainable into the future and meets the mental health care demand, a new generation of motivated and enthusiastic young doctors is needed to enter psychiatry. A recent study showed in a comprehensive international survey that only 4.5% of students were considering a career in psychiatry [3]. This number is not enough to meet the demand. Now more than ever, understanding where psychiatry has been and moving toward where it needs to be is essential. Moreover, investing in trainees and faculty to create work environments that promote intellectual curiosity, social connectivity, and meaning in the work is critical to sustaining the workforce and promoting longevity in psychiatry.

Balancing the science of medicine with the art has been an ongoing struggle for many fields. Both are critical to this specialty. Every physician must learn to gather data critical for decision making and discuss the pros and cons of different treatment options in a humble and honest way. Deeply ingrained in the specialty is the ability to connect with the human soul. It is through deep listening, and showing empathy and compassion that psychiatrists contribute most to the betterment of their patients. One of our biggest challenges is to combine the science with the art in a way that promotes individuals' passion for the work and sustainability in medicine as a career. Compounding these issues is the gradual clarity in understanding how the practice of medicine affects students, residents, and faculty. Despite the significant personal reward, many struggle with symptoms of burnout, depression, disillusionment, and even suicidal thinking. The state that medicine is in at this time must be acknowledged and opportunities sought to address this distress.

*Corresponding author, *E-mail address:* Lmaclea1@hfhs.org

https://doi.org/10.1016/j.ypsc.2021.05.014
2667-3827/21/

Despite the concerns regarding stress and burnout in health care, this is an exciting time to be in psychiatry. Now, more than ever, with advances in neurosciences and technology, there is opportunity to be building bridges with other fields of medicine to increase capacity to take care of the mentally ill. New innovations such as artificial intelligence and neurostimulation techniques are driving further change and creating additional training opportunities. Advances in substance use treatment, suicide prevention, and neuroscience offer an opportunity for additional cutting-edge training experiences.

This article discusses the evolution of psychiatry, focusing specifically on the current vulnerabilities affecting the psychiatric workforce and future educational trends within the field. This article reflects on where the authors believe psychiatry has been and where it is going. It explores current training attitudes, the culture of medicine, the assessment of clinician well-being, advances in technology, supervision challenges, and the practice trends in psychiatry. It makes some specific recommendations for psychiatry departments to meet the needs of their trainees and faculty so that they are prepared for the current and future state of psychiatry. It organizes these strategies into the domains of (1) clinician well-being and (2) education and training.

DISCUSSION

Training Attitudes

The American Medical Association and the Health Resources and Services Administration have identified an extreme shortage of psychiatrists in the United States. [4]. Recruitment into psychiatry has been an ongoing challenge for many decades, resulting in not having enough psychiatrists to care for the aging population. In recent times, the level of psychiatric morbidity in the population has not decreased, nor has the demand for psychiatrists. Instead, with ever-changing social conditions, research shows not only an overall increased prevalence of mental illness but also a growth in suicide rates [5,6]. There are many factors that could be contributing to recruitment challenges into the field. Brockington and Mumford [7] named a few, including manageable but not reversible disorder, negative stigma, a belief that psychiatry is unscientific, lower income potential, and antipsychiatry sentiment. In contrast, many who enter the field voice a strong personal concern for the mentally ill. A study by Walton [8] showed that students who choose psychiatry are more reflective and responsive to abstract ideas, liked complexity, and were tolerant of ambiguity. Scher and colleagues' [9] work showed that students entering psychiatry appreciated its holistic approach and the opportunity to know patients in depth. However, negative attitudes toward psychiatry and psychiatrists may be well ingrained before students even enter medical school. Denigrating fictional images of mental illness appear frequently in the media. These portrayals do little to convince the public that people with mental illness are not violent or that they can recover. Media images of psychiatry are equally negative, with images depicting treatments as oppressive and controlling and mental health professionals as unethical, exploitive, and mentally deranged [10]. In the 1930s, when the neurosciences were still in their infancy, the field relied on psychology and the social sciences contributing to the understanding of patients [11]. This situation led to separation from a more structural neurology approach, and the decision to break away from neurology set a historical precedent when psychiatry became the first medical specialty without ties to a particular organ. One byproduct of this was the moving away of patients with dementia, developmental disability, and substance use disorders in favor of those with trust issues, low self-esteem, and neurosis. In the last 50 years, there has been gradual and steady growth back toward the biological aspects of mental illness. Some clinicians would argue this paradigm shift has been critical to secure the future of the field as a respected specialty.

Outside of psychiatry, the world of medicine seems to be changing too. Medical schools have gone to holistic admission processes, opening up medicine to a diverse group of applicants. This approach aligns with psychiatry's desire to increase diversity, equity, and inclusivity within the field. Considering the national shortage of psychiatrists, there is an increased movement to collaborate and train our primary care colleagues to manage straightforward mental health concerns, leaving the more complex cases for psychiatrists. There is also a movement away from hierarchical medicine and toward valuing every member of the team, including students and residents. Generationally, both groups want to contribute to the care of the patients, and the medical world is slowly adjusting and moving toward a culture of caring and support and away from one of shame and blame. Training attitudes in psychiatry require the development of settings that encourage self-reflective processes in which trainees become aware of their own cultural assumptions, biases, and their personal struggles. Understanding and respecting the diverse backgrounds of patients and colleagues requires attitudes of curiosity and humility. To build empathy across cultures and generations, trainees need to tolerate uncertainty and ambiguity and build their self-awareness. All of this can only be fostered in a culture that is supportive of individual growth and learning needs.

Culture of Medicine

The culture of medicine continues to be an impediment to overall progress. Once a well-respected career, now many bright young people experience burnout before they even complete their medical training. In the United States, burnout has reached rampant levels with more than one-half of physicians experiencing symptoms [12]. Broadly, burnout is a combination of exhaustion, cynicism, and perceived inefficacy resulting from long-term job stress [13].

The consequences of burnout are not limited to the personal well-being of the health care workers; many studies have shown that provider burnout is detrimental to patient care and correlates with lower patient satisfaction [14,15]. Clinically, burnout can interfere with an individuals' ability to establish rapport, sort through diagnostic dilemmas, and work through complex treatment decision making [16]. Burnout can also result in greater job turnover, early retirement, and a reduction in clinical hours, which likely contributes to the national concern regarding physician shortages [17]. There have been many identified causes of burnout, including too many bureaucratic tasks and increasing mechanization of practice [18]. Specific to psychiatry, Lambert and colleagues [19] report a high number of challenging patients, depressing work conditions, job stress, and low morale among staff as the reasons doctors are leaving the field. Other factors that contribute to burnout within psychiatry include a lack of administrative support and validation, low pay, responsibility without corresponding authority, and too much paperwork and bureaucracy [20]. Additional factors could also contribute to burnout in psychiatry and should be considered, including risk of violence, limited resources, crowded inpatient wards, and an increasing culture of blame creeping into the mental health services [21].

Surprisingly, even with high levels of distress reported, psychiatrists continue to report high levels of job satisfaction [22]. Being valued, task variety, and having support in their role were some factors that contributed to job satisfaction [20]. The relative risk of specialty choice regret is also reported to be lower among psychiatric trainees than among those training in internal medicine [23]. Furthermore, clinical specialty areas with the highest prevalence of resident physicians experiencing symptoms of burnout mirror those of practicing physicians [24]. These finding suggest that increased burnout among physicians in specific specialties may be related, in part, to the unique characteristics of the work intrinsic to each specialty. Psychiatry uses and celebrates specific personal qualities that can be protective, such as high levels of empathy. The training environment is also typically caring and supportive, emphasizing self-reflection and self-compassion.

In contrast, these same qualities can also create stress for psychiatrists. Psychiatrists as a professional group are particularly prone to stress [25]. Specific stressors within the field include overwork, perceived stigma, relationships with other staff, inadequate resources, and working with violent patients. Jovanovic and colleagues [26] found that those who work with chronically ill patients are more emotionally exhausted than others. Patient suicide is also an important occupational hazard for psychiatrists. The personal stress brought on by this event is significant. Chemtob and colleagues [27] showed that psychiatrists experience feelings of anger and guilt, low self-esteem, and intrusive thoughts of the suicide and that 57% of psychiatrists reported experiencing posttraumatic stress symptoms after a patient suicide. Younger psychiatrists were more affected by a patient suicide than their older, more experienced colleagues [28]. Kumar and colleagues [29] describe the personal nature of the relationship between patients and their psychiatrists. This relationship can evoke emotions such as a need to rescue the patient; a sense of failure or frustration when the patient fails to improved or respond to treatment; and, at times, a desire to escape the feelings of grief, loss, and fear when a patient's mental health declines despite the clinician's greatest efforts [30].

However, the personality features that attract students to psychiatry, such as openness and empathy, may also be the same traits that predispose them to burnout and make them prone to internalize stressful experiences [29]. The training experience may also play a significant role in the causation of stress and burnout. Psychiatric trainees are more closely involved with people's inner worlds and personal difficulties than other disciplines, which could result in more self-doubt, anxiety, and fatigue [31]. Even after adjusting for individual differences, country differences in burnout rates, and years in training, 3 work-related factors remained associated with severe burnout in psychiatry trainees: long working hours, lack of clinical supervision, and not having regular time to rest [26]. These issues need to be acknowledged by the residency program and addressed actively in supervision. In particular, an emphasis on healthy coping, appreciation for a job well done, and mentorship may play an important role in the eventual outcome of chronic stress [32,33].

It is with this in mind that psychiatry needs to build on and create interventions that will protect its workforce. There is some evidence that lifestyle factors and paying attention to one's nonprofessional life may have a protective effect [34]. There is also evidence that teaching is associated with decreased burnout by increasing the sense of professional accomplishment. This idea aligns with the work done by Shanafelt and colleagues [35] that found that clinicians who spent less than 20% of their time in work they found most meaningful had an increase in risk for burnout. There is still work to be done to continue to promote learning environments that allow trainees to blossom by emphasizing qualities such as empathy, self-compassion, and curiosity and showing that the profession cares about them as much as it cares about the patients. The external stressors caused by rapidly changing ways of service delivery, the widening gaps between the way residents are trained and the way they practice, and the increasingly complex administrative and legal frameworks must also be remembered [36].

Furthermore, it is important to consider the causes but equally important to develop strategies to combat burnout. Doing so means involving leadership, encouraging work-life integration, creating resources that allow self-care and stress management, and encouraging peer support. Another central way involves connecting clinicians with the reasons they entered medicine and creating learning environments that build trust and allow open dialogue about the pain points that drive distress. Educators need to celebrate the art of medicine and emphasize healing as just as important as curing. Validating uncertainty, encouraging beginners minds, acknowledging grief and loss as part of medicine, and emphasizing effective patient communication and centricity brings clinicians closer to the vision of who they want to be in medicine [33].

Assessment of Clinician Well-Being

In 2017, the Accreditation Council for Graduate Medical Education mandated that accredited programs and institutions develop wellness programming for both residents and faculty focused on preventing and mitigating burnout within residency programs [37]. This requirement came after burnout research showed that medical students enter medical school with less burnout and improved quality of life compared with same-age controls and, by year 2 of medical school, have reduced quality of life and burnout [38]. Similarly, medical students enter medical school with high degrees of empathy, which gradually decline throughout medical school [39]. Research shows that depression and suicidal ideation, plans, and attempts are noted to be high in trainees with burnout and decline with recovery from it [40,41]. Burnout may also lead to increased alcohol or drug use, which can negatively affect patient care [42].

Creating mechanisms for residents and faculty to measure their well-being is essential. It shows that you care enough to ask but it is also the first step to creating strategies for change. There are many tools that might be considered, but having national comparative data is particularly helpful. Data gathering should be followed by conversations with colleagues about the specific pain points in order to understand the key drivers. These strategies are seldom a one-size-fits-all recipe, even within the same institution, and are highly dependent on the department. There are particular issues related to psychiatry that need to be addressed as a plan is developed. Developing the plan in collaboration with resident input can also be a key to success.

Advances in Technology

Within medicine, there is a huge variation in learner preferences. Biomedical research data doubles every 20 years; thus, medical professionals must be able to constantly review material and update their knowledge base [43]. Most current trainees in medicine are from the millennial generation, and most attending physicians are either baby boomers or from Generation X [44]. The millennial generation, also known as Generation Y, refers to those born between 1982 and 2004 [45]. A study by Nimjee and colleagues [46] showed that baby boomers, Generation X, and millennials were all able to adopt newer technologies, but all experienced a phase of adjustment. Regardless of the depth of adjustment, embracing change is something everyone struggles with. Work by Ludviga and Sennikova [47] suggested that the response to change is different and dependent on the generation. Nimjee and colleagues [46] showed that baby boomers may be key influencers in the process of managing and steering change. This point speaks to the importance of senior faculty in adopting technology early so that those they mentor will adapt more quickly. These advances in technology will only continue over time, so developing an environment that not only welcomes but also accepts change as a natural part of personal growth is essential. In the context of these technology changes comes opportunity for growth and the acknowledgment that the old way is not necessarily the best way. New technology allows us to collaborate with colleagues across the nation, find information more quickly, and improve personal independence. If approached with openness, technology can break down walls.

Although the Accreditation Council for Graduate Medical Education outlines for psychiatry residency training programs the expected content of their education curriculum, many questions remain about how best to teach relevant knowledge, skills, and attitudes [48]. Current literature on curricula highlights the importance of maintaining a clinical focus with a balance between didactic content and process issues. Adult learning theory supports the need for teaching sessions to have an interactive, practical, and real-world context in order to engage learners and solidify knowledge [49]. Modern learners are not just interested in the what but also in the how and the why. Awaad and colleagues [50] found that the use of a process-oriented approach, especially for affectively potent topics such as culture, diversity, religion, and spiritually, resulted in a positive change in perceived competency and clinical practice for residents. This approach is predicated on a belief that clinicians have blind spots, anxieties, and sensitivities that may impede clinical care, and that, by exploring and seeking to understand their unspoken biases, clinical care can be enhanced. Integrating more interactive teaching methods such as process-oriented education, objective structured clinical examinations, standardized patients, role playing, virtual learning platforms, live patient testimonial, and interdisciplinary clinician panels into psychiatry educational curriculum needs further research but shows promise in engaging learners and improving competency.

Supervision Challenges

There is also a need to not only explore how clinicians teach but also the learning environment in which they teach. How can supervisors engage their adult learners and create learning environments that promote caring, support, and trust? Supervision has often been considered a unique learning experience for psychiatric trainees. It offers an effective platform for trainees to reflect on their practice, and supports development of competence and professional identity [51]. In light of the known importance of clinical supervision, it is surprising that almost 15% of trainees did not receive regular weekly supervision (or did not perceive it as such) [52]. With advances in thought and newer technology, gone is the discuss-after-you-see-the-patient model; supervision can now be in real time.

Generationally, the millennials grew up in environments in which their emotions were protected and their schedules were largely dictated by so-called helicopter parents. [53] Many of the struggles of previous generations were absent from their childhoods, and, with that, the growth that people experience because of hardship. As a result, some within this generation can be perceived as entitled. However, this generation values connectedness, teamwork, free expression, and work-life flexibility [54]. Honoring these values, supervision in this current time requires approaching these trainees thoughtfully and with sensitivity. When giving feedback, emphasizing the intent helps the trainees not only to take better care of patients but also to grow as individuals. Reminding trainees that medicine is a calling and not a job may be helpful in inspiring learners to meet the professional expectations set by the patients. Patients literally call on clinicians at their greatest need and to answer this call requires commitment and dedication. Acknowledging what is important in their lives and working with the trainees to find happy work-life integration is essential to their well-being. Millennials' emphasis on work-life balance can be one of their greatest contributions to medicine in working toward the restoration of work-life balance for all. Supervisors' own levels of burnout have the potential to adversely affect the learning environment by modeling burnout to residents', placing residents at greater risk for burnout [23].

The Current and Future Practice of Psychiatry

Mastery of knowledge and acquisition of technical skills are the core foundation of formal medical training, but it is clear that these achievements are not enough [55]. Teaching psychiatry trainees to self-assess their verbal and nonverbal cues and simultaneously regulate their own reactions takes practice. An increased ability to engage in self-reflection and self-regulation strengthens these abilities [56]. Mindfulness is one way to promote the development of these skills. It is understood as a present moment, purposeful, and nonjudgmental form of directing attention [57]. A study by Grepmair and colleagues [58] showed that the promotion of mindfulness in psychotherapy training can positively affect the course of treatment in patients. In addition to being present, it is also the ability to make sound decisions with professionalism that defines a good doctor [59]. Preparing residents to become independent

TABLE 1
Final Recommendations

	Clinician Well-Being	Education and Training
Training attitudes	• Create well-being programming that not only actively addresses the causes of burnout but promotes resilience • Acknowledge the impact of generational differences and work with trainees to create learning environments that allow good work-life integration	• Recognize the impact of stress and burnout on medical students and create psychiatry rotations that provides supportive supervision in caring learning environments
Culture of medicine	• Create a culture that shows respect, appreciation, collaboration, and transparency through open communication between trainees and faculty	• Enhance the perception of psychiatrists as good role models for trainees and the efficacy of psychiatric treatment with the goal of improving recruitment into psychiatry as a career
Assessment of clinical well-being	• Create a process to measure trainee and faculty well-being • Create mechanisms to manage resident workload, duty hours, self-care, and team building • Remove barriers to the use of mental health services by trainees and faculty by creating a streamlined process for care that is confidential and free	• Teach trainees to recognize stress, burnout, and depression in themselves and their colleagues and encourage them to use mental health services
Advances in technology	• Provide education and clear guidance on the appropriate use of technology and media in the clinical setting	• Role model the use of technology in patient care and in educational activities
Supervision challenges	• Invest in the well-being of supervisors, recognizing their role in creating learning environments that provide caring and support	• Create programming specific to patient suicide that focuses on support and validation with a goal of dissipating feelings of guilt, blame, and isolation • Develop mentoring processes that role model healthy coping behaviors and support good work-life integration • Develop process groups to help train residents in effective communication and professional identity

(continued on next page)

TABLE 1
(continued)

	Clinician Well-Being	Education and Training
Practice trends in psychiatry	• Teach about the art of medicine and emphasize and celebrate these qualities in training: self-compassion, mindfulness, empathy, deep listening, growth mindset, and self-awareness	• Train psychiatric residents in multiple medical settings through creating innovative training opportunities, particularly in primary care, pediatrics, obstetrics/gynecology, geriatrics, and palliative medicine using mental health expertise in diverse medical settings • Use non–mental health specialty settings to teach nonpsychiatrists how to screen for mental illnesses; provide initial treatment and education regarding when to refer for mental health specialty care • Provide psychiatric residents with culturally appropriate skills for dealing with patients who are disadvantaged and underserved and issues related to racism, unconscious bias, microaggressions, diversity, equity, and inclusion • Expand the research and education of psychiatry residents in neuroscience with the goal of bringing future advances into clinical practice • Integrate curriculum focused on the advances in areas such as pain, genetics, suicide prevention, trauma care, ethics, medication compliance, the use of artificial intelligence, and advanced psychopharmacology

decision makers dedicated to their patients is central to clinical education. Learning to handle clinical dilemmas while developing one's professional identity is essential to becoming a good psychiatrist.

Now, more than ever, because of the massive expansion of knowledge, residents need to be facile in using technology to quickly extract information from trusted sources. Topics such as evidence-based treatments, research design, interpretation of data, and ethics help to inform residents about up-to-date practices within the specialty. The expansion into neuroscience has opened new doors to other treatments beyond psychotherapy, psychopharmacology, and electroconvulsive therapy into neurostimulation techniques such as transcranial magnetic stimulation. There is also growing interest and use of complementary medical and natural supplement approaches as alternative strategies to psychopharmacology. In addition, the recognition of training in cultural psychiatry to support a diverse society is key to the effort to understand the impact of race, religion, and culture on mental health. Further understanding of specific populations such as immigrants, refugees, and ethnocultural groups needs additional research. There needs to be an emphasis on understanding the disparities in the delivery of mental health services to vulnerable populations.

Recently, there has been a quick adoption of emerging technology and rapid growth of the use of virtual platforms. Many clinicians have found the use of telemedicine to be acceptable, and patients voiced appreciation for the use of technology to continue and engage in care.

An emphasis on research that invests greater scientific effort into studies of cause and pathophysiology of major brain disorders is also needed. The number of research-intensive departments of psychiatry is small, and only 20% of the nation's medical schools participate in National Institutes of Health–sponsored research [60]. At present, there are too few psychiatrists who have completed research fellowships, too few mentors, and an overly rigid approach to graduate medical education with inadequate flexibility to allow the integration of research training into clinical training [61]. There are tremendous opportunities to conduct research into the cause of mental illness and develop selective and indicated preventive intervention for people at high risk for mental illness across the lifecycle, thereby enhancing the public health impact of modern psychiatric treatment. Psychiatry can also improve both assessment and treatment strategies via a deeper understanding of genetics, pathophysiology, functional neuroanatomy, and neuropsychopharmacology, allowing the development of more personalized interventions. The opportunity to develop and implement models of mental health service delivery that have public health relevance will further psychiatry's reach and allow it to combat stigma against the mentally ill.

Not forgetting the specialty's roots, it is also important to acknowledge that teaching skills in providing psychotherapy remains critical to clinicians' identity as psychiatrists. Over the years, the depth of training in psychotherapy continues to shrink. Often, the teaching and supervising of therapy cases is relegated to part-time clinical faculty [62]. As a result of all of the advances, it is easy for residents to move away from why they entered medicine. Psychiatry is still an area in which the art of medicine remains critical. Skills such as empathy, compassion, and listening continue to be central to residents' success in connecting with patients. Research also shows that connecting to these skills helps to build continued sustainability in medicine [62]. It is these relationships that drive satisfaction and meaning in the work that psychiatrist do. This area is also key to the health and wellness of trainees and psychiatry faculty. In addition, the development and maintenance of competence in trainees depends on self-directed learning, which, in turn, depends on self-assessment. Although Lynn and colleagues [63] showed that self-assessment did not correlate with academic mastery, honest and thoughtful self-assessment could help residents have greater insight into their well-being and encourage connecting with available mental health resources.

SUMMARY

Psychiatry is an integral part of the practice of medicine, and it is important that the specialty approaches its workforce holistically, providing the support that they need in order to find long-term happiness in the field. Psychiatry needs to be careful that it does not lose its roots: it must celebrate the art of medicine through deep listening, empathy, and compassion. Educators need to develop an active awareness of burnout, should incorporate a well-being curriculum into the general didactics, and should codevelop interventions for both preventive and mitigating burnout (Table 1). Program leadership should consider workload, mentorship, and team-building exercises to manage conflict resolution and make an effort to create caring and supportive learning environments. Reducing working hours and regular supervision could represent a way of reducing severe burnout. Helping trainees to create a defined boundary between work and home has been shown to be helpful [64]. It is important for faculty to model and demonstrate self-care and self-awareness and to support residents in identifying coping strategies that they find most useful. Psychiatrists need to be creative in thinking of ways to build connectivity with each other and the system as a whole. This work needs to be intentional to continue to recruit into the field and retain those already practicing psychiatry. This period is an exciting time to be in psychiatry, and embracing the advances as opportunities will solidify the specialty's role in medicine. Incorporating novel treatment approaches, growing the research foundation, and embracing developing technology are all critical to the future of psychiatry.

CLINICS CARE POINTS

- Programs should continuously update and integrate scientific advances in teaching curriculum.
- Faculty should ensure supervision appropriate to the level of training.
- Burnout mitigation should be addressed at the program level and during clinical rotations.

DISCLOSURE

The authors have nothing to disclose.

REFERENCES

[1] Demyttenaere K, Bruffaerts R, Posada-Villa J, et al. Prevalence, severity, and unmet need for treatment of mental

disorders in the World Health Organization World Mental Health Surveys. JAMA 2004;291:2581–90.
[2] Rusch N, Angermeyer MC, Corrigan PW. Mental illness stigma: concepts, consequences, and initiatives to reduce stigma. Eur Psychiatry 2005;20:529–39.
[3] Farooq K, Lydall GJ, Malik A, et al, ISOSCCIP Group. Why medical students choose psychiatry – a 20 country cross-sectional survey. BMC Med Educ 2014;14:12.
[4] Bureau of Health Workforce, Health Resources and Services Administration, US Department of Health and Human Services. Designated health professional shortage areas statistics. 2020. Available at: https://data.hrsa.gov/Default/GenerateHPSAQuarterlyReports. Accessed September 7, 2020.
[5] National Institute of Mental Health. Statistics: mental illness. 2019. Available at: https://www.nimh.nih.gov/health/statistics/mental-illness.shtml. Accessed September 7, 2020.
[6] Curtin SC, Warner M, Hedegaard H. Increase in suicide rate in the United States, 1999-2014. NCHS Data Brief 2016;241:1–8.
[7] Brockington I, Mumford D. Recruitment into psychiatry. Br J Psychiatry 2002;180:307–12.
[8] Walton HJ. Differences between physically-minded and psychologically-minded medical practitioners. Br J Psychiatry 1966;112:1097–102.
[9] Scher ME, Carline JD, Murray JA. Specialization in psychiatry: what determines the medical student's choice pro or con? Compr Psychiatry 1983;24: 459–68.
[10] Stuart H. Media portrayal of mental illness and its treatments: what effect does it have on people with mental illness? CNS Drugs 2006;20:99–106.
[11] Detre T. The future of psychiatry. Am J Psychiatry 1987; 144:621–5.
[12] Kane L. Medscape national physician burnout, depression & suicide report 2019 2019. Available at: https://www.medscape.com/slideshow/2019-lifestyle-burnout-depression-6011056. Accessed September 7, 2020.
[13] Maslach C, Jackson SE, Leiter MP. Maslach burnout inventory manual. 3rd edition. Palo Alto (CA): Consulting Psychological Press; 1996.
[14] Shanafelt TD, Balch CM, Bechamps G, et al. Burnout and medical errors among American surgeons. Ann Surg 2010;251:995–1000.
[15] Halbesleben JR, Rathert C. Linking physician burnout and patient outcomes: exploring the dyadic relationship between physicians and patients. Health Care Manage Rev 2008;33:29–39.
[16] Ishak WW, Lederer S, Mandili C, et al. Burnout during residency training: a literature review. J Grad Med Educ 2009;1:236–42.
[17] Shanafelt TD, Mungo M, Schmitigen J, et al. Longitudinal study evaluating the association between physician burnout and changes in professional work effort. Mayo Clin Proc 2016;91:422–31.
[18] Reith TP. Burnout in United States healthcare professionals: a narrative review. Cureus 2018;10:e3681.
[19] Lambert TE, Turner G, Fazel S, et al. Reasons why some UK medical graduates who initially choose psychiatry do not pursue it as a long-term career. Psychol Med 2006;36:679–84.
[20] Clark GH Jr, Vaccaro JV. Burnout among CMHC psychiatrists and the struggle to survive. Hosp Community Psychiatry 1987;38:843–7.
[21] Deahl M, Turner T. General psychiatry in no-man's land. Br J Psychiatry 1997;171:6–8.
[22] Rathod S, Roy L, Ramsay M, et al. A survey of stress in psychiatrists working in the Wessex region. Psychiatr Bull R Coll Psychiatr 2000;24:133–6.
[23] Dyrbye LN, Burke SE, Hardeman RR, et al. Association of clinical specialty with symptoms of burnout and career choice regret among US resident physicians. JAMA 2018;320:1114–30.
[24] Shanafelt TD, Hasan O, Dyrbye LN, et al. Changes in burnout and satisfaction with work-life balance in physicians and the general US working population between 2011 and 2014. Mayo Clin Proc 2015;90: 1600–13.
[25] Thomsen S, Soares J, Nolan P, et al. Feeling of professional fulfilment and exhaustion in mental health personnel: the important of organizational and individual factors. Psychother Psychosom 1999;68: 157–64.
[26] Jovanovic N, Podlesek A, Volpe U, et al. Burnout syndrome among psychiatric trainees in 22 countries: risk increased by long working hours, lack of supervision, and psychiatry not being first career choice. Eur Psychiatry 2016;32:34–41.
[27] Chemtob CM, Hamada RS, Bauer G, et al. Patients' suicides: frequency and impact on psychiatrists. Am J Psychiatry 1998;145:224–8.
[28] Prabhakar D, Balon R, Anzia JM, et al. Helping psychiatry residents cope with patient suicide. Acad Psychiatry 2014;38:593–7.
[29] Kumar S, Hatcher S, Huggard P. Burnout in psychiatrists: an etiological model. Int J Psychiatry Med 2005;35: 405–16.
[30] Meier DE, Back AL, Morrison RS. The inner life of physicians and care of the seriously ill. JAMA 2001;286:3007–14.
[31] Hoop JG. Hidden ethical dilemmas in psychiatric residency training: the psychiatry resident as dual agent. Acad Psychiatry 2004;28:183–9.
[32] Holloway F, Szmukler G, Cardon J. Support systems. 1. Introduction. Adv Psychiatr Treat 2000;6:226–35.
[33] Prabhakar D, MacLean L, Akinyemi E. Suicide and suicidal behaviors: supervising adverse outcomes. In: De Golia SG, Corcoran KM, editors. Supervision in psychiatric practice: practical approaches across Venues and providers. Washington, DC: American Psychiatric Association Publishing; 2019. p. 359–68.
[34] Garfinkel PE, Bagby RM, Schuller DR, et al. Predictors of success and satisfaction in the practice of psychiatry: a preliminary follow-up study. Can J Psychiatry 2001;46: 835–40.

[35] Shanafelt TD, West CP, Sloan JA, et al. Career fit and burnout among academic faculty. Arch Intern Med 2009;169:990–5.

[36] Kumar S. Burnout in psychiatrists. World Psychiatry 2007;6:186–9.

[37] Accreditation Council Graduate Medical Education. Improving physician well-being, restoring meaning in medicine. Available at: https://www.acgme.org/What-We-Do/Initiatives/Physician-Well-Being. Accessed September 21, 2020.

[38] Dyrbye LN, Harper W, Moutier C, et al. A multi-institutional study exploring the impact of positive mental health on medical students' professionalism in an era of high burnout. Acad Med 2012;87:1024–31.

[39] Dyrbye LN, Massie FS Jr, Eacker A, et al. Relationship between burnout and professional conduct and attitudes among US medical students. JAMA 2010;304:1173–80.

[40] Martin F, Poyen D, Bouderlique E, et al. Depression and burnout in hospital health care professionals. Int J Occup Environ Health 1997;3:204–9.

[41] Dyrbye LN, Thomas MR, Massie FS, et al. Burnout and suicidal ideation among U.S. medical students. Ann Intern Med 2008;149:334–41.

[42] Ahola K, Honkonen T, Pirokola S, et al. Alcohol dependence in relation to burnout among the Finnish working population. Addiction 2006;101:1438–43.

[43] Davies K, Harrison J. The information-seeking behavior of doctors: a review of the evidence. Health Info Libr J 2007;24:78–94.

[44] Padiyath A, Bolin E, Daily J. Recommendations for Millennials on successfully navigating medical training. MedEdPublish. 2019. Available at: https://doi.org/10.15694/mep.2019.000143.1. Accessed September 21, 2020.

[45] Howe N, Strauss W. Millennials rising: the next great generation. 3rd edition. New York: Vintage Books; 2000.

[46] Nimjee T, Miller E, Solomon S. Exploring generational differences in physicians' perspectives on the proliferation of technology within the medical field: a narrative study. Healthc Q 2020;23:53–9.

[47] Ludviga I, Sennikova I. Organizational change: generational differences in reaction and commitment. In: 9th International Scientific Conference "Business and Management 2016." Vilnius, Lithuania: Vilnius Gediminas Technical University; 2016. p. bm.2016.10. Accessed July 1, 2020.

[48] Accreditation Council for Graduate Medical Education. Psychiatry: psychiatry requirements and FAQs 2020. Available at: https://www.acgme.org/Specialties/Program-Requirements-and-FAQs-and-Applications/pfcatid/21/Psychiatry. Accessed September 7, 2020.

[49] Clapper TC. Beyond Knowles: what those conducting simulation need to know about adult learning theory. Clin Simul Nurs 2010;6:e7–14.

[50] Awaad R, Ali S, Salvador M, et al. A process-oriented approach to teaching religion and spirituality in psychiatry resident training. Acad Psychiatry 2015;39:654–60.

[51] Falender CA, Sharfranske EP. Clinical supervision: a competency-based approach. Washington, DC: American Psychological Association; 2004.

[52] Julyan TE. Educational supervision and the impact of workplace-based assessments: a survey of psychiatry trainees and their supervisors. BMC Med Educ 2009;9:51.

[53] Espinoza C, Ukleja M, Rusch C. Managing the Millennials: discover the core competencies for managing today's workforce. Hoboken (NJ): John Wiley & Sons; 2010.

[54] Howell LP, Joad JP, Callahan E, et al. Generational forecasting in academic medicine: a unique method of planning for success in the next two decades. Acad Med 2009;84:985–93.

[55] Wallace AG. Educating tomorrow's doctors: the thing that really matters is that we care. Acad Med 1997;72:253–8.

[56] Craig PE. Sanctuary and presence: an existential view on the therapist's contribution. Humanistic Psychol 1986;14:22–8.

[57] Kabat-Zinn J. Mindfulness-based interventions in context: past, present, and future. Clin Psychol (New York) 2003;10:144–56.

[58] Grepmair L, Mitterlehner F, Loew T, et al. Promotion of mindfulness in psychotherapists in training: preliminary study. Eur Psychiatry 2007;22:485–9.

[59] Inui TS. A flag in the wind: educating for professionalism in medicine. Washington, DC: Association of American Medical Colleges; 2003.

[60] National Institute of Mental Health, National Institutes of Health. The National Institute of Mental Health Strategic Plan Goals. 2008. Available at: https://www.nimh.nih.gov/about/strategic-planning-reports/index.shtml. Accessed June 28, 2020.

[61] Reynolds CF 3rd, Lewis DA, Detre T, et al. The future of psychiatry as clinical neuroscience. Acad Med 2009;84:446–50.

[62] Mohl PC, Lomax J, Tasman A, et al. Psychotherapy training for the psychiatrist of the future. Am J Psychiatry 1990;147:7–13.

[63] Lynn DJ, Holzer C, O'Neill P. Relationships between self-assessment skills, test performance, and demographic variables in psychiatry residents. Adv Health Sci Educ Theor Pract 2006;11:51–60.

[64] Sherman MD, Thelen MH. Distress and professional impairment among psychologists in clinical practice. Prof Psychol Res Pr 1998;29:79–85.

Advances in Psychiatry and Behavioral Health 1 (2021) 229–237
ADVANCES IN PSYCHIATRY AND BEHAVIORAL HEALTH

Clinical Psychology Training

Past, Present, and Future

Lisa R. Miller-Matero, PhD, ABPP[a,*], Nora Coultis, MS[b], Anissa J. Maffett, MA[b], Brittany A. Haage, MS[b], Sai B. Narotam, MS[b], Kellie M. Martens, PhD[c]
[a]Behavioral Health and Center for Health Policy & Health Services Research, Henry Ford Health System, 1 Ford Place, 1C, Detroit, MI 48202, USA; [b]Behavioral Health, Henry Ford Health System, 1 Ford Place, 1C, Detroit, MI 48202, USA; [c]Behavioral Health and Bariatric Surgery, Henry Ford Health System, 1 Ford Place, 1C, Detroit, MI 48202, USA

KEYWORDS
• Clinical psychology • Training • Technology • Board certification • Integrated care • Culture

KEY POINTS
- Training in clinical psychology has substantially grown over time.
- Recent key areas of growth include specialty training, integrated care, multiculturalism, and technology.
- Future research should focus on effectiveness of training components so that training experiences can be better tailored.

INTRODUCTION

Earning a doctorate in clinical psychology requires years of extensive training in mental health and behavior. Graduate school begins with years of coursework as well as clinical experiences known as practica, which allow students to gain direct clinical experience conducting psychological services while receiving close supervision from licensed psychologists. Typically, the final year of the graduate program is a year-long, full-time psychology internship, where the focus is primarily training in clinical services. Following the doctoral degree, trainees often complete a postdoctoral fellowship to gain additional supervised experience before independent licensure as a psychologist.

Training in clinical psychology, including coursework, and practicum, internship, and fellowship experiences, has changed over time. This article reflects on several key areas of recent growth in clinical psychology, including specialties/board certification, integrated care, technology, and multiculturalism. For each of these areas, the article reviews the history of the topic, how training in this area is delivered, and areas for future directions.

SPECIALTIES AND BOARD CERTIFICATION

The American Psychological Association (APA) Commission for the Recognition of Specialties and Subspecialties in Professional Psychology (CRSSPP) defines a specialty as an "area of psychological practice which requires advanced knowledge and skills acquired through an organized sequence of education and training." [1] Specialty training is obtained following a graduate education in psychology [2]. Specialty board certification, or documented competence in a defined area of practice, not only indicates breadth and depth of professional skills but also reflects a personal motivation that goes beyond what is required of licensure [2].

The history of specialization began when the APA established a certification committee in 1919; however, it was not until 1986 that the APA developed procedures to formally recognize specialties [1]. The CRSSPP was

*Corresponding author, *E-mail address:* LMatero1@hfhs.org

https://doi.org/10.1016/j.ypsc.2021.05.013
2667-3827/21/

established in 1995 and resulted in the formation of numerous specialties (Table 1) [1]. In addition to the CRSSPP, the American Board of Professional Psychology (ABPP) coordinates specialty boards [2,3]. The ABPP also conducts competency-based examinations and certifies specialists [2,3]. Historically, specialization and subsequent board certification have not been regarded as necessary in professional psychology [2,4]. However, there has been increased pressure for specialization and board certification as an indicator of competence because of the emphasis on improving the quality of patient care in the era of health care reform [2,5].

Training in Specialties and Board Certification

According to the ABPP, only 3337 psychologists were board certified by 2011, which represented a 1% increase compared with the previous decade [4,5]. Similarly, only 4% of psychologists were board certified by 2017 [6,7]. The rate of board certification may indicate the lack of exposure to experiential training during graduate school because specialties are generally considered to be achieved at the postdoctoral level [5]. Despite continued low rates of board certification, there have been many advances in training that encourage specialization. First, it is estimated that more than half of doctoral programs now offer specialized training, the most common of which are child, health psychology, neuropsychology, and family [8]. Belonging to a specialized track may include completion of certain coursework, research, and/or practica. Doctoral programs also place great emphasis on clinical experience through practica and externships where trainees can explore specialty interests outside of their academic institutions [9]. In addition, the Association of Psychology Postdoctoral and Internship Centers (APPIC) continues to add accredited internship sites with various specialties [9,10]. The APA and APPIC developed guidelines to improve the current specialty training model [2,10]. Changes included adopting a

TABLE 1
Recognized Specialties in Professional Psychology

Specialties	Year of Initial Recognition	ABPP Board Certification
Clinical neuropsychology	1996	Yes
Industrial-organizational psychology	1996	Yes
Clinical health psychology	1997	Yes
Psychoanalysis	1998	Yes
School psychology	1998	Yes
Clinical psychology	1998	Yes
Clinical child and adolescent psychology	1998	Yes
Counseling psychology	1998	Yes
Behavioral and cognitive psychology	2000	Yes
Forensic psychology	2001	Yes
Couple and family psychology	2002	Yes
Geropsychology	2010	Yes
Police and public safety psychology	2013	Yes
Sleep psychology	2013	No
Rehabilitation psychology	2015	Yes
Group psychology and group psychotherapy	2018	Yes
Serious mental illness psychology	2019	No
Clinical psychopharmacology	2020	No

Data from the American Psychological Association (APA) and American Board of Professional Psychology (ABPP).

developmental model that focuses on foundational, functional, and professional growth in training [2,10]. These guidelines have also been adopted by postdoctoral residency programs and aid in the identification of competencies and standards for attainment within specialty areas [2,10]. To improve the competency-based training model (ie, education, training, and experience), encourage board certification, and increase awareness of this process, the ABPP developed the Early Entry Program [10]. The goal of the program is to increase board certification and to expand diversity among board-certified specialists by allowing graduate students, interns, and postdoctoral fellows to begin the process of filing credentials [10]. There are also numerous divisions within the APA that offer information about specialties and more easily promote advances in specialty areas [10].

Despite these resources, the most beneficial resource for learning about specialized postdoctoral training opportunities comes from informal and formal professional contacts [11]. Compared with supervisors in clinical practice, fewer graduate academic advisors are board certified because many believe that board certification is not relevant to their professional goals [12]. Thus, they may be less likely to provide education on the credentialing process. Even within doctoral internships, programs have a great deal of autonomy with regard to didactic training and may not include education on the board certification process [13]. In contrast, postdoctoral fellowships are designed for continuing professional education and obtaining specialization [5,11], and, therefore, are likely to be where most of the specialty and board certification training occurs.

Future Directions

Although there is debate on the importance of board certification, the current and evolving health care climate supports specialization and credentialing [2]. As such, it is essential for educators, training directors, and supervisors to discuss the steps to credentialing as a part of professional development [10]. Mentors may consider becoming board certified themselves to communicate the importance of competency within a specialty [10]. There are also recommendations that preparation for board certification be integrated into internship and postdoctoral training programs [5]. Accreditation and specialty boards could also offer resources for training, such as funding or scholarships for preparation materials (eg, APA, APPIC), mentorship opportunities that connect current and previous trainees, and counsel from other professionals who have been through the credentialing process [11]. In addition, there is limited research examining the impact of board certification on psychological services and health outcomes [5]. Future research could elucidate the potential benefits and limitations of board certification on the services provided by psychologists.

INTEGRATED CARE

In psychology, integrated care is commonly defined as integrating psychological services in medical settings (ie, team-based rounds, meetings, and collaborating in patient care) [14]. Integrated care is classified into 6 levels, ranging from no or minimal collaboration to fully integrated models [15]. Common terms used to describe levels of integrated care include colocated, collaborative, and partially or fully integrated.

Early documentation of integration was in 1962 by Kaiser-Permanente, where a psychologist was placed in multiple primary care clinics [16], resulting in a 62% decrease in medical use by individuals who presented with unexplained physical symptoms. This early integration could perhaps explain why primary care is the most common medical setting in which psychological services are integrated. As such, much of the research on satisfaction and effectiveness of integrated care models is in a primary care setting. First, patients and physicians are overwhelmingly satisfied with having integrated services available [17–20]. Second, integrating behavioral health services into primary care increases access and use of behavioral health services regardless of age, gender, race/ethnicity, and insurance type [18,21,22]. Third, integrated care improves patient mental health outcomes, including depression [23,24] and anxiety [25,26]. Not only has integrated care improved psychiatric outcomes, it benefits physical health as well, including improvements in diabetes, medication adherence, blood pressure, cholesterol level, smoking cessation, weight management, and chronic pain [27–34]. In addition, because of these benefits, integrated care has resulted in a reduction of health care costs [35–37].

Training in Integrated Care

Historically, there has been a lack of standardized training in integrated care [38]. Thus, the APA created a task force to develop recommendations for training [39]. The task force contacted 1180 training programs and 230 (19.5%) responses were received. Of these, 48% indicated they provided training for integrated care at the doctoral level, 55% reported this at the internship level, and 31% endorsed training at the postdoctoral level. However, the type or quality of training in integrated care at these levels were not evaluated. Recommendations from the task force included that the APA (1) support advanced ways to train in topics essential to integrated care (ie, management of illness); (2) continue to educate the public, health care professionals, policy makers, and health care administrators regarding integrated care; (3) encourage educational programs to investigate relationships between physical and mental health; (4) focus on advocacy efforts that allow for funding of education and training; and (5) evaluate educational and training efforts in integrated care.

Although there is not a universally accepted model for training in integrated care, there are training opportunities across various levels of training, including doctorate programs, internships, postdoctoral fellowships, and as a psychologist. Nearly half of graduate programs that offer specialized training reported having a health-focused track, which is where training related to integrated care commonly occurs (ie, a course in primary care or psychopharmacology) [8,40–42]. Graduate students can also elect to complete a practicum in integrated care, where the student receives supervision for providing psychological services in a medical setting and works alongside other medical professionals [43]. Through a practicum experience, there may be opportunities to attend case conferences, didactics, and team meetings that provide additional training in integrated care in areas such as chronic pain, heart disease, weight loss management, and ethical concerns [44,45].

Internship and postdoctoral fellowship opportunities offer intensive supervised clinical experiences. Although the experiences may be similar to a practicum, interns and fellows are typically full time, have greater responsibilities and workload, and often have more autonomy [39]. Internships and fellowships that offer experiences in integrated care tend to be health systems, academic medical centers, and the Department of Veterans' Affairs (VA); the VA has offered integrated care training for approximately 50 years [46]. Licensed psychologists are encouraged to attend continuing education courses in integrated care, which could provide updated knowledge on integrated care practices, as well as consult with other psychologists [47,48].

Future Directions

As the demand for integrated care increases, so does the demand for training; thus, specific training opportunities for trainees and established psychologists need to be available. Although there has been substantial growth in training opportunities, there is no standardized training suggested for graduate programs, internships, fellowships, or for licensed psychologists. Further, current opportunities have not been systematically evaluated to determine whether they produce competency in integrated care. Therefore, future research evaluating the feasibility and effectiveness of integrated care is needed.

TECHNOLOGY

Psychological interventions have historically been implemented face to face; however, barriers such as cost, transportation, time conflicts/scheduling, and childcare may impede the adherence to attending appointments [49,50]. Technological advances allow alternative delivery methods of therapeutic services [49] and have increased patient access to psychological services [51]. Telehealth can be defined as the fusion of technology with the delivery of health services [52] and comes in many forms, such as smartphone apps, social media, wearable technology, phone interventions, computerized or Internet-delivered interventions, and videoconferencing [49,52].

Biofeedback, implemented around 1977, was one of the first advances in technology for psychology [49]. Wearable technology (ie, pedometers) and telephone interventions (ie, smoking cessation) followed in 1940s to 1950s and 1980s, respectively [49,53]. However, the recent mobile phone technology (ie, text messaging and applications) led to a quick emergence of numerous technology-based interventions [49].

Training in Technology

As technologies for psychological interventions continue to develop, training in this area is needed [52,54,55]. The Joint Task Force for the Development of Telepsychology Guidelines for Psychologists [51] developed 8 main guidelines for practicing telepsychology. The first guideline addresses the need for psychologists to demonstrate their competence in providing telepsychology services and continue to receive necessary training in telepsychology. However, there is a lack of documented guidelines for training programs, and there is no consensus for developing and implementing training in telepsychology [52,55]. Thus, there is a need for specific training in provision of telepsychology services and competencies unique to this growing area of clinical psychology [55].

Future Directions

There are several challenges and related future directions for training in telepsychology. First, there are systemic and administrative barriers that inhibit the ability to develop and provide adequate, standardized training in telepsychology. Regulations for providing technology-based psychological services vary by state [52,56]. In addition, billing, reimbursement, and licensure requirements hinder the universal application of telehealth [54]. The effect of COVID-19 (coronavirus disease 2019) on the use of telehealth services has provided some assistance in that insurance companies have made temporary allowances for telehealth services [57]. More standardized governmental and insurance policies could increase access to telehealth and the ability to provide training in this area.

Second, telepsychology presents unique ethical concerns regarding informed consent, confidentiality, and mandatory reporting [52,56]. Although there are ethical guidelines and standards for those aspects in traditional psychological services, technological services add a complexity that would require additional adaptation to those ethical considerations [56]. Furthermore, with technology continuously changing, additional adaptations will likely be needed [56]. Thus, training in ethical issues unique to telepsychology could improve patient care and prevent ramifications because licensing authorities can enforce penalties for violations of the ethics code for telepsychology services [58].

MULTICULTURALISM

With the racial and ethnic makeup of the United States becoming increasingly diverse over the past few decades [59], there has been a call for psychologists to be prepared to work with individuals of diverse backgrounds. The Commission on Accreditation defines diversity as being composed of numerous concepts, including age, race and ethnicity, gender and gender identify, sexual orientation, socioeconomic status, and religion [60]. Various definitions have been provided over the years to operationalize multicultural competence [61–63]; however, cultural awareness, cultural knowledge, and cultural skills are 3 elements of multicultural competence that have been deemed essential [63,64].

Growing sentiment about the ethical and moral obligation to recognize diversity has been reflected in the evolution of professional guidelines and training objectives. Before the 1960s, multicultural considerations in psychology were mostly nonexistent [65,66]. It was not until the 1960 to 1970s, considered the birth of the multicultural movement, that the role of diversity in theory, research, and practice was formally addressed [66]. Soon thereafter, the APA published Guidelines for Providers of Psychological Services to Ethnic, Linguistic, and Culturally Diverse Populations [67], which was followed by the publication of the Guidelines for Research in Ethnic Minority Communities in 2000 and the Guidelines on Multicultural Education, Training, Research, Practice, and Organization Change for Psychologists in 2003 [68,69].

Training in Multicultural Considerations

Formalized coursework addressing minority mental health considerations was sparse before the mid-1980s, with less than half of programs offering a course specifically addressing minority populations [70,71]. In 1986, the APA accreditation standards included mandatory multicultural education, although programs were largely left on their own to incorporate requirements [68,69,72]. Following this, the number of programs requiring formal coursework grew exponentially [73].

At present, APA accreditation continues to mandate that students receive training in multiculturalism and diversity [74]. APA guidelines include knowledge about various dimensions of diversity (eg, race, ethnicity, language, sexual orientation, gender, age, disability, class status, education, religious/spiritual orientation, other cultural dimensions); knowledge of one's own dimensions of identity (eg, worldview); an understanding broader social systems (eg, racism, systemic discrimination, marginalization), and knowledge of relevant research regarding evidence-based, culturally adapted interventions. Beyond this, academic institutions and training programs have been given latitude on how to address these guidelines. Consequently, little uniformity exists among programs. However, graduate students report receiving multicultural education from a multitude of sources (ie, courses, research, mentorship, clinical experiences) [75], and students report overall satisfaction with the infusion of diversity in their training [76]. More than half of students reported diversity being integrated into coursework, and 83% of advanced students reported multicultural training through clinical experiences. However, most students indicated that they had no experience in research focused on diversity and did not receive mentorship from minority faculty. Various training strategies currently used in the field include lecture, group discussion, immersive experiences, therapeutic role play, journaling, exposure to diverse individuals, service learning opportunities, and case vignettes [77]. However, there is limited information on the time spent on topics or range of topics covered. Further, students report a desire for diversity-related issues to be more intentionally incorporated throughout training [76].

Doctoral internships and postdoctoral fellowships remain areas of growth. To date, most of the research evaluating educational practices pertaining to multicultural competence has focused on graduate training. Thus, understanding of the training opportunities available during predoctoral and postdoctoral training is limited. Nonetheless, promising evidence indicates that students may make significant gains in both knowledge and skill while on internship and fellowship because trainees have often deemed internship sites to be more conducive to fostering multicultural competence than their academic institutions [78]. Effective strategies may include diversity-themed didactics and seminars and diverse student recruitment efforts [79].

Overall, several limitations make it difficult to fully conceptualize the state of diversity training within clinical psychology training programs. Although trainees are exposed to a wide variety of educational experiences, very little research has been conducted to decide which modalities are effective in building the skills needed for autonomy. In the context of a dearth of research, some evidence has shown the effectiveness of specific methods on self-perceived competence. For example, programs with diversity committees or courses based on specific theoretic approaches (eg, tripartite model of cultural competency) seem to be beneficial [76,80]. Clinical experience and supervision have also been found to be integral to training, particularly for minority trainees [81,82].

Future Directions

One area for growth is ensuring that trainees are provided comprehensive training in all spheres of diversity. When asked to define diversity, students tend to disproportionately focus on ethnicity, race, and culture [75]. A similar lack of breadth has been reported in other studies, and training programs may benefit from expanding the focus of training to address underrepresented backgrounds, such as disability status and lesbian, gay, bisexual, transgender, queer, intersex, asexual, and agender (LGBTQIA) identities, spiritual and religious issues, and issues related to social justice and health disparities [76,83,84].

At present, there is insufficient information on the effectiveness of specific strategies in fostering multicultural competence. Studies that have sought to examine the impact of training on multicultural competence have relied primarily on self-reported competence rather than skill [77,85]. Future research examining the most effective strategies will help determine the best direction for training. Future studies should also extend past graduate training institutions and allocate attention to examining the most effective strategies in doctoral internships and postdoctoral fellowship training. As such, clinical psychology may benefit from having evidence-based training, skills-based assessments, and specific competency benchmarks across different levels of training [75,85–88].

SUMMARY

There has been a great deal of growth in what is needed, and desired, for training in clinical psychology. Although historically the doctorate has been focused on generalized training and specialization began during fellowship, it seems that specialization now often begins during graduate school. In addition, as society has changed, various gaps in training have been recognized (ie, integrated care, multiculturalism, and technology) and methods have been developed to fill these gaps in an effort to train competent psychologists. One challenge of implementing new training is that graduate programs, internships, and fellowships already have many requirements to meet (often because of rigorous APA accreditation standards), and it becomes difficult to integrate new education modules. Although much of this additional training could be (and currently often is) achieved outside of coursework either as a formal didactic/workshop or integrated into clinical experiences and supervision, there is a need to be creative to address the needs of trainees. Future directions include finding additional ways to provide essential training in these key areas.

DISCLOSURE

The authors have nothing to disclose.

REFERENCES

[1] APA. Specialties, subspecialities, and proficiencies in professional psychology. 2020. Available at: https://www.apa.org/ed/graduate/specialize. Accessed November 7, 2020.

[2] Kaslow NJ, Graves CC, Smith CO. Specialization in psychology and health care reform. J Clin Psychol Med Settings 2012;19(1):12–21.

[3] ABPP. Learn about specialty boards 2020. Available at: https://www.abpp.org/Applicant-Information/Specialty-Boards.aspx. Accessed November 7, 2020.

[4] Dattilio F. Board Certification in Psychology: Is It Really Necessary? Prof Psychol Res Pr 2002;33:54–7.

[5] Robiner WN, Dixon KE, Miner JL, et al. Board Certification in Psychology: Insights from Medicine and Hospital Psychology. J Clin Psychol Med Settings 2012;19(1):30–40.

[6] ABPP. ABPP Directory. 2017. Available at: www.abpp.org/i4a/member_directory/feSearchForm.cfm?directory_id=3. Accessed November 7, 2020.

[7] Lin L, Christidis P, Stamm K. A look at psychologists' specialty areas. Monitor Psychol 2017;48(8).

[8] Perry KM, Boccaccini MTJCPS, Practice. Specialized training in APA-accredited clinical psychology doctoral programs: Findings from a review of program websites. Clinical Psychology: Science and Practice 2009;16(3): 348–59.

[9] Belar CD. Graduate education in clinical psychology. "We're not in Kansas anymore". Am Psychol 1998; 53(4):456–64.

[10] Cox DR. Board certification in professional psychology: promoting competency and consumer protection. Clin Neuropsychol 2010;24(3):493–505.

[11] Logsdon-Conradsen S, Sirl K, Battle J, et al. Formalized postdoctoral fellowships: A national survey of postdoctoral fellows. Prof Psychol Res Pr 2001;32(3):312–8.

[12] Crowley SL, Lichtenberg JW, Pollard JW. Board Certification in Counseling Psychology. Couns Psychol 2012; 40(6):944–58.

[13] Zuckerman SE, Weisberg RB, Silberbogen AK, et al. A National Survey on Didactic Curricula in Psychology Internship Training Programs. Train Educ Prof Psychol 2019;13. https://doi.org/10.1037/tep0000279.

[14] James LC. Integrating clinical psychology into primary care settings. J Clin Psychol 2006;62(10):1207–12.

[15] Heath B, Wise Romero P, Reynolds K. A standard framework for levels of integrated healthcare. Washington, DC: SAMHSA-HRSA Center for Integrated Health Solutions; 2013.

[16] Masters KS, Stillman AM, Browning AD, et al. Primary Care Psychology Training on Campus: Collaboration Within a Student Health Center. Prof Psychol Res Pr 2005;36(2):144–50.

[17] Funderburk JS, Sugarman DE, Maisto SA, et al. The description and evaluation of the implementation of an integrated healthcare model. Fam Syst Health 2010; 28(2):146–60.

[18] Miller-Matero LR, Dykuis KE, Albujoq K, et al. Benefits of integrated behavioral health services: The physician perspective. Fam Syst Health 2016;34(1):51–5.

[19] Miller-Matero LR, Khan S, Thiem R, et al. Integrated primary care: patient perceptions and the role of mental health stigma. Prim Health Care Res Dev 2018;20:1–4.

[20] Pomerantz A, Cole BH, Watts BV, et al. Improving efficiency and access to mental health care: combining integrated care and advanced access. Gen Hosp Psychiatry 2008;30(6):546–51.

[21] Guck T, Guck A, Badura-Brack A, et al. No-Show Rates in Partially Integrated Models of Behavioral Health Care in a Primary Care Setting. Families, Syst Health 2007;25: 137–46.

[22] Horevitz E, Organista KC, Arean PA. Depression Treatment Uptake in Integrated Primary Care: How a "Warm Handoff" and Other Factors Affect Decision Making by Latinos. Psychiatr Serv 2015;66(8):824–30.

[23] Linde K, Sigterman K, Kriston L, et al. Effectiveness of psychological treatments for depressive disorders in primary care: systematic review and meta-analysis. Ann Fam Med 2015;13(1):56–68.

[24] Santoft F, Axelsson E, Öst LG, et al. Cognitive behaviour therapy for depression in primary care: systematic review and meta-analysis. Psychol Med 2019;49(8):1266–74.

[25] Butler M, Kane RL, McAlpine D, et al. Does Integrated Care Improve Treatment for Depression?: A Systematic Review. J Ambul Care Manage 2011;34(2):113–25.

[26] Roy-Byrne P, Craske MG, Sullivan G, et al. Delivery of evidence-based treatment for multiple anxiety disorders in primary care: a randomized controlled trial. J Am Med Assoc 2010;303(19):1921–8.

[27] Bogner HR, de Vries HF. Integration of depression and hypertension treatment: a pilot, randomized controlled trial. Ann Fam Med 2008;6(4):295–301.

[28] Bogner HR, de Vries HF. Integrating type 2 diabetes mellitus and depression treatment among African Americans: a randomized controlled pilot trial. Diabetes Educ 2010;36(2):284–92.

[29] Katon WJ, Lin EH, Von Korff M, et al. Collaborative care for patients with depression and chronic illnesses. N Engl J Med 2010;363(27):2611–20.

[30] Miller-Matero LR, Hecht L, Miller MK, et al. A brief psychological intervention for chronic pain in primary care: A pilot randomized controlled trial. Pa Med 2021 pnaa444.

[31] Piper ME, Baker TB, Mermelstein R, et al. Recruiting and engaging smokers in treatment in a primary care setting: developing a chronic care model implemented through a modified electronic health record. Transl Behav Med 2013;3(3):253–63.

[32] Sadock E, Auerbach SM, Rybarczyk B, et al. Evaluation of integrated psychological services in a university-based primary care clinic. J Clin Psychol Med Settings 2014; 21(1):19–32.

[33] Schütze R, Slater H, O'Sullivan P, et al. Mindfulness Based Functional Therapy: A preliminary open trial of an integrated model of care for people with persistent low back pain. Front Psychol 2014;5:839.

[34] Von Korff M, Katon WJ, Lin EH, et al. Functional outcomes of multi-condition collaborative care and successful ageing: results of randomised trial. Bmj 2011;343:d6612.

[35] Wahass SH. The role of psychologists in health care delivery. J Fam Commun Med 2005;12(2):63–70.

[36] Bruns D, Mueller K, Warren PA. Biopsychosocial law, health care reform, and the control of medical inflation in Colorado. Rehabil Psychol 2012;57(2):81–97.

[37] Lemmens LC, Molema CC, Versnel N, et al. Integrated care programs for patients with psychological comorbidity: A systematic review and meta-analysis. J Psychosom Res 2015;79(6):580–94.

[38] Talen M, Fraser JS, Cauley K. From soup to nuts: Integrating clinical psychology training into primary healthcare settings. Families, Syst Health 2002;20:419–29.

[39] Cubic B, Neumann C, Kearney L, et al. Report of the primary care training task force to the APA board of educational Affairs. Washington, DC: American Psychological Association; 2011.
[40] Kenkel MB, DeLeon PH, Mantell EO, et al. Divided No More: Psychology's Role in Integrated Health Care. Can Psychology/Psychologie canadienne 2005;46(4): 189–202.
[41] O'Donohue WT, Cummings NA, Cummings JL. The unmet educational agenda in integrated care. J Clin Psychol Med Settings 2009;16(1):94–100.
[42] McDaniel S, Belar C, Schroeder C, et al. A training curriculum for professional psychologists in primary care. Prof Psychol Res Pr 2002;33:65–72.
[43] Moye J, Brown E. Postdoctoral training in geropsychology: Guidelines for formal programs and continuing education. Prof Psychol Res Pr 1995;26(6):591–7.
[44] Bray JH. Training Primary Care Psychologists. J Clin Psychol Med Settings 2004;11(2):101–7.
[45] Twilling LL, Sockell ME, Sommers LS. Collaborative practice in primary care: Integrated training for psychologists and physicians. Prof Psychol Res Pr 2000;31(6):685–91.
[46] Spruill J. Interprofessional health care services in primary care settings: Implications for the education and training of psychologists. Washington, DC: Am Psychol Assoc 1998.
[47] McDaniel SH, Hargrove DS, Belar CD, et al. Recommendations for education and training in primary care psychology. In: Frank RG, McDaniel SH, Bray JH, Heldring M, editors. Primary care psychology. Washington, DC: American Psychological Association; 2004. p. 63–92.
[48] Anderson GL, Lovejoy DW. Predoctoral training in collaborative primary care: An exam room built for two. Prof Psychol Res Pr 2000;31(6):692–7.
[49] Arigo D, Jake-Schoffman DE, Wolin K, et al. The history and future of digital health in the field of behavioral medicine. J Behav Med 2019;42(1):67–83.
[50] Keefe FJ, Buffington ALH, Studts JL, et al. Behavioral medicine: 2002 and beyond. J Consult Clin Psychol 2002;70(3):852–6.
[51] APA. Guidelines for the practice of telepsychology. Am Psychol 2013;68(9):791–800.
[52] Perle J, Burt J, Higgins W. Psychologist and Physician Interest in Telehealth Training and Referral for Mental Health Services: An Exploratory Study. J Technol Hum Serv 2014;32:158–85.
[53] Cummins SE, Bailey L, Campbell S, et al. Tobacco cessation quitlines in North America: a descriptive study. Tob Control 2007;16(Suppl 1):i9–15.
[54] Camhi SS, Herweck A, Perone H. Telehealth Training Is Essential to Care for Underserved Populations: a Medical Student Perspective. Med Sci Educ 2020;1–4.
[55] McCord C, Saenz J, Armstrong T, et al. Training the next generation of counseling psychologists in the practice of telepsychology. Counselling Psychol Q 2015;28(3): 324–44.
[56] Eby M, Chin J, Rollock D, et al. Professional Psychology Training in the Era of a Thousand Flowers: Dilemmas and Challenges for the Future. Train Educ Prof Psychol 2011;5:57–68.
[57] Koonin LM, Hoots B, Tsang CA, et al. Trends in the Use of Telehealth During the Emergence of the COVID-19 Pandemic — United States, January–March 2020. MMWR Morb Mortal Wkly Rep 2020;69:1595–9.
[58] Maheu M, Pulier M, McMenamin J, et al. Future of Telepsychology, Telehealth, and Various Technologies in Psychological Research and Practice. Prof Psychol Res Pr 2012;43:613.
[59] Humes KR, Jones NA, Ramirez RR. Overview of race and Hispanic Origin: 2010. Washington, DC: US Census Bureau; 2011.
[60] APA. Standards of accreditation for health service psychology and accreditation operating procedures. Washington, DC: American Psychological Association, Commission on Accreditation; 2015.
[61] Mollah TN, Antoniades J, Lafeer FI, et al. How do mental health practitioners operationalise cultural competency in everyday practice? A qualitative analysis. BMC Health Serv Res 2018;18(1):480.
[62] Sue DW, Arredondo P, McDavis RJ. Multicultural counseling competencies and standards: A call to the profession. J Multicultural Couns Dev 1992;20(2):64–88.
[63] Sue DW, Bernier JE, Durran A, et al. Position Paper: Cross-Cultural Counseling Competencies. Couns Psychol 1982;10(2):45–52.
[64] Alizadeh S, Chavan M. Cultural competence dimensions and outcomes: A systematic review of the literature. Health Soc Care Community 2015;24.
[65] Korman M. National conference on levels and patterns of professional training in psychology: The major themes. Am Psychol 1974;29(6):441–9.
[66] McClincey S. Multicultural training in APA-accredited clinical psychology doctoral programs. Dissertation Abstr Int Section B: The Sci Eng 2018;78:7-B(E).
[67] APA. Guidelines for providers of psychological services to ethnic, linguistic, and culturally diverse populations. Am Psychol 1993;48(1):45–8.
[68] APA. Guidelines and principles for accreditation. Washington, DC: American Psychological Association; 2002.
[69] Manese J, Douce L, Croteau J, et al. Guidelines on Multicultural Education, Training, Research, Practice, and Organizational Change for Psychologists. Am Psychol 2003;58:377–402.
[70] Boxley R, Wagner NN. Clinical psychology training programs and minority groups: A survey. Prof Psychol 1971; 2(1):75–81.
[71] Bernal ME, Padilla AM. Status of minority curricula and training in clinical psychology. Am Psychol 1982;37(7): 780–7.
[72] Smith T, Constantine M, Dunn T, et al. Multicultural Education in the Mental Health Professions: A Meta-Analytic Review. J Couns Psychol 2006;53:132–45.

[73] Bernal ME, Castro FG. Are clinical psychologists prepared for service and research with ethnic minorities? Report of a decade of progress. Am Psychol 1994; 49(9):797–805.

[74] APA. Standards of accreditation for health service psychology and accreditation operating procedures. Washington, DC: American Psychological Association; 2019.

[75] Green D, Callands TA, Radcliffe AM, et al. Clinical psychology students' perceptions of diversity training: a study of exposure and satisfaction. J Clin Psychol 2009; 65(10):1056–70.

[76] Gregus S, Stevens K, Seivert N, et al. Student perceptions of multicultural training and program climate in clinical psychology doctoral programs. Train Educ Prof Psychol 2019;14.

[77] Benuto L, Casas J, o'Donohue W. Training Culturally Competent Psychologists: A Systematic Review of the Training Outcome Literature. Train Educ Prof Psychol 2018;12.

[78] Peters H, Krumm A, Gonzales R, et al. Multicultural Environments of Academic Versus Internship Training Programs: Lessons to Be Learned. J Multicultural Couns Dev 2011;39.

[79] Thurston I, Gray W, Pulgaron E. Going Above and Beyond: Exemplar Diversity Training in Pediatric Psychology. Clin Pract Pediatr Psychol 2015;3.

[80] Smith TB, Trimble JE. Multicultural education/training and experience: A meta-analysis of surveys and outcome studies. In: Smith TB, Trimble JE, editors. Foundations of multicultural psychology: research to inform effective practice, 8. Washington, D.C.: American Psychological Association; 2016. p. 21–47.

[81] Goode-Cross D. Those Who Learn Have a Responsibility To Teach": Black Therapists' Experiences Supervising Black Therapist Trainees. Train Educ Prof Psychol 2011; 5:73–80.

[82] Watkins JC, Hook J, Owen J, et al. Multicultural Orientation in Psychotherapy Supervision: Cultural Humility, Cultural Comfort, and Cultural Opportunities. Am J Psychother 2019;72:38–46.

[83] Treichler E, Crawford J, Higdon A, et al. Diversity and social justice training at the postdoctoral level: A scoping study and pilot of a self-assessment. Train Educ Prof Psychol 2020;14:126–37.

[84] Brawer P, Handal P, Fabricatore A, et al. Training and Education in Religion/Spirituality Within APA-Accredited Clinical Psychology Programs. Prof Psychol Res Pr 2002;33:203–6.

[85] Frisby CL, O'Donohue W, Benuto LT, et al. Conceptual and Empirical Issues in Training Culturally Competent Psychologists. In: Frisby C, O'Donohue W, editors. Cultural Competence in Applied Psychology. Springer; Cham 2018. pp 95-102.

[86] Fouad N, Grus C, Hatcher R, et al. Competency Benchmarks: A Model for Understanding and Measuring Competence in Professional Psychology Across Training Levels. Train Educ Prof Psychol 2009;3.

[87] Allen J. A Multicultural Assessment Supervision Model to Guide Research and Practice. Prof Psychol Res Pr 2007; 38:248–58.

[88] Neblett E. Diversity (Psychological) Science Training: Challenges, Tensions, and a Call to Action. J Soc Issues 2019;75.

Advances in Psychiatry and Behavioral Health 1 (2021) 239–245

ADVANCES IN PSYCHIATRY AND BEHAVIORAL HEALTH

Integrating Book Club in Psychiatric Education

Deepak Prabhakar, MD, MPH[a,*], Lisa MacLean, MD[b]

[a]Sheppard Pratt, 6501 North Charles Street, Baltimore, MD 21204, USA; [b]Henry Ford Health System, One Ford Place, 1C, Detroit, MI 48202, USA

KEYWORDS

• Curriculum • Book club • Residency

KEY POINTS

- Book club is one way to address knowledge gaps while engaging learners and fostering a sense of community.
- Identifying key knowledge gaps in advance can help the course director strategically choose books that fulfill curricular needs.
- The role of the faculty discussant as a facilitator and the resident leaders cannot be overemphasized; this activity does require effective role modeling to help bring skeptical participants on board.
- The benefits of book club can potentially reach beyond the growth of knowledge into areas like personal development and burnout prevention.

INTRODUCTION

As novel diagnostic and therapeutic strategies are introduced with the wave of ongoing advancements in the field of psychiatry, residency programs face challenges introducing additional content into annual didactic curriculum in a timely manner. Add to this the need to address curriculum, such as quality improvement [1], integrated medicine [2], neuroscience, wellness, diversity, and equity and inclusion [3], and most programs struggle with finding time within the yearly organized didactic curriculum to address all pertinent topics in appropriate depth. Meeting these rapidly changing requirements and having content experts to teach in diverse topic areas is another challenge for program leadership. Further, even though the value of group learning has been established for specific topics, the pedagogical pearls are still potentially underutilized, limiting its use to specific topics and sessions based on the comfort level of instructors.

A book club organized to help address curricular gaps has the potential of leveraging not only group learning but also maximizing the learning outcomes across multiple competencies instead of adding hours of didactics to address each and every new topic separately. Although textbooks and lectures can transmit information, by themselves they may not foster the development of self-directed and life-long learning. Book club is not necessarily a novel concept [4,5]; however, we believe it is underutilized or not used at all in psychiatric pedagogy. Book clubs have been used for a variety of purposes in other disciplines, including education, nursing, and pharmacy, to expand on identified gaps of knowledge and skills [3,4]. Haley and colleagues [6] also found that book club could be used in interprofessional education. One qualitative study found that the book club structure fostered critical, reflective inquiry and served as a mechanism for confronting assumptions, biases, and stereotypes in an urban setting. Geraci [7] found that book clubs allow

*Corresponding author, *E-mail address:* dprabhakar@sheppardpratt.org

https://doi.org/10.1016/j.ypsc.2021.06.002
2667-3827/21/

learners to interact socially with other cultures in a nonthreatening way toward developing reading, writing, critical thinking, and literacy discourse. In a study by Moore Mensah [3], a book club format was used to teach diversity, equity, and inclusion, and showed that the structure and theoretic foundation of a book club promotes change in beliefs, multicultural awareness, and transformative learning.

In addition, reading books can be fun. Learners gathering to share lessons learned in a group format is not only a welcome departure from the routine of day-to-day clinical work, it has the added advantage of opening new doors and development of insight into concepts that would otherwise be missed or may have taken several didactic sessions to develop. Furthermore, a group learning modality such as book club emphasizing the human aspects of medicine while underscoring the positive impact of physicians, not only on patient outcomes but also on the broader society, may help promote wellness by mitigating the risk of disillusionment and detachment often fostered by the tedious and impersonal aspects of the current health care environment [8,9]. There is also opportunity within this framework to build resident community and connectivity across residency years. Jordan and colleagues [10] showed how book club could positively contribute to the professional development of a trainee by promoting reflection and deliberate practice. Professional development can help mitigate burnout and has been identified as a strategy to build resilience within medicine [11]. The purpose of this article was to describe how one program incorporated book club successfully into their curriculum, explore the benefits of this approach, and offer insight into how other topics of interest, like quality improvement, integrated medicine, leadership, wellness and diversity, and equity and inclusion, could be incorporated into a psychiatry residency curriculum.

BACKGROUND

Fink's [12] Taxonomy of Significant Learning supports the use of book club as a meaningful way to add to a psychiatry training curriculum (Table 1). In this taxonomy, residents learn to connect their life experiences with content learned in their assigned books [12]. According to Fink [12], when types of learning in the taxonomy interact, like integration and caring, this creates synergy that produces lasting change for the learner. Creating connections between didactic content and examples of experiences is essential in educating psychiatry residents and maximizing their learning. Learners can compartmentalize knowledge they learn in courses, failing to make connections between related information and concepts. Reading about a clinical struggle, whether fictional or nonfictional, can create links between diseases and patient experiences. In addition, through a book club format, the presence of many ideas and voices lends itself to an expansion of thoughts and creates the opportunity for challenging one's ideas and assumptions. Books about patient or health care provider experiences allow the readers to reflect on the sensitive or shocking parts of the story in their home environment before the discussion, giving the readers time to think about their feelings and reactions [5]. There is also the potential secondary gain of expanding learners' love for literature. Overall, book clubs provide an intellectual nonjudgmental forum in which learners can share ideas, thoughts, feelings, and reactions to a book and thus serves as a great framework for adult learners to build cohesiveness, gather insights, and grow as individuals [13].

BOOK CLUB DESIGN

With this in mind, in 2017, program leadership at one institution met to design and discuss creating a 1-year curriculum for 24 residents using a book club framework. Book recommendations were solicited from the residents, and the program director made final selection based on the curricular application in consultation with the co-chairs of the resident book club. Ultimately, books were selected based on a core goal of building resident knowledge in key areas (Table 2). From there, a monthly book club was organized for all the residents (postgraduate years 1 through 4) in the psychiatry residency program to help address growing curricular needs, and foster group engagement and learning. The main learning activity was small group discussions whereby residents were encouraged to pick an excerpt to discuss during the 1-hour club meeting that met on didactic days. Book club was peer-directed but included a faculty instructor who acted as a facilitator and helped to focus learners toward the most important content areas and to ensure that the educational goals were met. The faculty instructor also helped the learner to make connections, encouraged residents to share personal experiences, and worked to clarify comments made by participants. The faculty also supplemented the discussion by providing personal examples of their past and current experiences.

Discussion was also supplemented with key articles that were closely tied to the specific texts and helped augment discussion with the aim of improving medical knowledge about specific topics. *Brain on Fire: My Month of Madness* [14] and *Concussion* [15] were selected to address curricular needs in neurosciences while also

TABLE 1
Fink's application of taxonomy of significant learning experiences to book club

Category	Taxonomy Description
Foundational knowledge	Understanding and remembering information and ideas
Application	Developing skills, engaging in thinking, managing projects
Integration	Connecting ideas, people, and realms of life
Human dimension	Learning about oneself and others
Caring	Developing new feelings, interests, and values
Learning how to learn	Becoming better learners, inquiring about a subject, and self-directive

supplementing the professionalism and ethics course series. *A Test of Will* [16] and *The Curious Incident of the Dog in the Night-Time* [17] were selected to help reinforce the curricula in child psychiatry and growth and development. *Being Mortal: Medicine and What Matters in the End* [18] was selected to help address curricular gaps related to end-of-life care. *Why Physicians Die by Suicide: Lessons Learned from Their Families and Others Who Cared* [19] was selected to explore in more depth physician suicide. Because these books were helping address key curricular elements, we were able to add an hour each month for book club discussion during the didactic schedule. This was considered a departure from the traditional approach of organizing interest-based activities after work hours or on weekends. These 6 texts were discussed over 12 months of didactics schedule.

Even though it was not a stated objective, we believed that the group format and reading quality text would foster wellness for our residents, and by orienting the discussion around the broader meaning of a physician's work would help mitigate the risk of professional stagnation, detachment, and ultimately burnout [9]. This across residency program intervention also promoted resident community across years of training. Because the format included all levels of training, the bimonthly discussions were diverse with regard to levels of expertise and life experiences. The discussions also provided a unique opportunity to create a safe space to explore different interpretations and opinions of the books.

TABLE 2
Six-month book club curriculum

Book Title	Topic Areas
Brain on Fire: My Month of Madness [14]	Neuroscience and patient experience
Concussion [15]	Neuroscience, traumatic brain injury, and ethics
A Test of Will [16]	Growth/development and resilience
The Curious Incident of the Dog in the Night-Time [17]	Autism and family dynamics
Being Mortal: Medicine and What Matters in the End [18]	End-of-life care and systems of care
Why Physicians Die by Suicide: Lessons Learned from Their Families and Others Who Cared [19]	Physician suicide and wellness

Overall, the residency book club was well received. Not only were residents able to read the assigned text consistently, but they also took advantage of the supplemental material to help improve knowledge pertaining to these specific topics. At the end of 1 year, residents felt that their participation in book club would positively alter aspects of their practice. Residents also highlighted the clinical and social relevance of the topics covered in addition to the growing appreciation of the need for reflective listening and the central role of patient experience in a book club format. Because there was no knowledge test at the end of this activity, we cannot be certain about the specific improvement in medical knowledge; however, both the training director's observations as well as resident feedback were reflective of growing appreciation of nuances pertaining to the diagnosis and clinical management of anti-N-methyl D-aspartate (NMDA) encephalitis, mild traumatic brain injury, chronic traumatic encephalopathy (CTE), autism, and Tourette syndrome. As a result of the positive feedback, the decision was made to continue the program, which is now currently in its fourth year.

OTHER CONSIDERATIONS

There are several other factors that should be considered when implementing similar interventions. Initially, some residents were concerned about the cost and time commitment. We addressed this by spreading the books over 1 year of didactic schedule as opposed to assigning 6 months for 6 texts; further, residents were able to purchase these texts using the book funds that are made available each year to residents, thereby mitigating the negative cost implications. Because we organized these discussions during didactics, it eliminated the need to take time out of personal family time. The role of the faculty discussant as a facilitator and the resident leaders cannot be overemphasized, this activity does require effective role modeling to help bring skeptical participants on board in reading the text. After all, a book club discussion is only helpful if participants have all read the text and come prepared to discuss.

In the next section, we describe each text in brief with accompanying session details. This section was included in the article to help readers consider the purpose and gains of a particular book choice for a resident book club. For example, if the primary focus is to advance resident knowledge in diversity, equity, and inclusion topics, picking a book in this sphere and adding a scientific article could help to build on a body of knowledge and get residents talking about challenging concepts or issues.

BOOK DESCRIPTIONS AND SESSION DETAILS

The 6 books described as follows allow the reader to understand more fully how a book might be selected, what focus a teaching session might look like, and how a book club framework can be used in medical education. The first book was *Brain on Fire: My Month of Madness* by Susannah Cahalan. This book was about a young woman's struggle and ultimately recovery from NMDA encephalitis, which not only helped cover elements of neuroscience curriculum, it also added valuable discussion around first-hand patient experience going through psychotic episodes and her interaction with the medical community. Through her experience, Ms Cahalan's narrative helped participants understand the helplessness associated with waking up alone in a hospital room, strapped to her bed, and unable to move or speak; unfortunately, an experience not so uncommon for many of our patients. The text helped residents appreciate the patient experience of hallucinations, waves of hopelessness and fluctuating trust as a large team of doctors spent 30 days *and more than a million dollars* to find an explanation for Ms Cahalan's presentation. This book helped us address the curricular gap about a novel condition, NMDA encephalitis, while emphasizing the importance of bedside examinations and compassionate interactions with patients in crisis. In addition, for our residents, the book helped highlight the skeptical attitude toward mental health by the community and other medical specialties. The book club discussion was supplemented by the seminal article [20] on NMDA encephalitis that residents were required to have read before the discussion.

Concussion by Jeanne Marie Laskas is about a pathologist, Dr Bennet Omalu, from Nigeria, who brought forward the impact of concussions and CTE to public conscious through his persistent effort. As he discovered that Mike Webster, a famous football player, might have experienced significant mental deterioration due to the trauma his brain endured from playing the game, he also realized that he was up against a mammoth of denial fostered by the business and the culture surrounding American football. This book helped address the curricular elements related to mild traumatic brain injury and CTE. Of note, the text generated discussion not only about the medical aspects of mild traumatic brain injury and CTE, but also the discussion was reflective of appreciation of medical ethics and professionalism; residents identified and discussed the importance of being aware of conflicts of interest and the potential negative impact that this may have on clinical decision making. The discussion about CTE was supplemented by a case report that was one of the few published by Dr Omalu's group [21]. Furthermore, leveraging Dr Omalu's personal story, the book club discussion underscored elements related to acculturation, personal and professional growth, and vulnerability; given the recent emphasis on physician burnout, this discussion was especially timely and valuable.

A Test of Will by Diane Shader Smith is about a young high school boy with Tourette disorder, attention deficit hyperactivity disorder, and obsessive-compulsive disorder, and his struggles to "fit in." Even though he spent time around people who knew about his condition, Will was confronted with differential reactions based on their appreciation of his challenges. Will's coach provoked him, his peers ridiculed him, his teacher made excuses for him, and his therapist pushed him to identify himself outside of his disorder. For our residents, the text highlighted the need of educating patients and those around them. Especially in child psychiatry to make an effective change in the child's environment at home and in school with participation from appropriate stakeholders was reinforced through this book. We also reviewed the American Academy of Child and Adolescent Psychiatry practice parameters for tic disorders to help augment discussion about screening, diagnosis, and management of tic disorders [22]. This specific book club discussion complemented our child psychiatry didactic curriculum.

The Curious Incident of the Dog in the Night-Time by Mark Haddon is about an autistic child who has a pet rat and finds a sense of comfort around animals. As he puts on his detective hat to solve the mystery of who killed his neighbor's dog, he comes across hidden lies and secrets about his family. Being someone who struggles with understanding human behaviors, relationships, and social cues, he embarks on a journey to escape the frightening truth. As the story unfolds, book club participants were able to empathize and better learn the impact of psychosocial factors on child development through the eyes of the character. Videos were shared during this session to better understand the presentation of autism spectrum disorder. Moreover, those who were interested and available for a follow-up wellness event to this session attended *The Curious Incident of the Dog in the Night-Time* Broadway touring show based on this text. This book club helped augment the didactic curriculum on child development and autism.

Being Mortal: Medicine and What Matters in the End by Atul Gawande was chosen to help introduce end-of-life issues to our curriculum. The text highlights a common conflict for physicians serving patients who are at the end of their lives, whether to focus on prolonging life or making life meaningful. Gawande is a surgeon and he illustrates various issues pertaining to palliative medicine from his personal and professional experience. The text helped our residency group appreciate the life patterns of declining vitality with aging and disease. Residents were able to identify with the potential role that physicians may play in end-of-life discussions, many were able to reflect from personal experiences with a loved one, and some were even able to identify with Gawande's experience of physicians keeping information from patients when they know the outlook is bleak. To further enhance the discussion, residents reviewed an article focusing on why physicians do not have conversations about poor prognosis with their patients, learning that patients with terminal conditions often spend 2 months in the hospital before someone mentions hospice [23]. The discussion also encouraged residents to be supportive of one another when approaching difficult end-of-life treatment and care issues pertaining to their own near and dear ones. After all, when dealing with loss and mortality, isolation can be a coping mechanism with significant negative consequences for those involved.

Finally, *Why Physicians Die by Suicide: Lessons Learned from Their Families and Others Who Cared* by Michael F. Myers was a good way to introduce the exploration of the sensitive yet important topic of physician suicide. In this text, Dr Myers, a psychiatrist and a specialist in physician health, provides his unique insights into why so many physicians die by suicide and explores the topic in an engaging and informative text that combines powerful personal narratives of survivors and bereaved loved ones with helpful clinical observations and research. Suicide is a complex subject and to make matters worse, even though physician suicide has been a concern for several decades, to date, it remains one of the most under-researched and taboo areas in medicine. The residents were able to see that the stigma that prevents help-seeking behavior is even more profound in physicians who live in a culture that does not promote, and at times inadvertently discourages, those who seek treatment. The book was supplemented with a book review article [24]. The residents also discussed specific ways they can contribute and make a difference as colleagues, teachers, and clinicians.

SUMMARY

The primary focus of this curriculum was the acquisition of increased knowledge in diverse topics using a book club, a self-directed learning format. We believe a well-planned book club can potentially provide a platform not only for enhancing medical knowledge, but also can help develop competency in empathic listening, system-based issues, and ethics and professionalism. Conceivably, programs could develop a 4-year curriculum consisting of 6 books annually and include diverse topics of interest allowing programs to meet the growing curricular demands outlined by the Accreditation Council for Graduate Medical Education. The creation of a book club is a feasible, innovative, interactive strategy that promotes group cohesion, nurtures personal and professional development, and has the potential to expand knowledge in key topic areas.

CLINICS CARE POINTS

- Books for discussion can be selected from topics addressing knowledge gaps identified during clinical rotations.
- Books addressing patient experience should be included to enhance clinical care.
- Text addressing self-care and wellness can help facilitate professional growth and development of learners in otherwise busy clinical environments.
- Books addressing systems of care should be included to help facilitate broader understanding of health care.

ACKNOWLEDGMENTS

The authors acknowledge the book club discussions and many contributions of psychiatry residents at Henry Ford Health System that influenced the development of this article.

DISCLOSURE

The authors have nothing to disclose.

REFERENCES

[1] Arbuckle MR, Weinberg M, Cabaniss DL, et al. Training psychiatry residents in quality improvement: an integrated, year-long curriculum. Acad Psychiatry 2013;37:42–5.
[2] Reardon CL, Bentman A, Cowley DS, et al. General and child and adolescent psychiatry resident training in integrated care: a survey of program directors. Acad Psychiatry 2015;39:442–7.
[3] Moore Mensah F. Confronting assumptions, biases, and stereotypes in preservice teachers' conceptualizations of science teaching through the use of book club. J Res Sci Teach 2009;46:1041–66.
[4] Chappell A, Dervay K. Leadership book club: an innovative strategy to incorporate leadership development into pharmacy residency programs. Hosp Pharm 2016;51:635–8.
[5] Plake KS. Book club elective to facilitate student learning of the patient experience with chronic disease. Am J Pharm Educ 2010;74:37.
[6] Haley J, Carlson McCall R, Zomorodi M, et al. Interprofessional collaboration between health sciences librarians and health professions faculty to implement a book club discussion for incoming students. J Med Libr Assoc 2018;107:403–10.
[7] Geraci PM. Promoting positive reading discourse and self-exploration through a multi-cultural book club. J Correct Educ (Glen Mills) 2003;54:54–9.
[8] Slavin SJ, Chibnall JT. Finding the why, changing the how: improving the mental health of medical students, residents, and physicians. Acad Med 2016;91:1194–6.
[9] Shanafelt TD, Hasan O, Dyrbye LN, et al. Changes in burnout and satisfaction with work-life balance in physicians and the general US working population from 2011 to 2014. Mayo Clin Proc 2015;90:1600–13.
[10] Jordan J, Bavolek RA, Dyne PL, et al. A virtual book club for professional development in emergency medicine. West J Emerg Med 2020;22:108–14.
[11] Patel RS, Sekhri S, Bhimandadham NN, et al. A review of strategies to manage physician burnout. Cureus 2019;11:e4805.
[12] Fink LD. Creating significant learning experiences: an integrated approach to designing college courses. San Francisco: Jossey-Bass; 2003.
[13] Flood J, Lapp D. Teachers book clubs: establishing literature discussion groups for teachers. Read Teach 1994;47:574–6.
[14] Cahalan S. Brain on fire: my month on madness. New York: Simon & Schuster; 2012.
[15] Laskas JM. Concussion. New York: Random House; 2015.
[16] Shader Smith D. A test of Will. Diane Shader Smith; 2002.
[17] Haddon M. The curious incident of the dog in the nighttime. New York: Vintage Books; 2003.
[18] Gawande A. Being mortal: medicine and what matters in the end. New York: Metropolitan Books; 2014.
[19] Myers MF. Why physicians die by suicide: lessons learned from their families and others who cared. Michael F. Myers; 2017.
[20] Dalmau J, Lancaster E, Martinez-Hernandez E, et al. Clinical experience and laboratory investigations in patients with anti-NMDAR encephalitis. Lancet Neurol 2011;10:63–74.
[21] Raji CA, Merrill DA, Barrio JR, et al. Progressive focal gray matter volume loss in a former high school football

player: a possible magnetic resonance imaging volumetric signature for chronic traumatic encephalopathy. Am J Geriatr Psychiatry 2016;24:784–90.

[22] Murphy TK, Lewin AB, Storch EA, et al. American Academy of Child and Adolescent Psychiatry (AACAP) Committee on Quality Issues (CQI). Practice parameter for the assessment and treatment of children and adolescents with tic disorders. J Am Acad Child Adolesc Psychiatry 2013;52:1341–59.

[23] Mack JW, Smith TJ. Reasons why physicians do not have discussions about poor prognosis, why it matters, and what can be improved. J Clin Oncol 2012;30:2715–7.

[24] MacLean L, Prabhakar D. Why physicians die by suicide: lessons learned from their families and others who cared. J Am Acad Child Adolesc Psychiatry 2017;56:P898–9.

Printed and bound by CPI Group (UK) Ltd, Croydon, CR0 4YY
08/05/2025
01864715-0006